Data Driven Insights in Healthcare

Data Driven Insights in Healthcare

Guest Editors

Victor R. Prybutok
Gayle Linda Prybutok

MDPI • Basel • Beijing • Wuhan • Barcelona • Belgrade • Novi Sad • Cluj • Manchester

Guest Editors
Victor R. Prybutok
Department of Information Technology and Decision Sciences
University of North Texas
Denton
USA

Gayle Linda Prybutok
Department of Rehabilitation and Health Services
University of North Texas
Denton
USA

Editorial Office
MDPI AG
Grosspeteranlage 5
4052 Basel, Switzerland

This is a reprint of the Special Issue, published open access by the journal *Healthcare* (ISSN 2227-9032), freely accessible at: https://www.mdpi.com/journal/healthcare/special_issues/N23J7XDBRZ.

For citation purposes, cite each article independently as indicated on the article page online and as indicated below:

Lastname, A.A.; Lastname, B.B. Article Title. *Journal Name* **Year**, *Volume Number*, Page Range.

ISBN 978-3-7258-5841-5 (Hbk)
ISBN 978-3-7258-5842-2 (PDF)
https://doi.org/10.3390/books978-3-7258-5842-2

Contents

About the Editors

Victor R. Prybutok

Victor R. Prybutok is the G. Brint Ryan Endowed Professor and Regents Professor of Decision Sciences in the Department of Information Technology and Decision Sciences at the University of North Texas, where he has served since 1991. He served as President of the Decision Sciences Institute from May 2024 to April 2025 and currently serves as the immediate Past President. His research focuses on data analytics, quality management, and decision sciences applied to healthcare and service delivery. Dr. Prybutok holds American Society for Quality professional certifications as a Certified Quality Engineer, Certified Quality Auditor, Certified Manager of Quality and Organizational Excellence, and is an American Statistical Association Accredited Professional Statistician. He played a pivotal role in creating the MS in Advanced Data Analytics degree at the University of North Texas, designed with an interdisciplinary analytics core that enables healthcare and other programs to incorporate data-driven insights. His work emphasizes mining large data sets to discover actionable insights that improve healthcare practice and delivery. Dr. Prybutok has received numerous honors, including the 2018 Decision Sciences Institute Lifetime Distinguished Educator Award and the 2017 American Society for Quality Gryna Award. He served as Vice Provost for Graduate Education and Dean of the Toulouse Graduate School from 2017 to 2025, where he championed the development of data analytics programs and increased visibility for graduate research across multiple disciplines.

Gayle Linda Prybutok

Gayle Linda Prybutok is an Associate Professor in Health Services Administration at the University of North Texas, where she has served since 2016. She holds a PhD in Information Science with an emphasis on Health Informatics and is a registered nurse in Texas. Dr. Prybutok designed and developed the MS in Health Services Administration program and the PhD in Health Services Research, including the innovative Health Data Analytics concentration that applies data-driven approaches to healthcare management. Her research interests center on health communication and education, healthcare quality improvement, Internet-based health communication, mobile health, and health disparities. She has published extensively on data-driven insights in healthcare, including research on cyberchondria, COVID-19 information framing, online health information seeking behaviors, and subjective cognitive decline in older adults. Dr. Prybutok received the College of Health and Public Service Distinguished Teaching Award in 2018 and CLEAR Outstanding and Exemplary Online Course and Instructor Awards. She served as an Early Career Reviewer for the National Institutes of Health and is Vice President for Student Liaison and Director of the Doctoral Student Consortium for the Southwest Decision Sciences Institute. Her work emphasizes using data analytics and exploratory research methods to generate actionable insights that improve healthcare delivery and patient outcomes.

Preface

As Guest Editors of this Reprint, we are pleased to present this collection of research that explores the transformative potential of data-driven approaches in healthcare. The motivation for assembling this body of work stems from a fundamental recognition that, while theory-driven research remains essential, the vast repositories of healthcare data now available offer unprecedented opportunities to discover insights that can directly improve patient care and healthcare delivery systems.

This Reprint addresses a critical need in contemporary healthcare research: bridging the gap between observational data and actionable knowledge. The healthcare sector generates massive volumes of data daily, yet the systematic exploration of these data sets to uncover meaningful patterns and relationships remains an underutilized approach. The studies compiled here demonstrate that data exploration is not merely descriptive but can generate hypotheses, reveal unexpected associations, and provide evidence that informs both practice and future research directions.

This collection is intended for healthcare researchers, data scientists, practitioners, and policy makers who recognize that innovative analytical approaches including artificial intelligence, machine learning, and advanced data mining techniques can complement traditional research methodologies. We hope these works inspire readers to consider how their own data assets might yield valuable insights when subjected to rigorous exploratory analysis.

The research presented represents diverse healthcare contexts and analytical methods, unified by a commitment to extracting meaningful knowledge from empirical observations. We trust this Reprint will serve as both a resource and a catalyst for advancing data-driven discovery in healthcare.

Victor R. Prybutok and Gayle Linda Prybutok
Guest Editors

healthcare

MDPI

Editorial

Data-Driven Insights in Healthcare

Victor R. Prybutok [1,*] and Gayle L. Prybutok [2]

[1] Department of Information Technology and Decision Sciences, G. Brint Ryan College of Business, University of North Texas, Denton, TX 76203, USA
[2] Department of Rehabilitation and Health Services, College of Health and Public Service, University of North Texas, Denton, TX 76203, USA
* Correspondence: victor.prybutok@unt.edu; Tel.: +01-940-565-4767

1. Introduction

We are pleased to present this Special Issue, which is a curated collection of research that showcases the transformative power of data-driven approaches in healthcare. The healthcare sector generates vast amounts of observational data daily, yet systematic exploration of these datasets to uncover meaningful patterns remains underutilized. The rapid advancement of digital health technologies, including electronic health records, medical imaging systems, wearable devices, and genomic sequencing platforms, has led to an exponential growth in healthcare data availability [1]. In addition, data from routine clinical practices offer unique opportunities to complement evidence from randomized controlled trials, particularly for understanding treatment effectiveness in diverse patient populations and real-world clinical settings [2,3]. However, ensuring the quality and appropriate use of these observational datasets remains a persistent challenge that requires systematic attention [4,5]. The collection in this Special Issue demonstrates that while theory-driven research remains essential, data exploration can generate hypotheses, reveal unexpected associations, and provide evidence that directly informs practice and future research directions.

The ten contributions assembled in this Special Issue span diverse healthcare contexts and analytical methodologies, unified by a commitment to extracting actionable knowledge from empirical observations. These publications employ innovative techniques, including artificial intelligence, machine learning, natural language processing, advanced statistical modeling, operations research, and exploratory data analytics, to address critical challenges in healthcare delivery, quality improvement, and patient outcomes [6]. The integration of these data-driven methodologies supports the need for future research and application regarding how healthcare systems can leverage observational evidence to inform clinical decision-making and policy development [7].

2. Artificial Intelligence and Machine Learning for Clinical Prediction

The Special Issue opens with three contributions that demonstrate the power of artificial intelligence and advanced analytical methods for clinical prediction and decision support. Halwani and Halwani (contribution 1) present "Prediction of COVID-19 Hospitalization and Mortality Using Artificial Intelligence," employing decision trees, support vector machines, and random forest algorithms to predict hospital mortality among COVID-19 patients. Their analysis of data from King Abdulaziz University Hospital in Saudi Arabia achieved predictive accuracy rates of 76–82%, with hospital stay duration, D-Dimers, alkaline phosphatase, bilirubin, lactate dehydrogenase, C-reactive protein, and ferritin identified as significant mortality predictors. This work illustrates how AI tools can enhance early identification of high-risk patients and support clinical decision-making during pandemic situations.

Alasmari (contribution 2) provides a comprehensive scoping review titled "A Scoping Review of Arabic Natural Language Processing for Mental Health," examining NLP techniques applied to mental health detection in Arabic-speaking populations. Following the PRISMA-ScR framework, this review identifies the effectiveness of various approaches, with transformer-based models such as AraBERT and MARBERT achieving superior performance with accuracy rates up to 99.3% and 98.3%, respectively. The review highlights how NLP can analyze social media data to detect depression and suicidality, demonstrating the potential of these techniques for population-level mental health surveillance in linguistically diverse contexts.

Chang, Ryu, Choi, Kwon, and Kim (contribution 3) present "A Comparative Study of Hospitalization Mortality Rates between General and Emergency Hospitalized Patients Using Survival Analysis," employing Kaplan–Meier survival estimation and Cox proportional hazards models to analyze four years of data from the Korean National Health Insurance Services. Their analysis reveals distinct determinants of mortality risk between general inpatients and emergency admissions, with geographic factors and institutional characteristics such as physician and nurse staffing ratios, bed capacity, and emergency bed availability showing differential effects. This work demonstrates how survival analysis techniques can accommodate censored medical data characteristics often overlooked by conventional regression approaches.

3. Data-Driven Quality Improvement and Healthcare Standards

Two articles explore how data-driven methodologies can enhance healthcare quality standards and establish evidence-based benchmarks. Richardson, Penumaka, Smoot, Panaganti, Chinta, Guduri, Tiyyagura, Martin, Korvink, and Gunn (contribution 4) present "A Data-Driven Approach to Defining Risk-Adjusted Coding Specificity Metrics for a Large U.S. Dementia Patient Cohort," analyzing 487,775 hospitalization records to develop risk-adjusted metrics for assessing medical coding specificity. Using logistic regression models incorporating patient and facility characteristics, combined with Poisson binomial modeling, they created benchmarks enabling healthcare facilities to assess coding practices against industry standards. With an AUC of 0.727 for principal dementia diagnoses, their approach demonstrates how data-driven methods can identify facilities that over- or under-specify diagnoses, ultimately contributing to improved patient care quality and healthcare system reliability.

Velev, Velazquez-Sosa, Lebien, Janwa, and Roche-Lima (contribution 5) provide "Modeling Multivariate Distributions of Lipid Panel Biomarkers for Reference Interval Estimation and Comorbidity Analysis," employing Gaussian Mixture Models to derive reference intervals directly from large-scale, real-world laboratory data from Puerto Rico. Their methodology enables separation of healthy and pathological subpopulations without relying on diagnostic codes, producing sex- and age-stratified reference intervals for total cholesterol, LDL, HDL, and triglycerides. By examining selective mortality patterns and constructing comorbidity implication networks, they explain counterintuitive age trends in lipid values and characterize interdependencies between conditions, demonstrating how population-specific reference intervals can be derived without recruiting healthy cohorts.

4. Healthcare Operations Research and Resource Optimization

Two contributions employ operations research methodologies to optimize healthcare resource allocation and workforce management. Mystakidis, Koukaras, Koukaras, Kaparis, Stavrinides, and Tjortjis (contribution 6) present "Optimizing Nurse Rostering:

A Case Study Using Integer Programming to Enhance Operational Efficiency and Care Quality," developing a comprehensive integer programming model for nurse scheduling in oncology departments. Their model integrates constraints including legal work hours, staff qualifications, and personal preferences to generate equitable and efficient schedules. Implementation in a clinical setting revealed significant improvements in scheduling efficiency, staff satisfaction, workload distribution, and compliance with work-hour regulations, demonstrating how operations research techniques can enhance both operational excellence and staff well-being in acute care settings.

Clapper, ten Hove, Bekker, and Moeke (contribution 7) provide "Team Size and Composition in Home Healthcare: Quantitative Insights and Six Model-Based Principles," developing six model-based principles to guide managerial decisions regarding home healthcare team structure. Through extensive data analysis and mathematical modeling based on real-life scenarios, they demonstrate that efficiency improves with team size but with diminishing returns, while team manageability becomes increasingly complex as size grows. Their work provides estimates for travel time based on team size and territory, establishes upper bounds for full-time contract fractions to avoid split shifts, and concludes that ideally sized teams should serve at least several hundred care hours weekly. This research exemplifies how quantitative modeling can inform practical workforce planning decisions.

5. Technology-Enabled Healthcare and Behavioral Insights

Two articles examine how technology shapes health-seeking behaviors and social interactions in healthcare contexts. Boyce, Harun, G. Prybutok, and V. Prybutok (contribution 8) present "The Role of Technology in Online Health Communities: A Study of Information-Seeking Behavior", employing partial least squares structural equation modeling with multi-group and importance-performance map analysis to examine technology's role in online health communities. Their cross-sectional survey identifies ease of site navigation and interaction with other members as the most beneficial technology-related factors influencing information-seeking processes. The findings provide actionable insights for developing and managing online health communities and for healthcare professionals seeking to disseminate relevant information to individuals with chronic illnesses such as COPD.

Chen, Hsu, and Rahman (contribution 9) provide "From Mandate to Choice: How Voluntary Mask Wearing Shapes Interpersonal Distance Among University Students After COVID-19," examining the association between voluntary protective behaviors and social interactions in post-mandate Taiwan. Through an online interpersonal distance simulation with 100 university students, they employed four-way ANOVA to reveal that mask-wearing individuals maintain significantly greater interpersonal distances, suggesting heightened risk perception, while masked targets elicit smaller distances, possibly due to safety signaling. Gender differences emerged in both protective behavior adoption (72% of females versus 44% of males) and spatial preferences, offering insights into how voluntary behavioral adaptations continue shaping social norms after mandate removal.

6. Research Infrastructure and Data Governance

The Special Issue concludes with a perspective on research infrastructure challenges. Landi, D'Ambrosio, Faggion, Rocchi, Paganin, Lain, Ceci, and Giannuzzi on behalf of the EPIICAL Consortium (contribution 10) present "Sharing Data and Transferring Samples Within Pediatric Clinical Studies: How to Overcome Challenges and Make Them a Science Opportunity." This perspective examines the EPIICAL project's establishment of a dedicated Working Group to navigate ethical and regulatory complexities of international pediatric clinical studies involving HIV-infected children. The consortium developed well-structured informed consent and assent templates, data sharing agreements, and material transfer agreements to regulate sample transfers among partners and sites across European and non-European boundaries. This contribution highlights how structured governance frameworks and expert support can transform regulatory challenges into opportunities for advancing pediatric clinical research.

7. Conclusions

The contributions assembled in this Special Issue collectively demonstrate that data-driven discovery in healthcare extends far beyond descriptive analysis. These works show how systematic exploration of observational data using diverse methodologies, from artificial intelligence and machine learning to operations research and behavioral modeling, can generate actionable insights that improve patient care, enhance operational efficiency, establish evidence-based standards, and inform policy decisions.

As healthcare systems continue generating unprecedented volumes of data through digital transformation initiatives [1,6], the approaches showcased in this Special Issue provide both inspiration and practical guidance for researchers, practitioners, and policy-makers seeking to extract maximum value from their data assets. The successful translation of data-driven insights into improved patient outcomes requires not only sophisticated analytical methods but also robust data governance frameworks, quality assurance mechanisms, and ethical oversight [2,4]. We hope this collection serves as a catalyst for continued innovation in data-driven healthcare research and practice.

Author Contributions: V.R.P. and G.L.P. contributed equally to the conceptualization, curation, and writing of this editorial. All authors have read and agreed to the published version of the manuscript.

Conflicts of Interest: The authors declare no conflicts of interest.

List of Contributions:

1. Halwani, M.A.; Halwani, M.A. Prediction of COVID-19 Hospitalization and Mortality Using Artificial Intelligence. *Healthcare* **2024**, *12*, 1694. https://doi.org/10.3390/healthcare12171694.
2. Alasmari, A. A Scoping Review of Arabic Natural Language Processing for Mental Health. *Healthcare* **2025**, *13*, 963. https://doi.org/10.3390/healthcare13090963.
3. Chang, H.; Ryu, S.; Choi, I.; Kwon, A.E.; Kim, J. A Comparative Study of Hospitalization Mortality Rates between General and Emergency Hospitalized Patients Using Survival Analysis. *Healthcare* **2024**, *12*, 1982. https://doi.org/10.3390/healthcare12191982.
4. Richardson, K.; Penumaka, S.; Smoot, J.; Panaganti, M.R.; Chinta, I.R.; Guduri, D.P.; Tiyyagura, S.R.; Martin, J.; Korvink, M.; Gunn, L.H. A Data-Driven Approach to Defining Risk-Adjusted Coding Specificity Metrics for a Large U.S. Dementia Patient Cohort. *Healthcare* **2024**, *12*, 983.
5. Velev, J.; Velázquez-Sosa, L.; Lebien, J.; Janwa, H.; Roche-Lima, A. Modeling Multivariate Distributions of Lipid Panel Biomarkers for Reference Interval Estimation and Comorbidity Analysis. *Healthcare* **2025**, *13*, 2499. https://doi.org/10.3390/healthcare13192499.
6. Mystakidis, A.; Koukaras, C.; Koukaras, P.; Kaparis, K.; Stavrinides, S.G.; Tjortjis, C. Optimizing Nurse Rostering: A Case Study Using Integer Programming to Enhance Operational Efficiency and Care Quality. *Healthcare* **2024**, *12*, 2545. https://doi.org/10.3390/healthcare12242545.
7. Clapper, Y.; ten Hove, W.; Bekker, R.; Moeke, D. Team Size and Composition in Home Healthcare: Quantitative Insights and Six Model-Based Principles. *Healthcare* **2023**, *11*, 2935. https://doi.org/10.3390/healthcare11222935.
8. Boyce, L.; Harun, A.; Prybutok, G.; Prybutok, V.R. The Role of Technology in Online Health Communities: A Study of Information-Seeking Behavior. *Healthcare* **2024**, *12*, 336. https://doi.org/10.3390/healthcare12030336.
9. Chen, Y.-L.; Hsu, C.-W.; Rahman, A. From Mandate to Choice: How Voluntary Mask Wearing Shapes Interpersonal Distance Among University Students After COVID-19. *Healthcare* **2025**, *13*, 1956. https://doi.org/10.3390/healthcare13161956.

10. Landi, A.; D'Ambrosio, F.; Faggion, S.; Rocchi, F.; Paganin, C.; Lain, M.G.; Ceci, A.; Giannuzzi, V., on behalf of the EPIICAL Consortium. Sharing Data and Transferring Samples Within Pediatric Clinical Studies: How to Overcome Challenges and Make Them a Science Opportunity. *Healthcare* **2024**, *12*, 2473. https://doi.org/10.3390/healthcare12232473.

References

1. Rahman, M.A.; Moayedikia, A.; Wiil, U.K. Editorial: Data-Driven Technologies for Future Healthcare Systems. *Front. Med. Technol.* **2023**, *5*, 1183687. [CrossRef] [PubMed]
2. Lighterness, A.; Adcock, M.; Scanlon, L.A.; Price, G. Data Quality-Driven Improvement in Health Care: Systematic Literature Review. *J. Med. Internet Res.* **2024**, *26*, e57615. [CrossRef] [PubMed]
3. Barbieri, D.; Chudy-Onwugaje, K.; Langel, J.; Peluso, M.J.; Torres, L.; Kelly, J.D.; Deter, H. Real-World Data and Real-World Evidence in Healthcare in the United States and European Union. *Bioengineering* **2024**, *11*, 784. [CrossRef]
4. Alam, M.A.; Sajib, M.R.U.Z.; Rahman, F.; Ether, S.; Hanson, M.; Sayeed, A.; Akter, E.; Nusrat, N.; Islam, T.T.; Raza, S.; et al. Implications of Big Data Analytics, AI, Machine Learning, and Deep Learning in the Health Care System of Bangladesh: Scoping Review. *J. Med. Internet Res.* **2024**, *26*, e54710. [CrossRef] [PubMed]
5. Ricotta, E.E.; Rid, A.; Cohen, I.G.; Evans, N.G. Observational Studies Must Be Reformed Before the Next Pandemic. *Nat. Med.* **2023**, *29*, 1903–1905. [CrossRef] [PubMed]
6. Elragal, A.; Elragal, H.; Habibipour, A. Healthcare Analytics—A Literature Review and Proposed Research Agenda. *Front. Big Data* **2023**, *6*, 1277976. [CrossRef] [PubMed]
7. Gershon, A.S.; Lindenauer, P.K.; Wilson, K.C.; Rose, L.; Walkey, A.J.; Sadatsafavi, M.; Anstrom, K.J.; Au, D.H.; Bender, B.G.; Brookhart, M.A.; et al. Informing Healthcare Decisions with Observational Research Assessing Causal Effect: An Official American Thoracic Society Research Statement. *Am. J. Respir. Crit. Care Med.* **2021**, *203*, 14–23. [CrossRef] [PubMed]

healthcare

MDPI

Article

Prediction of COVID-19 Hospitalization and Mortality Using Artificial Intelligence

Marwah Ahmed Halwani [1,*] and Manal Ahmed Halwani [2]

1 College of Business, King Abdulaziz University, Rabigh 21589, Saudi Arabia
2 Emergency Department, College of Medicine, King Abdulaziz University, Jeddah 21589, Saudi Arabia; mahalawani@kau.edu.sa
* Correspondence: mamhalwani@kau.edu.sa

Abstract: Background: COVID-19 has had a substantial influence on healthcare systems, requiring early prognosis for innovative therapies and optimal results, especially in individuals with comorbidities. AI systems have been used by healthcare practitioners for investigating, anticipating, and predicting diseases, through means including medication development, clinical trial analysis, and pandemic forecasting. This study proposes the use of AI to predict disease severity in terms of hospital mortality among COVID-19 patients. Methods: A cross-sectional study was conducted at King Abdulaziz University, Saudi Arabia. Data were cleaned by encoding categorical variables and replacing missing quantitative values with their mean. The outcome variable, hospital mortality, was labeled as death = 0 or survival = 1, with all baseline investigations, clinical symptoms, and laboratory findings used as predictors. Decision trees, SVM, and random forest algorithms were employed. The training process included splitting the data set into training and testing sets, performing 5-fold cross-validation to tune hyperparameters, and evaluating performance on the test set using accuracy. Results: The study assessed the predictive accuracy of outcomes and mortality for COVID-19 patients based on factors such as CRP, LDH, Ferritin, ALP, Bilirubin, D-Dimers, and hospital stay (p-value ≤ 0.05). The analysis revealed that hospital stay, D-Dimers, ALP, Bilirubin, LDH, CRP, and Ferritin significantly influenced hospital mortality ($p \leq 0.0001$). The results demonstrated high predictive accuracy, with decision trees achieving 76%, random forest 80%, and support vector machines (SVMs) 82%. Conclusions: Artificial intelligence is a tool crucial for identifying early coronavirus infections and monitoring patient conditions. It improves treatment consistency and decision-making via the development of algorithms.

Keywords: artificial intelligence; clinical decision support systems; predictive tools; disease severity; mortality

1. Introduction

A virus is an infectious microbe with a unique genome and protein layer that can reproduce within live cells. By hijacking host cells, these tiny, potent viruses can cause significant health issues [1]. SARS-CoV-2, a new coronavirus, belongs to a larger family of pathogenic viruses that target the respiratory system of humans. It was discovered in 2002 and caused mild infection in China [2]. The seventh strain of SARS-CoV-2, COVID-19, emerged in December 2019, causing respiratory problems and having high transmission rates among species [3]. COVID-19, induced by SARS-CoV-2, has resulted in widespread morbidity and mortality [4]. Despite immunizations, there is a need to prevent morbidity and death from severe COVID-19, especially among vulnerable groups [5]. Evidence points to a vicious loop of immunological dysfunction, endothelial damage, complement activation, and microangiopathy, making these processes critical [6].

In January 2020, the WHO labeled it a public health emergency of international concern (PHEIC) because of its lethal effect on human life [7]. The World Health Organization

(WHO) proclaimed COVID-19 a worldwide pandemic on 11 March 2020 [8]. COVID-19 swept over the world in 2020, infecting over 623 million people and causing over 6 million fatalities globally, as well as more than 5 million hospitalizations in the United States by 1 September 2022 [9]. Pandemics and epidemics are characterized by the spread of infectious diseases over a specific period, leading to significant morbidities and mortalities. The SARS epidemic, which infected over 8096 individuals and resulted in over 770 deaths, had greatly devastating effects [10]. Over 213 nations and territories have been affected by the pandemic since its first outbreak in China, infecting more than 98,529,820 people and killing more than 2,116,101 people. The World Health Organization has declared COVID-19 a pandemic, and experts are formulating measures to mitigate its impact on human health and the economy [11].

COVID-19 has a substantial impact on healthcare systems, particularly in patients with acute respiratory syndrome (ARS), necessitating early prognosis for innovative therapies and better results, especially in those with comorbidities [12]. RT-PCR is the standard method for detecting COVID-19 patients as early as possible for effective therapy and containment [13]. Advances in alternative diagnostic technologies are required to speed up detection and treatment, as healthcare professionals and medical personnel are limited, leading to radiologists' becoming overburdened [14]. In conjunction with COVID-19-related outcomes, the scientific community has widely supported artificial intelligence (AI), a concept encompassing computer systems capable of completing tasks that would otherwise require human intelligence [15].

AI specialists recommend creating ML and DL approaches to help radiologists diagnose pneumonia using imaging modalities and chest scans, which would enable physicians to better combat the disease [16,17]. Using computer algorithms to discover data regularities and categories them, ML is an AI branch with the potential for achieving high prediction accuracy and scalability, especially in fast-paced scenarios like the COVID-19 pandemic, which requires models that can adapt to changing data sources [18].

Classification and regression accuracy are improved with deep learning approaches because the latter have autonomous learning and feature representation capabilities, thereby eliminating the need for human expertise [19]. The development of auxiliary tools for detecting COVID-19-infected humans is crucial. Computer Tomography (CT) and chest X-ray (CXR) images of the lungs are linked to COVID-19 detection [20]. AI systems have been used by healthcare practitioners since 1976 for investigating, anticipating, and predicting diseases, including medication development, clinical trial analysis, and pandemic forecasting [21].

Considering the continually altering COVID-19 due to vaccination and viral mutations, there is an unmet clinical need for a prediction tool based on robust characteristics. Despite advancements in COVID-19 detection, there is no risk prediction model for early disease severity identification. Recent models and artificial networks have high sensitivity and specificity for predicting morbidity and mortality, but they rely on genetic susceptibility, requiring screening for multiple mutations that do not apply to the general population. The current study develops a risk prediction model for COVID-19 outcomes using artificial networks and minimal routine laboratory indices, focusing on admission to the Emergency Department to enhance its value in clinical practice.

2. Literature Review

Globally, about 25 million COVID-19 fatalities have been documented, and patients may require intensive care for up to four weeks, which puts a strain on healthcare systems. Prediction models can help clinical decision-making. A study conducted by Sharma et al. in 2020 examines the prediction of COVID-19 using machine learning and big data, taking into account all important factors. It was discovered that some algorithms have weak prediction patterns, resulting in inverted anticipated values. From 30 January to 30 May 2020, the study used two classification methods for Indian COVID-19 cases, as well as a population index. The Bayes point machine and logistic regression algorithms achieved the highest accuracy of 99.6% and 99.4%, respectively. The findings imply that anticipating future COVID-19 fatalities can aid in medical decision-making, particularly when immediate treatment is required [22].

A retrospective cohort analysis by Guan X et al., in 2021, of 1270 COVID-19 patients discovered that six major predictors of death were disease severity, age, high-sensitivity C-reactive protein (hs-CRP), lactate dehydrogenase (LDH), Ferritin, and interleukin-10. The simple-tree XGBoost model, which incorporated these characteristics, predicted death risk with over 90% accuracy and 85% sensitivity, with F1 scores more than 0.90 in both training and validation datasets. These findings might be useful in identifying high-risk situations [23]. The COVID-19 pandemic has raised worldwide healthcare demand, needing timely clinical evaluation. Using clinical data such as lymphocyte count, LDH, and CRP, Yan et al. predicted COVID-19 mortality with 90% accuracy. High LDH levels signal a need for emergency medical intervention. This offers a rule for prioritizing high-risk patients [24].

Supervised learning algorithms have been widely used in predicting COVID-19 results. Studies have been demonstrated on clinical data such as demographics, comorbidities, and test findings. These models can predict hospitalization and mortality risks with high accuracy. Maghdid et al. used a CNN-based model to analyze chest X-rays and CT images, reaching high prediction accuracy for severe COVID-19 patients [25]. The study based on generative adversarial networks (GANs) offers a data-efficient deep network for detecting COVID-19 on CT images. This technology makes more CT scans available while also estimating the parameters of convolutional and fully linked layers using synthetic and augmented data. The GAN-based deep learning model outperforms conventional models for COVID-19 detection, with ResNet-18 and MobileNetV2 performing best on the COVID-19 and Mosmed datasets, respectively [26]. Wynants and colleagues examined 145 models for COVID-19 prognosis, including 23 that predicted death. They discovered significant bias, imprecise reporting, and no external validation. As a result, the employment of these anticipated models is not encouraged in current practice [27].

COVID-19 has resulted in the prevalence of low-quality clinical prediction models. More actions are needed to serve patients in all areas of healthcare by building model development frameworks. The potential of AI in predicting COVID-19 hospitalization and mortality is intriguing, but issues with data quality, model interpretability, and generalizability must be solved before it can be fully utilized.

3. Materials and Methods

Research Ethics Committee boards approved a study, waived written informed consent, and de-identified patient data to avoid confidentiality breaches.

Patient cohorts: A cross-sectional study was conducted after approval from the Research Ethics Committee of King Abdulaziz University (KAU), Saudi Arabia. The study used sequential sampling approaches to include 50 Real-Time Polymerase Chain Reaction (RT-PCR)-positive COVID-19 patients from KAU's coronavirus isolation wards. Medical records were collected and analyzed by clinical teams. The results of RT-PCR were obtained from electronic medical records using approved TaqMan One-Step Kits. Positive results on the last-performed test confirmed diagnosis for patients with multiple assays.

Demographic and clinical information: Demographic information about each patient was gathered, including age, gender, symptoms, white blood cell and lymphocyte counts, comorbidity status, and history of COVID-19 exposure. Information on patients' mechanical breathing, intense medical treatment, death progression, admission and discharge times, and illness severity were all recorded based on symptom records, clinical findings, and chest X-rays. A pre-designed form was used to record each patient's demographic information, including age and gender, signs and symptoms, illness severity (mild, moderate, severe), and laboratory findings. Furthermore, the length of the hospital stay and the outcome, whether the patient recovered or died, were reported. Treatment information and clinical results were tracked over the following weeks until discharge (Table S1).

Predictive analysis: Predictive analytics, a subset of advanced analytics, uses historical data, statistical algorithms, and machine learning techniques to forecast future occurrences or outcomes. Through the examination of data patterns, trends are identified, and future behavior or events are predicted. Historical data serve as the basis for training forecasting models in this area. These models are then used to extrapolate predictions from new or unpublished data. Predictions range from simple binary outcomes such as positive or negative responses to complex scenarios involving multiple possible outcomes. In the current study, the steps outlined in the following paragraphs were followed to predict disease severity in terms of hospital mortality among COVID-19 patients. The study recorded demographic details, signs and symptoms, disease severity (Table 1), as well as laboratory findings such as Bilirubin, AST, ALT, phosphomonoesterases, GGT, protein, CRP, D-Dimers, white blood cells, platelets, LDH, prothrombin time, and Ferritin (ng/mL) (Table 2).

Table 1. COVID-19 patients' demographics and baseline characteristics.

Variables		
Age (Mean ± SD)	50.9 ± 15.09	
Hospital Stay (Days)	14.6 ± 2.8	
	Frequency	Percentages (%)
Gender		
Male	28	56.0
Female	22	44.0
Disease Severity		
Mild	17	34.0
Moderate	23	46.0
Severe	7	14.0
Critical	3	6.0
Sign and Symptoms		
Fever	24	48.0
Cough	18	36.0
Sore throat	12	24.0
Diarrhea	12	24.0
Fatigue	19	38.0
Nausea	8	16.0
Abdominal pain	5	10.0
Outcome		
Death	6	12.0
Survived	44	88.0

Table 2. Baseline laboratory.

Laboratory Parameters	Normal Range	Mean ± SD	Minimum	Maximum	Range
White blood cell × 10^9/L	3.5–9.5	11.91 ± 12.9	0.741	76.6	75.85
Platelets × 10^9/L	125–350	220.0 ± 80.5	40.0	418.0	378.0
CRP (mg/L)	<3	60.18 ± 83.01	0.10	322.13	322.03
LDH (U/L)	140 to 280	296.98 ± 163.01	155.0	1044.0	889.0

Table 2. *Cont.*

Laboratory Parameters	Normal Range	Mean ± SD	Minimum	Maximum	Range
Ferritin (ng/mL)	12 to 300	479.89 ± 436.07	8.0	1675	1667
D-Dimers (mg/L)	>0.5	438.59 ± 443.0	0.2	1600.0	1599.8
Alkaline phosphatase (ALP), (U/L)	44–147	85.12 ± 23.64	40.0	135.00	95.0
Gamma-glutamyl transferase (GGT), (U/L)	0–30	40.12 ± 16.54	10.0	79.0	69.0
Alanine transaminase (ALT), (U/L)	7–50	33.28 ± 11.12	17.0	60.0	43.0
Aspartate aminotransferase (AST), (U/L)	15–40	38.64 ± 13.93	18.0	75.0	57.0
Bilirubin (mg/dL)	<0.3	0.63 ± 0.32	0.2	1.4	1.2
Prothrombin time/sec	10–13/sec	11.6 ± 1.47	8.0	14.0	6.0
Calcium (mg/dL)	8.5 to 10.2	8.8 ± 0.33	8.0	9.6	1.6
Potassium (mEq/L)	3.5–5	4.05 ± 0.80	2.9	8.8	5.9

Data preprocessing:

a. Data cleaning and transformation: The data were cleaned through the handling of missing values. Missing values in the dataset were handled by using a boxplot. Records lacking essential data points were excluded from the analysis to maintain the models' integrity. The categorical variables were coded according to categorical variables, and the quantitative variables' missing values were replaced by their mean. The outcome variable (hospital mortality) was properly labeled as death = 0 or survival = 1. All the baseline investigations, clinical symptoms, and laboratory findings were labeled as predictors.
b. Dataset splitting: The data were divided into training and testing sets, with the training set used for model development and the testing set reserved for performance evaluation. To optimize the models' hyperparameters and enhance generalizability, a 5-fold cross-validation technique was applied. This approach helps minimize variance and bias in the models' performance.

Machine learning algorithms:

The algorithms used in the study were decision trees, SVM, and random forest.

Hyperparameters:

a. Decision trees: The model's hyperparameters include a maximum depth of 10 and a minimum sample split of 2. The criterion used for measuring the quality of splits is Gini impurity.
b. Support vector machines (SVMs): The model used a radial basis function (RBF) kernel, which is effective in high-dimensional spaces. The regularization parameter was set to 1.0, balancing the trade-off between maximizing the margin and minimizing classification errors. The kernel coefficient \(\gamma\) was set to 'scale'. This helps in capturing the non-linear relationships in the data. The tolerance for stopping criteria was set to 0.001. A 5-fold cross-validation was performed to ensure robustness and prevent overfitting.
c. Random forest: The model used 100 trees, balancing computational efficiency and model performance. The maximum depth of each tree was set to none, allowing trees to grow until all leaves were pure or until all leaves contained less than the minimum samples required to split. The minimum number of samples required to split an internal node was set to 2. The model used the Gini impurity criterion to measure the quality of a split. Bootstrap samples were used when building trees to reduce overfitting. A 5-fold cross-validation was performed to tune the hyperparameters and validate the model's performance.

These hyperparameters were optimized to enhance the predictive accuracy of the SVM and random forest models in predicting COVID-19 patient mortality.

Training process:

The dataset is divided into training and testing sets, typically with an 80–20 split. Cross-validation, such as 5-fold cross-validation, is performed to tune hyperparameters and prevent overfitting. The model is then trained using the training set and validated using the validation set. Finally, the model's performance is evaluated on the test set using appropriate metrics, such as accuracy.

Technical characteristics of computer used:

The computer utilized for the analysis is equipped with an Intel Core i7-9700K CPU, 32 GB DDR4 RAM, and an NVIDIA GeForce RTX 2080 Ti GPU. It also features 1 TB of SSD storage and runs on the Windows 10 Pro operating system. The software environment includes Python 3.8 as the programming language, with libraries such as Scikit-learn 0.24.2 for machine learning algorithms, Pandas 1.2.4 for data manipulation, NumPy 1.20.2 for numerical computations, and Matplotlib 3.4.2 and Seaborn 0.11.1 for data visualization. The analysis is conducted using the Jupyter Notebook 6.3.0 integrated development environment (IDE).

Block diagram:

The study follows a structured approach consisting of several key steps. First, data collection involves gathering patient data, including demographics, symptoms, and laboratory results. Second, data preprocessing entails cleaning and preparing the data for analysis. Third, feature selection identifies the key features that impact the prediction of COVID-19 outcomes. Fourth, model training is performed using the selected features to train machine learning models. Fifth, model evaluation assesses the models' performance using accuracy, precision, and recall metrics. Finally, the prediction phase involves using the trained models to predict outcomes for new patients (Figure 1).

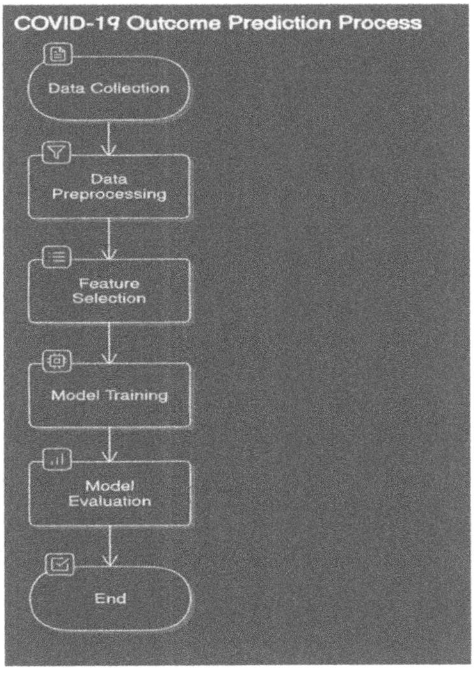

Figure 1. Block diagram of the study.

Statistical analysis: The data were entered and analyzed in SPSS. Mean ± standard deviation (SD) was calculated for quantitative variables and frequency/percentages for qualitative variables. The mean difference among laboratory findings for the outcome variables was calculated through an independent sample *t*-test. *p*-value < 0.05 was significant.

4. Results

4.1. Demographics and Baselines of COVID-19 Patients

The study included 50 patients, with an average age of 50.9 years (SD = 15.09). Patients stayed in the hospital for an average duration of 14.6 days (SD = 2.8). Gender distribution revealed 56.0% male and 44.0% female participants. Disease severity varied, with 34.0% experiencing mild symptoms, 46.0% moderate, 14.0% severe, and 6.0% critical conditions. Common symptoms included fever (48.0%), fatigue (38.0%), cough (36.0%), sore throat (24.0%), and diarrhea (24.0%). Less common symptoms were nausea (16.0%) and abdominal pain (10.0%). The majority of patients (88.0%) survived, while 12.0% unfortunately died due to COVID-19 (Table 1).

4.2. Laboratory Parameters in COVID-19 Patients

The analysis of laboratory parameters in the COVID-19 patients revealed significant details. The average white blood cell count was $11.91 \times 10^9/L$, indicating a broad range, predominantly above the normal threshold. The platelet count averaged $220.0 \times 10^9/L$, remaining within the expected range. However, the C-reactive protein (CRP) levels were notably elevated, averaging 60.18 mg/L, suggesting heightened inflammation. The lactate dehydrogenase (LDH) levels exhibited a mean of 296.98 U/L, indicating potential tissue damage. The Ferritin levels were also elevated, with a mean of 479.89 ng/mL, implying inflammation or iron overload. The D-Dimer levels showed an average of 438.59 mg/L, indicative of possible blood clot formation. While alkaline phosphatase (ALP), gamma-glutamyl transferase (GGT), alanine transaminase (ALT), and aspartate aminotransferase (AST) levels generally fell within normal ranges, the Bilirubin levels were slightly elevated, averaging 0.63 mg/dL. The prothrombin time and calcium levels remained within the expected parameters, while the potassium levels averaged 4.05 mEq/L, within normal limits (Table 2). There was a significant difference in CRP, LDH, Ferritin, ALP, Bilirubin, D-Dimers, and hospital stay, with a *p*-value < 0.05 (Table 3).

Table 3. Mean difference of laboratory findings among outcome variables (survival/death).

Laboratory Findings	Outcome	Mean ± SD	*p*-Value
WCC	Survival	10.81 ± 9.34	0.104
	Death	19.99 ± 28.37	
PLT	Survival	222.25 ± 72.39	0.605
	Death	203.83 ± 134.95	
CRP	Survival	51.17 ± 69.86	≤0.05 *
	Death	124.80 ± 139.48	
LDH	Survival	271.52 ± 102.10	≤0.001 **
	Death	483.67 ± 351.06	
Ferritin	Survival	439.42 ± 365.26	≤0.05 *
	Death	835.98 ± 819.24	
D-Dimers	Survival	332.47395 ± 345.07	≤0.001 **
	Death	1216.8 ± 271.52	
ALP	Survival	81.73 ± 22.25	≤0.001 **
	Death	110.00 ± 19.48	

Table 3. *Cont.*

Laboratory Findings	Outcome	Mean ± SD	*p*-Value
GGT	Survival	38.80 ± 16.88	0.127
	Death	49.83 ± 10.21	
ALT	Survival	32.68 ± 11.53	0.308
	Death	37.67 ± 6.53	
AST	Survival	37.70 ± 14.41	0.202
	Death	45.50 ± 7.31	
Bilirubin	Survival	0.60 ± 0.30	≤0.05 *
	Death	0.88 ± 0.39	
Prothrombin time	Survival	11.64 ± 1.40	0.641
	Death	11.33 ± 2.07	
Calcium	Survival	8.81 ± 0.35	0.595
	Death	8.73 ± 0.23	
Potassium	Survival	4.07 ± 0.83	0.665
	Death	3.92 ± 0.62	
Hospital stay	Survival	14.57 ± 2.96	≤0.001 **
	Death	23.00 ± 2.83	

p-value ≤ 0.05 * significant, *p*-value ≤ 0.01 ** strongly significant, results from independent sample *t*-test.

4.3. *Prediction of Mortality*

The hospital stay, D-Dimers, ALP, Bilirubin, LDH, CRP, and Ferritin levels were higher in COVID-19 patients indicated in Figure 2.

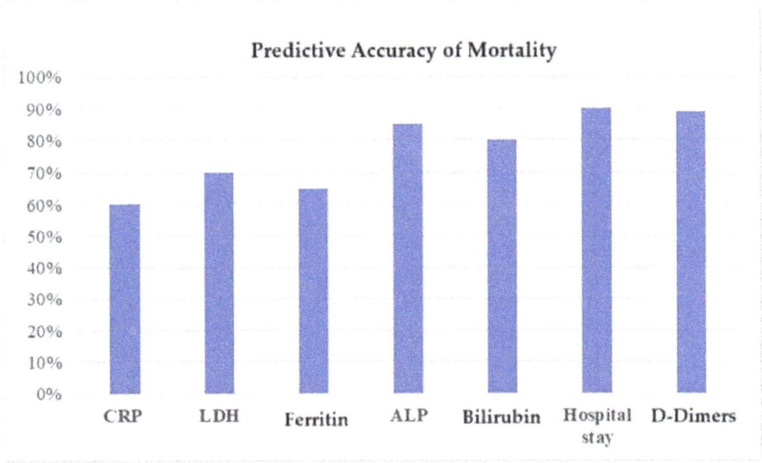

Figure 2. Predictive accuracy of mortality according to lab findings.

Increased levels indicated its association with mortality. The algorithm's accuracy was calculated and indicated high accuracy of the decision tree at 76%, random forest 80%, and SVM 82%; the decision tree was calculated, indicating a high decision tree (Table 4).

Table 4. Predictive accuracy of algorithms.

Algorithms	Accuracy (%)
Decision tree	76%
Random forest	80%
SVM	82%

4.4. Hypothetical Confusion Matrix for SVM

Table 5 shows that 41 patients survived, while 42 did not. The performance metrics of the model are as follows: sensitivity was 83.67%, specificity was 82.35%, positive predictive value (PPV) was 82.0%, negative predictive value (NPV) was 84.0%, and overall accuracy was 83%.

Table 5. Hypothetical confusion matrix for SVM.

Actual Findings	Results from SVM	
	Positive (Survived)	Negative (Died)
Positive (survived)	41	9
Negative (died)	8	42
Sensitivity	83.67%	
Specificity	82.35%	
Positive predicted value (PP V)	82.0%	
Negative predictive value (NPV)	84.0%	
Accuracy	83.0%	

The formula used to evaluate the diagnostic accuracy:

$$Accuracy = \frac{TP + TN}{TP + TN + FP + FN}$$

5. Discussion

The research included 50 patients with various illness severities, with the majority feeling fever, weariness, cough, sore throat, and diarrhea. The majority survived, with 56.0% males. The research of COVID-19 patients revealed laboratory measures, including an average white blood cell count that was higher than normal, a platelet count that was within the predicted range, raised C-reactive protein levels, probable tissue damage, ferritin levels, and D-Dimer levels. Other indicators, including alkaline phosphatase, gamma-glutamyl transferase, alanine transaminase, and aspartate aminotransferase, were typically within normal limits. Bilirubin levels were slightly higher, but prothrombin time, calcium, and potassium levels were within normal ranges.

The study conducted by Yaşar Ş et al. [28] demonstrates that, by utilizing AI, the prognosis of COVID-19 patients is mostly based on clinical characteristics such as vital signs and laboratory testing, which is also indicated in our work. The shortcoming of the previous study was that they did not use X-rays as a prediction for COVID-19 severity; this is also the limitation of our study. The work also emphasizes the feasibility of combining clinical information and laboratory values in a single system, offering a fresh viewpoint on prognostic AI systems. Acute respiratory distress syndrome affects 15% of patients, and more than half of ICU admissions are due to hypoxia or respiratory fatigue. Analysis using AI systems based on clinical data can predict disease development more accurately than clinical data alone, improving patient care by combining information from different sources [29]. The current study also emphasized the use of AI-based clinical prediction for the severity of COVID-19 to make it a predictive tool.

Early detection and treatment of COVID-19 disease is crucial for decreased mortality, especially for severely ill patients. Previous research using imaging data from COVID-19 patients has mostly focused on diagnosis rather than prognosis [30]. Prognostic models may forecast mortality, morbidity, and other outcomes, and they have real-world applications in patient identification, bed management, situational awareness, and resource allocation [31].

Computers are expected to play a crucial role in combating global health emergencies, with AI being extensively applied to predict clinical outcomes of hospitalization and mortality. AI is produced by computer systems capable of doing tasks that require human-like intellect, with machine learning playing a critical role in providing high prediction accuracy and scalability [32]. Substantial efforts from the scientific community have aimed to integrate AI, particularly machine learning, into predictive modeling for COVID-19-related outcomes [33]. ML and deep learning (DL) are key components of AI that use algorithms to learn and adapt from data. DL, a subset of machine learning, extracts complicated information using neural networks with numerous layers; it includes deep, deep belief, and recurrent learning [34]. This research introduced predicting COVID-19 diagnosis based on baseline demographics, comorbidities, vital signs, and lab findings. Predictive models can be used for diagnosis when the testing capacity is restricted, or they can be combined with clinical judgment. They uncover crucial clinical characteristics associated with positive diagnosis, giving information for effective patient stratification and population screening. The single-tree model's decision algorithm can be used in healthcare settings. The studies indicated acute respiratory distress syndrome (ARDS) and/or sepsis are strong markers of a positive COVID-19 diagnosis [35].

ML algorithms were associated with a positive COVID-19 diagnosis in both symptomatic and asymptomatic patients. Four models indicated age, lab results, comorbidities, vital signs, and hematologic characteristics as predictors of a positive diagnosis. Abnormal liver function tests, as well as low white blood cell count and hemoglobin levels, have previously been identified as indications of COVID-19 severity. These data may help predict the severity of COVID-19 [36]. The study's innovative use of machine learning classification may face significant challenges in model interpretability, which is essential for effective clinical decision-making. The complexity of these models can obscure the reasoning behind predictions. Moreover, by concentrating on comorbidities and their interactions with symptoms, the study may neglect other crucial factors, such as mental health, social determinants of health, and patient behavior, which also play a key role in COVID-19 outcomes.

Our results discovered that blood CRP, LDH, Ferritin, ALP, Bilirubin, and D-Dimer levels were the strongest predictive characteristic of COVID-19 diagnosis, which is consistent with earlier research identifying serum levels as a biomarker of clinical severity and poor prognosis. Numerous research has investigated the significance of biochemical and hematological indicators in COVID-19 to develop an algorithm for identifying poor prognosis, ventilation, and early intervention. Despite this, there is little agreement on this subject, and future studies should focus on regional biomarker profiles.

A comprehensive overview in a study conducted in 2021 found AI applications in the field of COVID-19 address various areas and have many benefits. In disease diagnosis, AI helps in the interpretation of various tests and symptoms and facilitates the rapid and accurate identification of infections. AI also contributes to patient monitoring by enabling continuous assessment and timely intervention. It plays a crucial role in determining the severity of a patient's condition and helps healthcare providers prioritize treatment strategies effectively. When processing imaging tests related to COVID-19, AI algorithms improve the analysis of radiological scans and enable the rapid detection of abnormalities indicative of infection by the virus. Epidemiology benefits from AI-driven predictive modeling, which helps to predict outbreaks, track trans-mission patterns, and develop targeted intervention strategies [37]. However, this paper's case studies may not be diverse enough, restricting a comprehensive understanding of AI's effectiveness across different healthcare systems. While ethical concerns such as data privacy and algorithmic bias are acknowledged, they are not thoroughly examined. Moreover, although the paper addresses emerging technologies and policy recommendations, it falls short of providing specific examples or actionable steps for AI implementation after the pandemic.

A deep learning system has been developed to predict the malignant progression of COVID-19 using clinical data and CT scans studied in 2020 in China. The system achieved an average AUC of 0.874 in a multicenter study. The system automatically identifies key indicators contributing to malignant progression, including Troponin, Brain natriuretic peptide, White cell count, Aspartate aminotransferase, Creatinine, and Hypersensitive C-reactive protein [38]. Another important study in 2020 conducted by Wynants et al. provided a detailed assessment of COVID-19 diagnosis and prognosis, assessing prediction models' accuracy and value in detecting suspected infections, forecasting patient outcomes, and identifying persons at increased risk of infection or hospitalization [39].

AI is currently being used to predict COVID-19 mortality and hospitalization by combining patient demographics, medical history, vital signs, and laboratory data. The objective is to identify high-risk individuals so that they can receive prompt medical treatment. Mortality studies employ comparable input factors, with an emphasis on illness severity and progression. Machine learning also predicts hospitalization and death, taking into account the interplay of these events [40].

Due to their excellent accuracy, machine learning algorithms, notably random forest, have been successful in predicting COVID-19-related hospitalization and mortality. Random forest operates by constructing multiple decision trees and aggregating predictions, effectively capturing complex data relationships [41]. Its versatility allows for handling diverse input variables without extensive pre-processing. Additionally, random forest provides insights into feature importance, aiding in identifying key predictors of COVID-19 outcomes. These analytical advantages make random forest a valuable tool in medical research and decision-making processes surrounding COVID-19 [42]. The study revealed the efficacy of predictive models in COVID-19 diagnosis, allowing for effective screening and patient classification. This is critical given the current pandemic's impact on huge populations, which necessitates more efficient testing resource allocation and improved patient care.

Another study examined clinical features and lab indicators in severe and non-severe COVID-19 patients, identifying significant differences in neutrophil-to-lymphocyte ratio, C-reactive protein, and lactate dehydrogenase. They developed a decision tree model that accurately predicted mortality in critically ill patients with 98% precision, helping prioritize treatment for high-risk individuals [43]. These findings were also comparable with our study, which also indicates that the tree predicts COVID mortality with good precision. However, a major shortcoming is the difficulty in generalizing AI models to different populations and settings. Models trained on specific datasets may not perform accurately when applied to new or diverse groups, leading to unreliable predictions.

Joaquim Carreras' study employed artificial intelligence (AI) to analyze celiac disease using a transcriptomic panel focused on autoimmune discovery. The AI models demonstrated exceptional accuracy, ranging from 95% to 100%, in predicting celiac disease based on the autoimmune gene panel. This highlights the models' effectiveness in distinguishing celiac disease patients from control subjects [44].

6. Conclusions

The gold-standard PCR test for COVID-19 is constrained by high turnaround times, a lack of specialized equipment, and low sensitivity, providing a challenge to global healthcare systems. NHS guidelines require testing of all emergency admissions, regardless of clinical suspicion, emphasizing the critical requirement for prompt and accurate COVID-19 exclusion in acute care settings. Our models have a strong predictive performance, making them suitable for screening COVID-19 diagnoses in emergency rooms. They help make rapid treatment decisions, guide safe patient streaming, and act as a pre-test for diagnostic molecular testing. Key benefit categories include viral-free individuals who were properly predicted to be COVID-19-negative. This strategy is extensively used in clinical practice. The clinically focused approach ruled out COVID-19 in enriched subpopulations that were more likely to test positive, proposing conclusive testing, comparable to the D-Dimer test for suspected deep-vein thrombosis and pulmonary embolism.

The integration of AI has significantly advanced the fight against COVID-19. From diagnosis to predicting outcomes to modeling future trends, AI has played a crucial role in interpreting data, improving patient care, and predicting outbreak dynamics. In addition, the application of ML models has significantly improved predictive accuracy and provided valuable insights into COVID-19-related hospital admissions and mortality rates. During a global health crisis, AI can improve public health and solve pandemic-related issues by improving decision-making and patient outcomes.

Until now, early detection models have mostly focused on radiological imaging evaluation. Few studies have evaluated routine laboratory tests, with studies to date including small numbers of patients with confirmed COVID-19, using PCR results for data labeling, and thus not ensuring disease freedom in so-called negative patients, as well as not being validated in the clinical population that is the target for their intended use.

7. Limitations of the Study

The use of small control cohorts during training is a shortcoming of this study since it fails to expose models to the breadth and range of alternate infectious and non-infectious diseases, including seasonal pathologies. Furthermore, while the application of artificial intelligence approaches for early detection has enormous potential, several published models are highly biased.

Supplementary Materials: The following supporting information can be downloaded at: https://www.mdpi.com/article/10.3390/healthcare12171694/s1. Table S1: COVID data.

Author Contributions: All of the authors contributed equally to the work. Conceptualization, M.A.H. (Marwah Ahmed Halwani); Validation, M.A.H. (Marwah Ahmed Halwani); Formal analysis, M.A.H. (Marwah Ahmed Halwani); Data curation, M.A.H. (Manal Ahmed Halwani); Writing—original draft, M.A.H. (Marwah Ahmed Halwani); Writing—review & editing, M.A.H. (Manal Ahmed Halwani). All authors have read and agreed to the published version of the manuscript.

Funding: This research received no external funding.

Institutional Review Board Statement: The study was conducted after approval from the Research Ethics Committee (REC), King Abdulaziz University, Saudi Arabia, under the NCBE Registration No: (HA-02-J-008, 11 April 2023), which allowed the authors to conduct the studies involving humans.

Informed Consent Statement: Informed consent was obtained from all of the subjects involved in the study.

Data Availability Statement: Data supporting reported results can be found, including links to publicly archived datasets analyzed or generated during the study.

Conflicts of Interest: The authors declare no conflicts of interest.

References

1. Domingo, E.J. Introduction to virus origins and their role in biological evolution. In *Virus as Populations*; Academic Press: Cambridge, MA, USA, 2020; pp. 1–33.
2. Kang, S.; Peng, W.; Zhu, Y.; Lu, S.; Zhou, M.; Lin, W.; Wu, W.; Huang, S.; Jiang, L.; Luo, X.; et al. Recent progress in understanding 2019 novel coronavirus (SARS-CoV-2) associated with human respiratory disease: Detection, mechanisms and treatment. *Int. J. Antimicrob. Agents* **2020**, *55*, 105950. [CrossRef] [PubMed]
3. Mohapatra, R.K.; Pintilie, L.; Kandi, V.; Sarangi, A.K.; Das, D.; Sahu, R.; Perekhoda, L. The recent challenges of highly contagious COVID-19, causing respiratory infections: Symptoms, diagnosis, transmission, possible vaccines, animal models, and immunotherapy. *Chem. Biol. Drug Des.* **2020**, *96*, 1187–1208. [CrossRef] [PubMed]
4. Mohan, B.; Nambiar, V.J. COVID-19: An insight into the SARS-CoV-2 pandemic originated at Wuhan City in Hubei Province of China. *J. Infect. Dis. Epidemiol.* **2020**, *6*, 146. [CrossRef]
5. Zhang, J.-j.; Dong, X.; Liu, G.-H.; Gao, Y.-D. Risk and protective factors for COVID-19 morbidity, severity, and mortality. *Clin. Rev. Allergy Immunol.* **2023**, *64*, 90–107. [CrossRef]

6. Ragnoli, B.; Da Re, B.; Galantino, A.; Kette, S.; Salotti, A.; Malerba, M. Interrelationship between COVID-19 and coagulopathy: Pathophysiological and clinical evidence. *Int. J. Mol. Sci.* **2023**, *24*, 8945. [CrossRef] [PubMed]
7. Wilder-Smith, A.; Osman, S. Public health emergencies of international concern: A historic overview. *J. Travel Med.* **2020**, *27*, taaa227. [CrossRef] [PubMed]
8. Zanke, A.A.; Thenge, R.R.; Adhao, V.S. COVID-19: A pandemic declared by the World Health Organization. *IP Int. J. Compr. Adv. Pharmacol.* **2020**, *5*, 49–57. [CrossRef]
9. Sohrabi, C.; Alsafi, Z.; O'neill, N.; Khan, M.; Kerwan, A.; Al-Jabir, A.; Iosifidis, C.; Agha, R. World Health Organization declares global emergency: A review of the 2019 novel coronavirus (COVID-19). *Int. J. Surg.* **2020**, *76*, 71–76. [CrossRef]
10. Yang, Y.; Peng, F.; Wang, R.; Guan, K.; Jiang, T.; Xu, G.; Sun, J.; Chang, C. The deadly coronaviruses: The 2003 SARS pandemic and the 2020 novel coronavirus epidemic in China. *J. Autoimmun.* **2020**, *109*, 102434. [CrossRef]
11. Adil, M.T.; Rahman, R.; Whitelaw, D.; Jain, V.; Al-Taan, O.; Rashid, F.; Munasinghe, A.; Jambulingam, P. SARS-CoV-2 and the pandemic of COVID-19. *Postgrad. Med. J.* **2021**, *97*, 110–116. [CrossRef]
12. Mallah, S.I.; Ghorab, O.K.; Al-Salmi, S.; Abdellatif, O.S.; Tharmaratnam, T.; Iskandar, M.A.; Sefen, J.A.N.; Sidhu, P.; Atallah, B.; El-Lababidi, R.; et al. COVID-19: Breaking down a global health crisis. *Ann. Clin. Microbiol. Antimicrob.* **2021**, *20*, 35. [CrossRef]
13. Lan, L.; Xu, D.; Ye, G.; Xia, C.; Wang, S.; Li, Y.; Xu, H. Positive RT-PCR test results in patients recovered from COVID-19. *JAMA* **2020**, *323*, 1502–1503. [CrossRef]
14. Fields, B.K.; Demirjian, N.L.; Gholamrezanezhad, A. Coronavirus Disease 2019 (COVID-19) diagnostic technologies: A country-based retrospective analysis of screening and containment procedures during the first wave of the pandemic. *Clin. Imaging* **2020**, *67*, 219–225. [CrossRef] [PubMed]
15. Piccialli, F.; Di Cola, V.S.; Giampaolo, F.; Cuomo, S. The role of artificial intelligence in fighting the COVID-19 pandemic. *Inf. Syst. Front.* **2021**, *23*, 1467–1497. [CrossRef] [PubMed]
16. Aruleba, R.T.; Adekiya, T.A.; Ayawei, N.; Obaido, G.; Aruleba, K.; Mienye, I.D.; Aruleba, I.; Ogbuokiri, B. COVID-19 Diagnosis: A Review of Rapid Antigen, RT-PCR and Artificial Intelligence Methods. *Bioengineering* **2022**, *9*, 153. [CrossRef] [PubMed]
17. Majumder, D.D. A unified approach to artificial intelligence, pattern recognition, image processing and computer vision in fifth-generation computer systems. *Inf. Sci.* **1988**, *45*, 391–431. [CrossRef]
18. Tsephe, R.; Makoele, L. Rethinking Pedagogy in the 4IR and Innovation-Driven Economy: Challenges and Opportunities. In Proceedings of the 18th International Technology, Education and Development Conference, Valencia, Spain, 4–6 March 2024; pp. 5042–5049.
19. Elshawi, R.; Maher, M.; Sakr, S. Automated machine learning: State-of-the-art and open challenges. *arXiv* **2019**, arXiv:1906.02287. [CrossRef]
20. Gudigar, A.; Raghavendra, U.; Nayak, S.; Ooi, C.P.; Chan, W.Y.; Gangavarapu, M.R.; Dharmik, C.; Samanth, J.; Kadri, N.A.; Hasikin, K.; et al. Role of artificial intelligence in COVID-19 detection. *Sensors* **2021**, *21*, 8045. [CrossRef]
21. Yang, Y.; Lure, F.Y.; Miao, H.; Zhang, Z.; Jaeger, S.; Liu, J.; Guo, L. Using artificial intelligence to assist radiologists in distinguishing COVID-19 from other pulmonary infections. *J. X-ray Sci. Technol.* **2021**, *29*, 1–17. [CrossRef]
22. Sharma, S.; Gupta, Y.K. Predictive analysis and survey of COVID-19 using machine learning and big data. *J. Interdiscip. Math.* **2021**, *24*, 175–195. [CrossRef]
23. Guan, X.; Zhang, B.; Fu, M.; Li, M.; Yuan, X.; Zhu, Y.; Peng, J.; Guo, H.; Lu, Y. Clinical and inflammatory features based machine learning model for fatal risk prediction of hospitalized COVID-19 patients: Results from a retrospective cohort study. *Ann. Med.* **2021**, *53*, 257–266. [CrossRef]
24. Yan, L.; Zhang, H.-T.; Goncalves, J.; Xiao, Y.; Wang, M.; Guo, Y.; Sun, C.; Tang, X.; Jing, L.; Zhang, M.; et al. An interpretable mortality prediction model for COVID-19 patients. *Nat. Mach. Intell.* **2020**, *2*, 283–288. [CrossRef]
25. Maghded, H.S.; Ghafoor, K.Z.; Sadiq, A.S.; Curran, K.; Rawat, D.B.; Rabie, K. A novel AI-enabled framework to diagnose coronavirus COVID-19 using smartphone embedded sensors: Design study. In Proceedings of the 2020 IEEE 21st International Conference on Information Reuse and Integration for Data Science (IRI), Las Vegas, NV, USA, 11–13 August 2020.
26. Serte, S.; Dirik, M.A.; Al-Turjman, F. Deep learning models for COVID-19 detection. *Sustainability* **2022**, *14*, 5820. [CrossRef]
27. Wynants, L.; Van Calster, B.; Collins, G.S.; Riley, R.D.; Heinze, G.; Schuit, E.; Bonten, M.M.J.; Dahly, D.L.; Damen, J.A.; Debray, T.P.A.; et al. Prediction models for diagnosis and prognosis of COVID-19: Systematic review and critical appraisal. *BMJ* **2020**, *369*, m1328. [CrossRef]
28. Yaşar, Ş.; Çolak, C.; Yoloğlu, S. Artificial intelligence-based prediction of COVID-19 severity on the results of protein profiling. *Comput. Methods Programs Biomed.* **2021**, *202*, 105996. [CrossRef]
29. Zhang, Z.; Navarese, E.P.; Zheng, B.; Meng, Q.; Liu, N.; Ge, H.; Pan, Q.; Yu, Y.; Ma, X. Analytics with artificial intelligence to advance the treatment of acute respiratory distress syndrome. *J. Evid.-Based Med.* **2020**, *13*, 301–312. [CrossRef] [PubMed]
30. Suri, J.S.; Agarwal, S.; Gupta, S.K.; Puvvula, A.; Biswas, M.; Saba, L.; Bit, A.; Tandel, G.S.; Agarwal, M.; Patrick, A.; et al. A narrative review on characterization of acute respiratory distress syndrome in COVID-19-infected lungs using artificial intelligence. *Comput. Biol. Med.* **2021**, *130*, 104210. [CrossRef] [PubMed]
31. Zhang, J.; Jun, T.; Frank, J.; Nirenberg, S.; Kovatch, P.; Huang, K.-L. Prediction of individual COVID-19 diagnosis using baseline demographics and lab data. *Sci. Rep.* **2021**, *11*, 13913. [CrossRef]

32. Badiola-Zabala, G.; Lopez-Guede, J.M.; Estevez, J.; Graña, M. Machine learning first response to COVID-19: A systematic literature review of clinical decision assistance approaches during pandemic years from 2020 to 2022. *Electronics* **2024**, *13*, 1005. [CrossRef]
33. Bilinski, A.; Emanuel, E.J. COVID-19 and excess all-cause mortality in the US and 18 comparison countries. *JAMA* **2020**, *324*, 2100–2102. [CrossRef]
34. Sjoding, M.W.; Taylor, D.; Motyka, J.; Lee, E.; Co, I.; Claar, D.; McSparron, J.I.; Ansari, S.; Kerlin, M.P.; Reilly, J.P.; et al. Deep learning to detect acute respiratory distress syndrome on chest radiographs: A retrospective study with external validation. *Lancet Digit. Health* **2021**, *3*, e340–e348. [CrossRef]
35. Kassirian, S.; Taneja, R.; Mehta, S. Diagnosis and management of acute respiratory distress syndrome in a time of COVID-19. *Diagnostics* **2020**, *10*, 1053. [CrossRef] [PubMed]
36. Aktar, S.; Talukder, A.; Ahamad, M.; Kamal, A.H.M.; Khan, J.R.; Protikuzzaman, M.; Hossain, N.; Azad, A.K.M.; Quinn, J.M.W.; Summers, M.A.; et al. Machine learning approaches to identify patient comorbidities and symptoms that increase the risk of mortality in COVID-19. *Diagnostics* **2021**, *11*, 1383. [CrossRef] [PubMed]
37. Tayarani, M. Applications of artificial intelligence in battling against COVID-19: A literature review. *Chaos Solitons Fractals* **2020**, *142*, 110338. [CrossRef]
38. Bai X, Fang C, Zhou Y, Bai S, Liu Z, Chen Q, Xu Y, Xia T, Gong S, Xie X, Song D. Predicting COVID-19 malignant progression with AI techniques. *MedRxiv*. [CrossRef]
39. Chen, J.H.; Asch, S.M. Machine learning and prediction in medicine—Beyond the peak of inflated expectations. *N. Engl. J. Med.* **2017**, *376*, 2507. [CrossRef]
40. Wang, A.; Li, F.; Chiang, S.; Fulcher, J.; Yang, O.; Wong, D.; Wei, F. Machine learning prediction of COVID-19 severity levels from salivaomics data. *arXiv* **2022**, arXiv:2207.07274v1.
41. Feng, C.; Kephart, G.; Juarez-Colunga, E. Predicting COVID-19 mortality risk in Toronto, Canada: A comparison of tree-based and regression-based machine learning methods. *BMC Med. Res. Methodol.* **2021**, *21*, 267. [CrossRef]
42. Shakibfar, S.; Nyberg, F.; Li, H.; Zhao, J.; Nordeng, H.M.E.; Sandve, G.K.F.; Pavlovic, M.; Hajiebrahimi, M.; Andersen, M.; Sessa, M. Artificial intelligence-driven prediction of COVID-19-related hospitalization and death: A systematic review. *Front. Public Health* **2023**, *11*, 1183725. [CrossRef] [PubMed]
43. Lv, C.; Guo, W.; Yin, X.; Liu, L.; Huang, X.; Li, S.; Zhang, L. Innovative applications of artificial intelligence during the COVID-19 pandemic. *Infect. Med.* **2024**, *3*, 100095. [CrossRef]
44. Carreras, J. Artificial intelligence analysis of celiac disease using an autoimmune discovery transcriptomic panel highlighted pathogenic genes including BTLA. *Healthcare* **2022**, *10*, 1550. [CrossRef]

healthcare

MDPI

Review

A Scoping Review of Arabic Natural Language Processing for Mental Health

Ashwag Alasmari [1,2]

[1] Computer Science Department, King Khalid University, Abha 62521, Saudi Arabia; aasmry@kku.edu.sa
[2] Center for Artificial Intelligence (CAI), King Khalid University, Abha 62521, Saudi Arabia

Abstract: Mental health disorders represent a substantial global health concern, impacting millions and placing a significant burden on public health systems. Natural Language Processing (NLP) has emerged as a promising tool for analyzing large textual datasets to identify and predict mental health challenges. The aim of this scoping review is to identify the Arabic NLP techniques employed in mental health research, the specific mental health conditions addressed, and the effectiveness of these techniques in detecting and predicting such conditions. This scoping review was conducted according to the PRISMA-ScR (Preferred Reporting Items for Systematic reviews and Meta-Analyses extension for Scoping Reviews) framework. Studies were included if they focused on the application of NLP techniques, addressed mental health issues (e.g., depression, anxiety, suicidal ideation) within Arabic text data, were published in peer-reviewed journals or conference proceedings, and were written in English or Arabic. The relevant literature was identified through a systematic search of four databases: PubMed, ScienceDirect, IEEE Xplore, and Google Scholar. The results of the included studies revealed a variety of NLP techniques used to address specific mental health issues among Arabic-speaking populations. Commonly utilized techniques included Support Vector Machine (SVM), Random Forest (RF), Decision Tree (DT), Recurrent Neural Network (RNN), and advanced transformer-based models such as AraBERT and MARBERT. The studies predominantly focused on detecting and predicting symptoms of depression and suicidality from Arabic social media data. The effectiveness of these techniques varied, with trans-former-based models like AraBERT and MARBERT demonstrating superior performance, achieving accuracy rates of up to 99.3% and 98.3%, respectively. Traditional machine learning models and RNNs also showed promise but generally lagged in accuracy and depth of insight compared to transformer models. This scoping review highlights the significant potential of NLP techniques, particularly advanced transformer-based models, in addressing mental health issues among Arabic-speaking populations. Ongoing research is essential to keep pace with the rapidly evolving field and to validate current findings.

Keywords: Natural Language Processing; Arabic-speaking populations; mental health

1. Introduction

Mental health disorders, often referred to as mental illnesses, are highly prevalent globally and pose a significant public health challenge [1]. These disorders include a variety of conditions like depression, anxiety, suicidal thoughts, bipolar disorder, and schizophrenia. Each of these conditions has the potential to negatively affect physical and overall well-being [2]. Mental health disorders are a widespread global issue, affecting millions of people suffering from one or more mental health disorders [1]. The early detection of mental illness can greatly benefit the progression and treatment of the disease.

Various text sources, such as social media messages, interview transcripts, and clinical notes, serve as mediums through which individuals express their moods and mental states. Natural Language Processing (NLP), a type of artificial intelligence (AI), has recently become crucial in analyzing and managing large-scale textual data. NLP facilitates information extraction, sentiment analysis, and emotion detection [3–5]. The detection of mental illness through textual data can be framed as a text classification or sentiment analysis task, employing NLP techniques to identify early indicators and facilitate early detection, prevention, and treatment strategies. The use of NLP for medical health intervention initially employed pre-packaged software tools [6], eventually progressing to more computationally intensive deep neural networks [7], particularly large language models like transformers [8]. These advanced methods help uncover meaningful trends in vast datasets. The proliferation of digital health platforms has made such data more accessible, enabling transformative studies on treatment fidelity [9], patient outcome estimation [10], the identification of treatment components [11], the evaluation of therapeutic alliances [12], and suicide risk assessment [13]. This evolution is generating excitement and apprehension regarding the use of conversational agents in mental health [14].

Despite the potential of NLP within the mental health domain, there remains a lack of comprehensive reviews that systematically identify and categorize the various Arabic NLP techniques employed, the specific mental health issues they target, and their effectiveness in predicting and detecting mental health problems. The existing literature often focuses on isolated studies or specific applications, leaving a gap in our understanding of the broader landscape of NLP in mental health research for the Arabic language. The Arabic language, with its rich morphology, diverse dialects, and unique cultural nuances, presents distinct challenges and opportunities for NLP-based mental health interventions [15]. Existing NLP tools and techniques developed for other languages may not directly translate to Arabic, necessitating tailored approaches. Furthermore, cultural factors and social contexts within Arabic-speaking communities play a vital role in how mental health is expressed and perceived, requiring culturally sensitive NLP methodologies.

This scoping review addresses the critical gap in the literature by focusing specifically on the use of NLP techniques for mental health interventions in the Arabic language. By focusing on the Arabic language context, this review aims to systematically map: (1) the types of NLP techniques used in Arabic mental health research; (2) the specific mental health problems targeted within Arabic-speaking populations; and (3) the effectiveness of these NLP approaches in predicting and detecting mental health issues.

1.1. Aims and Research Questions

This review aims to provide a comprehensive overview of the current state of research, identify key challenges and opportunities, and inform future directions for developing culturally appropriate and effective NLP-based mental health interventions for Arabic speakers. The following research questions (RQs) guided this review:

1. Which specific mental health conditions are primarily addressed in Arabic NLP research?
2. What are the most commonly employed NLP techniques in mental health research within the Arabic-speaking world?
3. What is the evidence for the effectiveness of these NLP techniques in detecting and predicting mental health issues within Arabic text data?

1.2. Literature Study

Arabic NLP for mental health has seen significant advancements, leveraging lexicon-based methods, deep learning models, and transformer architectures to detect mental health conditions like depression, anxiety, and suicidal ideation. Due to the complex structure of Arabic, including rich morphology, diacritics, dialectal variations, and limited labeled datasets, early studies relied on rule-based and statistical NLP approaches for sentiment analysis and psychological assessment. However, recent advancements in deep learning (CNNs, LSTMs) and transformer models (AraBERT, Arabic GPT, mBERT, XLM-RoBERTa) have improved the accuracy of mental health detection using social media, clinical records, and online counseling platforms.

Several studies have explored the landscape of digital mental health resources and the application of NLP in Arabic language. For example, ref. [16] systematically assessed the features, quality, and digital safety of Arabic mental health apps, revealing areas for improvement in design and content. Other reviews have focused on specific NLP techniques, such as recurrent neural networks for sentiment analysis [17], highlighting their effectiveness in navigating the complexities of the Arabic language. A broader examination of NLP in Arabic sentiment analysis [18] provided insights into challenges and advancements in the field. Furthermore, the automatic identification of hate speech in Arabic tweets has been explored, with [19] reviewing various classification techniques and feature engineering methods. However, despite these contributions, significant challenges persist, including the limited availability of labeled Arabic mental health datasets, the complexities posed by dialectal variations, and the cultural stigma surrounding open discussions of mental health.

The use of NLP for mental health has been more widely studied in English. Traditionally, articles on NLP for mental health focused on lexicon-based methods, N-grams, Hidden Markov Models (HMMs), and classical machine learning approaches (Naïve Bayes, SVM, etc.) for mental health detection. Articles on deep learning-based NLP for mental health involve deep learning architectures such as CNNs, RNNs, LSTMs, and BiLSTMs, which are more effective for text-based mental health detection. The application of transformer-based NLP to mental health articles involves the use of cutting-edge transformer models like BERT, AraBERT, GPT, and RoBERTa to enhance mental health prediction from text. A summary of recent articles is given in Table 1 below.

Table 1. List of relevant review studies in the landscape of NLP and mental health.

Articles (Journal, Year)	Language	Summary
"Natural Language Processing for Mental Health Interventions" (*Translational Psychiatry*, 2023) [20]	English	Reviews traditional NLP techniques such as lexicon-based sentiment analysis and feature engineering for mental health applications.
"Natural Language Processing Applied to Mental Illness Detection" (*npj Digital Medicine*, 2022) [21]	English	Discusses rule-based and statistical methods used for analyzing mental illness from text data.
"Screening for Depression Using Natural Language Processing: A Literature Review" (*Interactive Journal of Medical Research*, 2024) [22]	English	Explores traditional lexicon-based and keyword-based models in English and Arabic depression detection.
"Mental Health Stigma and Natural Language Processing: Two Enigmas Through the Lens of a Limited Corpus" (*IEEE Conference Publication*, 2022) [23]	English	Uses text classification techniques to identify mental health stigma in textual data.

Table 1. *Cont.*

Articles (Journal, Year)	Language	Summary
"Natural Language Processing and Social Determinants of Health in Mental Health Research: A Systematic Review"(*JMIR Mental Health*, 2025) [24]	English	Discusses deep learning methods to analyze social determinants of mental health from English-language textual data.
"Evaluation of ChatGPT for NLP-Based Mental Health Applications" (*arXiv preprint*, 2023) [25]	English	Evaluates ChatGPT's ability to classify stress, depression, and suicidality in English and Arabicdatasets.
"Large Language Models for Mental Health: A Systematic Review" (*arXiv preprint*, 2024) [26]	English	Reviews BERT, AraBERT, GPT-3, and RoBERTa in mental health applications across English and Arabic languages.

This paper is organized as follows. We first describe the methodology employed in this scoping review, including the search strategy, inclusion and exclusion criteria, and data extraction process. Subsequently, we present the results of our literature search, summarizing the key findings and identifying emerging trends in the application of NLP to mental health research within the Arabic-speaking world. Finally, we discuss the implications of these findings, highlighting the potential benefits and limitations of NLP in this context, and outline key areas for future research.

2. Methods

This scoping review followed the Preferred Reporting Items for Systematic Reviews and Meta-Analyses extension for Scoping Reviews (PRISMA-ScR) [27], a framework designed for transparency and reproducibility in scoping reviews. Unlike Systematic Literature Reviews (SLRs), which address narrow research questions, scoping reviews, using PRISMA-ScR, are ideal for exploring broad topics, identifying key concepts, summarizing evidence, and detecting research gaps [28]. Given the emerging nature of Arabic NLP for mental health, PRISMA-ScR facilitated a structured and comprehensive review. The PRISMA-ScR checklist guided our research questions, inclusion/exclusion criteria, literature search, and reporting, allowing us to capture the breadth of Arabic NLP applications without SLR's restrictive criteria. This framework also supports diverse study designs, crucial for understanding this interdisciplinary field. Thus, PRISMA-ScR ensured a rigorous and effective mapping of current advancements, challenges, and future directions in Arabic NLP for mental health.

2.1. Inclusion and Exclusion Criteria

Articles were eligible for inclusion if they were original and written in English, and they had to focus on the use of NLP in mental health research. Only studies conducted in Arabic-speaking countries or involving Arabic-speaking populations were included. Exclusion criteria included non-original research articles like systematic reviews, meta-analyses, editorials, article comments, and literature reviews. Additionally, studies were excluded if they did not focus on mental health, use NLP techniques, specify, or utilize NLP techniques, report on the effectiveness or impact of the interventions, or focus exclusively on mental health conditions without broader applicability to mental health interventions. Studies that did not involve Arabic language were also excluded. Table 2 shows the inclusion and exclusion criteria.

Table 2. Eligibility criteria.

Criteria	Inclusion	Exclusion
Study Type	Original research articles (e.g., empirical studies, case studies)	Reviews, meta-analyses, editorials, commentaries, letters to the editor, opinion pieces
Focus	Application of NLP techniques in mental health research	Studies not focusing on NLP applications in mental health
Language and Region	Studies conducted in Arabic-speaking countries or involving Arabic-speaking populations	Studies not conducted in Arabic-speaking countries or involving Arabic-speaking populations
Mental Health Focus	Studies addressing specific mental health issues (e.g., depression, anxiety, suicide ideation)	Studies not focusing on any specific mental health condition
Data Source	Studies utilizing Arabic text data (e.g., social media, clinical notes, patient records)	Studies utilizing Arabic text data (e.g., social media, clinical notes, patient records)
Publication	Published in peer-reviewed journals or conference proceedings	Unpublished studies, grey literature
Language of Publication	Studies published in English or Arabic	Studies published in other languages
NLP Technique Utilization	Studies that explicitly specify and utilize NLP techniques in their methodology	Studies that do not specify or utilize NLP techniques

2.2. *Information Sources and Study Selection*

To identify relevant studies, we conducted a comprehensive literature search across PubMed, ScienceDirect, IEEE, and Google Scholar for articles published up to December 30, 2024. Search terms were employed to locate potentially relevant studies, which were subsequently subjected to a rigorous selection process. The finalized search strategy can be found in Table 3. After removing duplicates, the title and abstract of all the articles were divided into two groups and screened independently by two reviewers using Covidence (https://www.covidence.org). Two reviewers (with a third acting as a judge) reviewed each potentially relevant abstract in the full text for eligibility criteria. Any disagreement was discussed with other reviewers to reach consensus.

Table 3. Search strings.

Databases	Search Strings
PubMed	("natural language processing" OR NLP OR "text analysis" OR "machine learning" OR "deep learning" OR transformers OR BERT OR GPT OR LSTM OR RNN OR CNN) AND ("mental health" OR depression OR anxiety OR schizophrenia OR "bipolar disorder" OR "mental illness" OR "psychological disorders" OR "emotional well-being" OR "mental wellness") AND (Arabic OR "Arabic language" OR "Arabic-speaking" OR "Modern Standard Arabic" OR "Arabic dialects" OR "Arabic text")
ScienceDirect	("natural language processing" OR NLP OR "machine learning" OR "deep learning") AND ("mental health" OR "psychological disorders") AND (Arabic OR "Arabic language")
IEEE	("natural language processing" OR NLP OR "text analysis" OR "machine learning" OR "deep learning" OR transformers OR BERT OR GPT OR LSTM OR RNN OR CNN) AND ("mental health" OR depression OR anxiety OR schizophrenia OR "bipolar disorder" OR "mental illness" OR "psychological disorders" OR "emotional well-being" OR "mental wellness") AND (Arabic OR "Arabic language" OR "Arabic-speaking" OR "Modern Standard Arabic" OR "Arabic dialects" OR "Arabic text")

Table 3. *Cont.*

Databases	Search Strings
Google Scholar	("natural language processing" OR NLP OR "text analysis" OR "machine learning" OR "deep learning" OR transformers OR BERT OR GPT OR LSTM OR RNN OR CNN) AND ("mental health" OR depression OR anxiety OR schizophrenia OR "bipolar disorder" OR "mental illness" OR "psychological disorders" OR "emotional well-being" OR "mental wellness") AND (Arabic OR "Arabic language" OR "Arabic-speaking" OR "Modern Standard Arabic" OR "Arabic dialects" OR "Arabic text")

No time frame was applied for all of the database's searches. The search string for ScienceDirect was shortened because the database only accepts search strings with a maximum of eight Boolean operators.

2.3. Data Extraction

To systematically capture the key characteristics of each included article, a summary table was developed. This table included author(s), publication year, study design, NLP techniques employed, mental health problems addressed, and the reported effectiveness of these techniques. Data extraction was conducted independently by two reviewers and verified by a third to ensure accuracy and consistency. The extracted information was then organized into a summary table, structured by research question, to demonstrate how each study contributed to answering the research questions.

2.4. Synthesis of Results

We conducted a thematic analysis to systematically categorize and analyze findings across the included studies. This approach identified recurring themes and patterns re-lated to NLP techniques in Arabic-speaking mental health research, including the specific mental health problems addressed and the reported effectiveness of NLP interventions. Two reviewers independently performed the thematic analysis, grouping similar as-sessment criteria into domains. Discrepancies were resolved through discussion with a third reviewer. For RQ1, we identified that the most frequently addressed mental health conditions in Arabic NLP research. A summary table was created to show the mental health conditions explored across the studies. For RQ2, we highlighted common NLP techniques, such as machine learning models and deep learning models, with a table presenting these techniques and their performance metrics like accuracy, precision, recall, and F1-score. For RQ3, the effectiveness of these techniques was evaluated by comparing their ability to detect and predict mental health conditions based on performance metrics across the studies.

3. Results

3.1. Search Results

The initial database search yielded 403 articles (Figure 1). After eliminating 31 duplicates, 312 records were excluded based on title and abstract screening. A thorough review of the remaining 53 articles was conducted, with 24 articles meeting all inclusion criteria and proceeding to the final analysis.

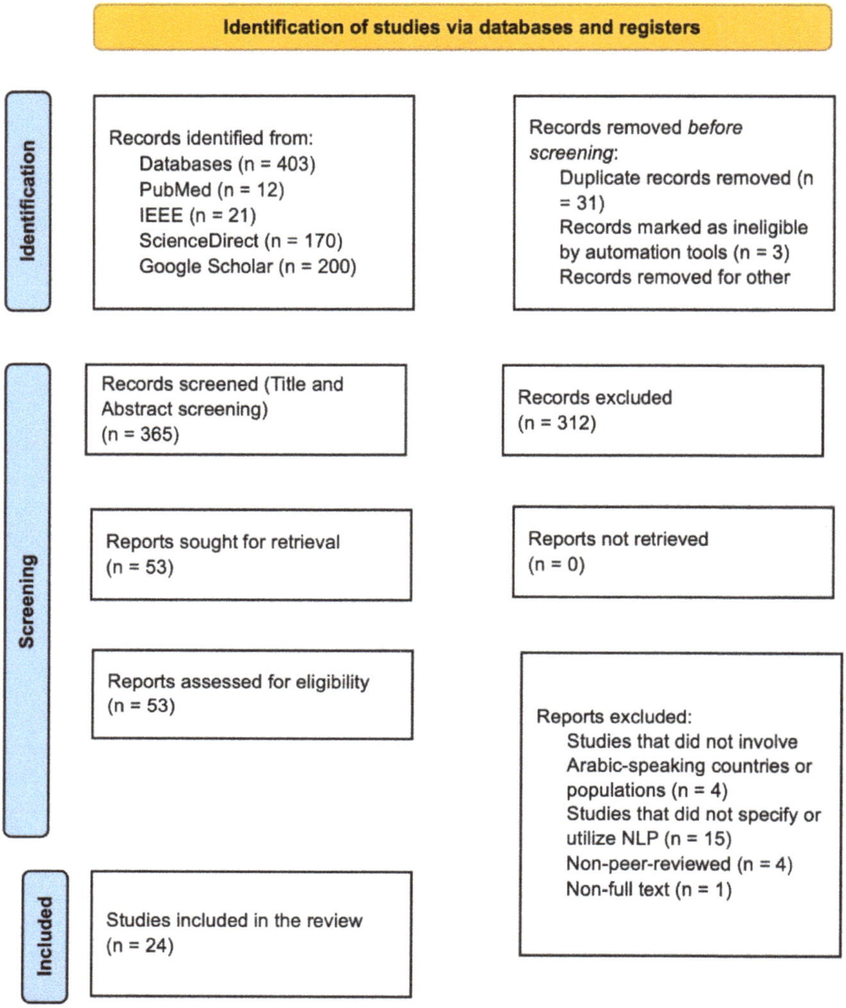

Figure 1. PRISMA flowchart showing the study selection process.

3.2. Results of Data Extraction

The study descriptor can be found in Table 4.

Table 4. Study descriptor.

Authors	Year	Study Design	NLP Techniques	Mental Health Problem(s)	Key Findings/Results
Abdulsalam et al. [29]	2024	Mixed	ML (Naïve Bayes, SVM, KNN, RF, XGBoost), Text Analysis, DL (AraBERT, AraELECTRA, AraGPT2)	Suicidal Thoughts	AraBERT (DL) achieved the highest performance (91% accuracy, 88% F1-score), outperforming other ML models. Among ML models, SVM and RF with character n-grams achieved 86% accuracy and a 79% F1-score.
Alabdulkreem [30]	2020	Quantitative	ML (RNN)	Depression	RNN model demonstrated effectiveness in detecting depression from 10,000 tweets (200 users).

Table 4. *Cont.*

Authors	Year	Study Design	NLP Techniques	Mental Health Problem(s)	Key Findings/Results
Alghamdi et al. [31]	2020	Quantitative	Text Analysis, ML (ArabDep lexicon)	Depression	Promising performance in predicting depression symptoms from posts (over 80% accuracy, 82% recall, 79% precision).
Alzoubi et al. [32]	2024	Quantitative	ML (Mutational Naïve Bayes, RF, Decision Tree, AdaBoost)	Depression	Mutational Naïve Bayes with TF-IDF achieved the highest accuracy (86%) in tweet classification.
Baghdadi et al. [33]	2022	Quantitative	DL (BERT, USE)	Suicidal Thoughts	BERT achieved a WSM of 95.26%; USE achieved a WSM of 80.2%.
Duwairi & Halloush [34]	2022	Quantitative	DL (CNN with Bi-LSTM)	Personality Disorders	Achieved a promising accuracy of 87% in classifying overlapping personality disorders.
Elmajali & Ahmad [35]	2024	Mixed	Pre-Trained Transformers (AraBERT, MARBERT)	Depression	AraBERT: 99.3% accuracy, 99.1% precision, 98.8% recall, 98.9% F1-score. MARBERT: 98.3% accuracy, 98.2% precision, 97.9% recall, 98% F1-score.
Almars [36]	2022	Quantitative	DL (Bi-LSTM)	Depression	Attention-based Bi-LSTM outperformed state-of-the-art ML models, achieving 83% accuracy.
Mezzi et al. [37]	2022	Quantitative	BERT, MINI	Depression, Suicidality, Panic Disorder, Social Phobia, Adjustment Disorder	Excellent performance in diagnosing multiple mental health conditions (over 92% accuracy, over 94% precision, recall, and F1-score). Tool positively evaluated by hospital staff for decision making and patient scheduling.
Sivakumar et al. [38]	2025	Mixed	m-Polar Neutrosophic Set, Applied Linguistics	Depression, Mood Change	Demonstrated improved detection of mood changes and depression using m-Polar Neutrosophic Set analysis.
Helmy et al. [39]	2025	Quantitative	Sentiment Analysis, Cross-Lingual NLP	Depression	Showed the effectiveness of sentiment analysis for detecting depression across Arabic and English tweets.
Saadany et al. [40]	2024	Mixed	Machine Translation, Cyber Risk Analysis	Depression, Mood Change	Highlighted risks of machine translation errors in detecting depression in Arabic mental health tweets.
Alaskar & Ykhlef [41]	2022	Quantitative	Machine Learning	Depression	Found that machine learning models effectively detect depression symptoms in Arabic tweets with high accuracy.
Rabie et al. [42]	2025	Quantitative	Machine Learning	Major Depressive Disorder	Developed a recognition model for predicting major depressive disorder in Arabic user-generated content with promising results.
Alatawi et al. [43]	2024	Quantitative	Sentiment Analysis, Empirical Analysis	Suicidality	Effective sentiment analysis for detecting suicidal ideation in Arabic online posts.
Alhuzali & Alasmari [44]	2024	Mixed	Foundational NLP Models, Question Answering	Mental Health Care Q&A	Evaluated the effectiveness of foundational NLP models in classifying Q&A in mental health care with promising results.
El-Ramly et al. [45]	2021	Quantitative	BERT Transformers, Deep Learning	Depression	BERT transformers showed high effectiveness in detecting depression in Arabic posts with strong accuracy.
Kumar & Singh [46]	2023	Mixed	Deep Learning, Explainable AI	Depression, Anxiety, Stress	Found deep learning and explainable AI models effective for detecting depression, anxiety, and stress in Arabic and English social media posts.
Hassib et al. [47]	2022	Quantitative	Transformers, Sentiment Analysis	Depression, Suicidality	Transformers were highly effective in detecting both depression and suicidal ideation in Arabic tweets.
Alghamdi & Alfalasi [31]	2020	Mixed	Machine Learning	Depression	Machine learning models predicted depression symptoms in Arabic psychological forums with good performance.
Bensalah et al. [48]	2024	Quantitative	AI, Mobile Apps, Sentiment Analysis	Mental Health Support	MindWave app uses AI and sentiment analysis to support mental health detection and intervention in both Arabic and English.

Table 4. *Cont.*

Authors	Year	Study Design	NLP Techniques	Mental Health Problem(s)	Key Findings/Results
Almouzini et al. [49]	2019	Mixed	Sentiment Analysis, Text Classification	Depression	Sentiment analysis effectively detected depression in Arabic Twitter users, demonstrating high accuracy in identifying depressive behavior.
Maghraby & Ali [50]	2022	Quantitative	Dataset Creation, Sentiment Analysis	Depression, Mood Changes	Developed a dataset for mood changes and depression in Modern Standard Arabic, showing its utility for NLP-based detection models.
Musleh et al. [51]	2022	Mixed	Machine Learning, Sentiment Analysis	Depression	Sentiment analysis using machine learning was effective in detecting depression from Arabic tweets with high classification accuracy.

Specifically, we have identified trends regarding the focus on specific mental health conditions, the types of NLP techniques used, and the effectiveness of these techniques over time.

Mental health conditions addressed: Depression was the most frequently studied mental health issue, appearing in 79% (19 out of 24) of studies. Suicidal thoughts were the focus in 16% (4 out of 24), while personality disorders, panic disorder, social phobia, and adjustment disorder were each studied in 4% (1 out of 24).

Trend in NLP techniques: Transformer-based models (e.g., AraBERT, MARBERT, BERT) were employed in 45% (11 out of 24) of the reviewed studies, highlighting their growing dominance in mental health-related Arabic NLP research. Traditional machine learning models (e.g., SVM, Naïve Bayes, RF) were used in 33% (8 out of 24) of studies, while deep learning architectures (e.g., Bi-LSTM, CNN with Bi-LSTM) were utilized in 20% (5 out of 24) of studies.

Effectiveness of NLP techniques: Studies that applied transformer models reported the highest accuracy, with AraBERT achieving 99.3% accuracy in depression detection and BERT achieving over 92% accuracy in diagnosing multiple mental health conditions.

The evolution of techniques over time: Earlier studies (2020) primarily used traditional ML models (RNN, lexicons) for depression detection. However, from 2022 onward, there was a shift towards deep learning and transformer-based models, which have demonstrated superior performance.

Figure 2 shows the evolution of NLP techniques in Arabic mental health research over time. It highlights the increasing adoption of transformer-based models (such as BERT and AraBERT) while traditional machine learning techniques have remained relatively stable. Deep learning methods like Bi-LSTM and CNN have also been consistently used.

3.3. Characteristics of Included Studies

This review included 24 studies employing various methods to explore the use of NLP techniques in addressing mental health problems. The studies focused on multiple mental health diseases, including depression, suicidal thoughts, and personality disorders. A range of NLP techniques were applied across the studies, including both classical machine learning models like Naïve Bayes, Support Vector Machine, K-Nearest Neighbor, Random Forest, XGBoost, and Mutational Naïve Bayes, as well as more advanced deep learning architectures such as AraBERT, AraELECTRA, AraGPT2, CNN with Bi-LSTM, Bi-LSTM, and the MARBERT transformer model. The studies demonstrated the effectiveness of these techniques in detecting and predicting mental health issues through various performance metrics.

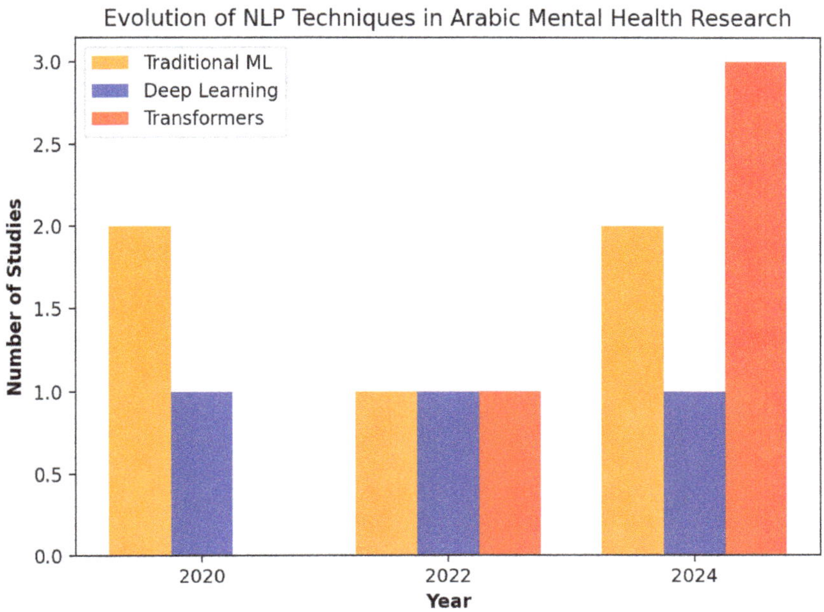

Figure 2. Trend of NLP techniques in Arabic mental health research (2020–2024).

3.4. Results of Included Studies: A Summary

3.4.1. Specific Mental Health Problems

The reviewed studies utilized NLP techniques to address specific mental health issues prevalent among Arabic-speaking populations. Abdulsalam et al. [29] focused on detecting suicidal thoughts in Arabic tweets. Alabdulkreem [30] aimed to predict depression symptoms in Arab women based on their tweets during the COVID-19 pandemic. Alghamdi et al. [31] explored NLP for predicting depression in Arabic text. Al-zoubi et al. [32] classified depression symptoms in Arabic tweets. Duwairi and Halloush [34] focused on detecting personality disorders among Arab Twitter users. Elmajali and Ahmad [35] aimed to detect depression symptoms in Arabic tweets using pre-trained transformers. Mezzi et al. [37] developed an intelligent tool to diagnose several mental health conditions in Arab-speaking patients, such as depression, suicidality, panic disorder, social phobia, and adjustment disorder. These studies collectively highlighted the diverse applications of NLP in addressing mental health issues specific to Arabic-speaking communities. Table 5 highlights the mental health conditions discussed in the included papers.

Table 5. The list of mental health conditions discussed.

Mental Health Condition	Studies Addressing the Condition
Depression	Abdulsalam et al. [29], Alabdulkreem [30], Alghamdi et al. [31], Alzoubi et al. [32], Elmajali & Ahmad [35], Almars [36], Sivakumar et al. [38], Helmy et al. [39], Saadany et al. [40], Alaskar & Ykhlef [41], Rabie et al. [42], Alhuzali & Alasmari [44], El-Ramly et al. [45], Kumar & Singh [46], Bensalah et al. [48], Almouzini et al. [49], Maghraby & Ali [50], Musleh et al. [51], Al-Musallam & Al-Abdullatif [52]
Suicidality	Abdulsalam et al. [29], Mezzi et al. [37], Alatawi et al. [43], Hassib et al. [47]
Panic Disorder	Mezzi et al. [37]
Social Phobia	Mezzi et al. [37]
Personality Disorders	Duwairi & Halloush [34]
Adjustment Disorder	Mezzi et al. [37]

3.4.2. Types and Effectiveness of NLP Techniques

Abdulsalam et al. [29] investigated the automatic detection of suicidal ideation in Arabic tweets, creating a novel dataset of such content. Their evaluation of various machine learning models, trained using word frequency and word embeddings, also explored the efficacy of pre-trained deep learning models. Among the machine learning approaches, Support Vector Machine (SVM) and Random Forest (RF) models, utilizing character n-grams, achieved the best results with 86% accuracy and a 79% F1-score. The AraBERT model demonstrated superior performance overall, achieving 91% accuracy and an 88% F1-score, significantly improving the detection of suicidal thoughts within their Arabic tweet dataset. In a related study, Alabdulkreem [30] used machine learning to predict depression symptoms from tweets posted by Arab women during the COVID-19 pandemic. Their research focused on developing a recurrent neural network (RNN) model for depression detection, evaluating its performance on a dataset of 10,000 tweets from 200 users. The results of this evaluation confirmed the model's effectiveness.

Alghamdi et al. [31] conducted an investigation into the utilization of NLP and machine learning methodologies for the prediction of depression from Arabic textual data, evaluating and comparing the efficacy of several approaches. The results of their study indicated promising performance metrics, with an accuracy exceeding 80%, a recall of 82%, and a precision of 79% in the identification of posts indicative of depressive symptomatology. Alzoubi et al. [32] collected 16,581 Arabic tweets from 1439 Arab Twitter users to determine whether the tweets expressed depression and to identify the symptoms they contained. They classified users as depressed or not and employed several machines learning algorithms, including DT, RF, Mutational Naïve Bayes, and AdaBoost, along with feature extraction methods such as Bag of Words (BOW) and TF-IDF. Their experiments showed that the Mutational Naïve Bayes algorithm with TF-IDF achieved the highest accuracy (86%) in tweet classification.

Baghdadi et al. [33] developed an Arabic tweet preprocessing algorithm comparing lemmatization, stemming, and other lexical analysis techniques. Their research involved conducting experiments using Twitter data gathered from online sources, which underwent annotation by five different annotators. This approach aimed to refine and optimize the preprocessing steps tailored for Arabic text. The study evaluated the effectiveness of their proposed dataset using advanced NLP models, including the Bidirectional Encoder Representations from Transformers (BERT) and Universal Sentence Encoder (USE). These models were assessed using a comprehensive set of performance metrics such as balanced accuracy, specificity, F1-score, IoU ROC curve analysis, Youden Index, NPV, and WSM. The results demonstrated notable achievements for the Arabic BERT models, which excelled with a highest recorded WSM of 95.26%. Conversely, the USE models achieved a WSM of 80.2%. These findings underscore the robustness and applicability of Arabic BERT models in effectively processing and analyzing Arabic tweets. Baghdadi et al.'s work [33] contributes valuable insights into enhancing the preprocessing and analysis of Arabic language data, particularly in leveraging state-of-the-art NLP techniques for improved performance across various evaluation metrics.

Duwairi and Halloush [34] proposed a novel multi-view fusion model based on deep learning algorithms to identify prevalent personality disorders among Arab Twitter users in an expert-driven approach. They addressed the lack of publicly available datasets focusing on personality disorders in Arabic by creating AraPerson, which comprises 8000 tweets and 8000 images annotated with the mental statuses of 150 users. This dataset was curated with input from domain experts and utilized regular expressions for data collection. Their study employed a baseline multi-view model combining a CNN with a Bi-LSTM to analyze textual and visual posts to detect personality disorders. In further experiments, they fused a DenseNet model with the Bi-LSTM, testing different vector combination techniques, including concatenation, addition, and multiplication. The highest reported accuracy achieved was 87%, indicating promising results despite the challenges of overlapping characteristics between the studied personality disorders. Elmajali and Ahmad [35] conducted research aimed at detecting nine depression symptoms, based on DSM-5 criteria, within Arabic tweets. Their approach leveraged pre-trained transformers such as AraBERT and MARBERT for tweet classification. To address dataset imbalance, they employed data augmentation techniques using ChatGPT, which included generating a 'normal' class to complement the depression symptom classes. Their study evaluated model performance using four critical metrics: accuracy, precision, recall, and F1 scores. The AraBERT model exhibited notably high performance, achieving an accuracy of 99.3%, a precision of 99.1%, a recall of 98.8%, and an F1-score of 98.9%. These metrics highlight the model's ability to accurately identify tweets expressing depression symptoms, with a low rate of misclassification.

MARBERT also performed strongly, achieving high scores across all metrics: 98.3% accuracy, 98.2% precision, 97.9% recall, and a 98% F1-score. These results highlight MABERT's effectiveness in capturing the nuances of depression symptom detection in Arabic tweets, albeit with slightly lower performance metrics compared to AraBERT.

Almars [36] conducted a study on depression analysis on Arabic social media content to discern user sentiments. They introduced a Bi-LSTM model augmented with an attention mechanism designed to effectively capture and weigh significant hidden features crucial for depression detection. This new deep learning architecture is designed to simultaneously identify key features and learn the weights of important words that strongly contribute to depression detection. Almars [36] collected a Twitter dataset comprising approximately 6000 tweets for their evaluation. The dataset was manually labeled by categorizing tweets as either expressing depression or not. Experimental results demonstrated that the proposed attention-based Bi-LSTM model surpassed existing state-of-the-art machine learning models in depression detection tasks. Specifically, the model achieved an accuracy of 83%, underscoring its effectiveness in accurately identifying depression-related content from Arabic social media posts. Mezzi et al. [37] conducted a study focused on the development of an intelligent instrument for mental health intent recognition within an Arabic-speaking patient population. Their methodology integrated the Bidirectional Encoder Representations from Transformers (BERT) model with the International Neuropsychiatric Interview (MINI). The evaluation at the Military Hospital of Tunis demonstrated the system's robust performance, with accuracy surpassing 92% and precision, recall, and F1-scores exceeding 94% in the diagnosis of mental health disorders, including depression, suicidality, panic disorder, social phobia, and adjustment disorder. The tool received positive feedback from medical personnel at the institution, who recognized its utility in clinical decision support and patient appointment scheduling within the context of high patient volume. Sivakumar et al. [38] explores Arabic text analysis by integrating applied linguistics with m-Polar Neutrosophic Set (m-PNS) to analyze mood changes and depression on social media. The authors propose a method for detecting mood shifts and depressive symptoms in Arabic social media posts using this advanced mathematical approach, enhancing the accuracy of mental health assessments in online Arabic communities. Helmy et al. [39] investigate cross-lingual sentiment analysis to detect depression in Twitter users, comparing the effectiveness of analyzing English and Arabic tweets. The researchers demonstrate how sentiment analysis can identify depressive behaviors, highlighting the challenges and variations between detecting depression in English versus Arabic posts.

Saadany et al.'s [40] research examines the cyber risks posed by critical machine translation errors, focusing on Arabic mental health tweets. The study uses a case study approach to illustrate how translation inaccuracies can impact the detection of mental health issues, specifically depression, in Arabic-language social media. Alaskar and Ykhlef [41] discuss the application of machine learning techniques for detecting depression from Arabic tweets. The authors utilize various algorithms to analyze Twitter data, focusing on the identification of depression-related content in Arabic social media. Rabie et al. [42] presents a recognition model for identifying major depressive disorder (MDD) in Arabic user-generated content. Using NLP and machine learning, the authors propose an effective approach for diagnosing MDD in Arabic-language online posts. Alatawi et al. [43] empirically analyze methods for detecting Arabic online suicidal ideation. The authors apply computational techniques to identify suicidal tendencies from online Arabic content, emphasizing the importance of early detection and intervention. Alhuzali and Alasmari [44] evaluate the effectiveness of foundational models for question-and-answer (Q&A) classification in mental health care, specifically for Arabic content. The authors analyze various models for their performance in addressing mental health queries and providing relevant responses. El-Ramly et al. [45] introduce CairoDep, a system for detecting depression in Arabic posts using BERT transformers. The study showcases the application of deep learning techniques to identify depressive content in Arabic social media and evaluates the system's performance in real-world scenarios. Kumar and Singh's [46] paper discusses explainable deep learning models for mental health detection in both English and Arabic social media posts. The authors explore how these models can interpret and explain the reasons behind detecting depression and other mental health issues in online content.

Among the included studies, Hassib et al. [47] which present AraDepSu, a model for detecting depression and suicidal ideation in Arabic tweets using transformers. The research highlights the use of advanced machine learning models to identify mental health issues in Arabic-language social media posts. Bensalah et al. [48] introduce the MindWave app, which leverages AI for mental health support in both English and Arabic. The authors highlight the app's capabilities in detecting mental health issues and providing support to users, focusing on its cross-lingual functionalities. Almouzini et al. [49] focus on detecting depressed users from Twitter data in Arabic. The authors use machine learning algorithms to analyze Arabic tweets, developing a model to detect depression based on linguistic and sentiment cues. Maghraby and Ali [50] introduce a dataset for mood changes and depression in Modern Standard Arabic. The authors provide a detailed description of the dataset, which includes annotated Arabic social media posts for use in mental health research and detection. Musleh et al.'s [51] research investigates sentiment analysis for detecting depression in Arabic tweets using machine learning. The authors apply various machine learning techniques to analyze the sentiments expressed in Arabic tweets and detect depressive symptoms based on linguistic patterns. Al-Musallam and Al-Abdullatif [52] explore the use of machine learning techniques to detect depression through the analysis of depressive Arabic tweets from Saudi Arabia. The authors propose a system that classifies tweets based on depressive content using a machine learning approach. By analyzing social media data, the study aims to contribute to the early detection of depression among Arabic-speaking individuals, particularly in the context of Saudi Arabia, using advanced computational methods to enhance mental health awareness and intervention. A summary table has been included that presents the effectiveness of each model in detecting mental health issues such as depression and suicidality (Table 6).

Table 6. Mapping research questions to relevant studies in Arabic NLP for mental health.

Research Question (RQ)	Respective Study
RQ1: Which specific mental health conditions are primarily addressed in Arabic NLP research?	Abdulsalam et al. [29] (Suicidal Thoughts) Alabdulkreem [30] (Depression) Alghamdi et al. [31] (Depression) Alzoubi et al. [32] (Depression) Duwairi & Halloush [34] (Personality Disorders) Sivakumar et al. [38] (Depression, Mood Change) Saadany et al. [40] (Depression, Mood Change) Alaskar & Ykhlef [41] (Depression) Rabie et al. [42] (Major Depressive Disorder) Alatawi et al. [43] (Suicidality) Alhuzali & Alasmari [44] (Mental Health Care Q&A) El-Ramly et al. [45] (Depression) Kumar & Singh [46] (Depression, Anxiety, Stress) Hassib et al. [47] (Depression, Suicidality) Alghamdi et al. [31] (Depression) Bensalah et al. [48] (Mental Health Support) Almouzini et al. [49] (Depression) Maghraby & Ali [50] (Depression, Mood Changes) Musleh et al. [51] (Depression)
RQ2: What are the most commonly employed NLP techniques in mental health research within the Arabic-speaking world?	Alzoubi et al. [32] (ML: Mutational Naïve Bayes, RF, Decision Tree, AdaBoost) Baghdadi et al. [33] (DL: BERT, USE) Elmajali & Ahmad [35] (Pre-trained Transformers: AraBERT, MARBERT) Almars [36] (DL: Bi-LSTM) Sivakumar et al. [38] (m-Polar Neutrosophic Set, Applied Linguistics) Helmy et al. [39] (Depression) Saadany et al. [40] (Machine Translation, Cyber Risk Analysis) Alaskar & Ykhlef [41] (Machine Learning) Rabie et al. [42] (Machine Learning) Alatawi et al. [43] (Empirical Analysis, Sentiment Analysis) Alhuzali & Alasmari [44] (Foundational NLP Models, Question Answering) El-Ramly et al. [45] (BERT Transformers, Deep Learning) Kumar & Singh [46] (Deep Learning, Explainable AI) Hassib et al. [47] (Transformers, Sentiment Analysis) Alghamdi et al. [31] (Machine Learning) Bensalah et al. [48] (AI, Mobile Apps, Sentiment Analysis) Almouzini et al. [49] (Sentiment Analysis, Text Classification) Maghraby & Ali [50] (Dataset Creation, Sentiment Analysis) Musleh et al. [51] (Machine Learning, Sentiment Analysis)

Table 6. *Cont.*

Research Question (RQ)	Respective Study
RQ3: What is the evidence for the effectiveness of these NLP techniques in detecting and predicting mental health issues within Arabic text data?	Abdulsalam et al. [29] (AraBERT, ML models: SVM, RF) Alabdulkreem [30] (RNN) Baghdadi et al. [33] (BERT, USE) Elmajali & Ahmad [35] (AraBERT, MARBERT) Mezzi et al. [37] (BERT, MINI) Sivakumar et al. [38] (m-Polar Neutrosophic Set) Helmy et al. [39] (Sentiment Analysis, Cross-Lingual NLP) Helmy et al. (sentiment analysis) Saadany et al. [40] (Highlighted risks of machine translation errors) Alaskar & Ykhlef [41] (High accuracy in detecting depression symptoms) Rabie et al. [42] (Demonstrates the effectiveness of machine learning) Alatawi et al. [43] (Demonstrates the effectiveness of sentiment analysis) Alhuzali & Alasmari [44] (Effectiveness of foundational models in mental health) El-Ramly et al. [45] (BERT transformers show high effectiveness) Kumar & Singh [46] (Effectiveness of deep learning and explainable AI models) Hassib et al. [47] (Transformers are effective in detecting both depression and suicidal ideation) Alghamdi et al. [31] (Machine learning predicts depression symptoms) Bensalah et al. [48] (AI-driven mobile apps (MindWave) can support mental health detection) Almouzini et al. [49] (Sentiment analysis for detecting depression) Maghraby & Ali [50] (Provides a dataset for mood changes and depression) Musleh et al. [51] (Effectiveness of sentiment analysis for depression detection)

4. Discussion

This scoping review revealed a diverse array of NLP techniques employed in mental health research among Arabic-speaking populations. These techniques ranged from traditional machine learning models to advanced deep learning and transformer-based models, each applied to address specific mental health issues prevalent in this demographic. The reviewed studies utilized various NLP techniques to analyze Arabic text data for mental health insights. Common techniques included SVM, RF, DT, and RNN. Advanced approaches such as BERT and its Arabic variants, AraBERT and MARBERT, were also prominently featured. Notably, AraBERT and MARBERT demonstrated superior performance due to their ability to capture contextual nuances in the Arabic language. Unique approaches included the use of Bi-LSTM models augmented with attention mechanisms to enhance feature extraction, as seen in Almars [36].

Arabic presents unique linguistic challenges, such as rich morphology, complex diacritization, dialectal variations, and script ambiguity, which significantly affect NLP performance [53]. Traditional machine learning methods like SVM and Random Forest depend on hand-crafted feature extraction, which struggles to capture these complexities.

In contrast, transformer-based models such as AraBERT and MARBERT leverage deep contextualized embeddings, making them more effective for mental health applications. Key challenges in Arabic NLP include morphological richness, where transformer models like AraBERT effectively learn contextual representations to reduce feature sparsity, and diacritization, where transformers handle ambiguity better than traditional models [54]. Dialectal variations and code-switching, common in Arabic social media, are also better managed by transformer-based architectures like MARBERT, which enhances performance in sentiment and emotion classification tasks [55]. Therefore, transformer-based models offer significant improvements in the accuracy and generalizability of Arabic NLP for mental health tasks. We have incorporated these justifications into the revised manuscript, along with relevant references.

The studies predominantly focused on detecting and predicting symptoms of depression and suicidality from Arabic social media data. For instance, Abdulsalam et al. [29] and Alghamdi et al. [31] aimed to identify depression symptoms, while Abdulsalam et al. [29] also targeted suicidal thoughts. Other mental health issues addressed included personality disorders, as explored by Duwairi and Halloush [34], and a broader range of conditions, such as panic disorder, social phobia, and adjustment disorder, as seen in the work by Mezzi et al. [37]. The effectiveness of these NLP techniques varied, with several studies reporting high accuracy and strong performance metrics. Abdulsalam et al. [29] found that SVM and RF models achieved an accuracy of 86% and a 79% F1 score in detecting suicidal thoughts, with AraBERT further enhancing the accuracy to 91% and F1 score to 88%. Alabdulkreem [30] reported the successful application of an RNN model in predicting depression from tweets. Alzoubi et al. [32] demonstrated that a combination of the Mutational Naïve Bayes algorithm and TF-IDF features achieved an accuracy of 86% in classifying depression-related tweets. Baghdadi et al. [33] highlighted the robust performance of Arabic BERT models, achieving a weighted sum metric (WSM) of 95.26%, underscoring their efficacy in processing Arabic tweets. The studies collectively highlighted the potential of NLP techniques in accurately detecting and predicting mental health issues from Arabic text data, with transformer models showing particularly promising results due to their advanced language processing capabilities. These findings highlight the versatility and potential of NLP techniques in addressing mental health issues in Arabic-speaking populations. Integrating advanced models like AraBERT and MARBERT represents a significant advancement in the field, offering higher accuracy and deeper insights into mental health patterns.

Arabic mental health datasets, especially those from social media, often face challenges such as data sparsity [56], dialectal variation, imbalanced classes, and noisy text, which can lead to overfitting in traditional machine learning models like SVM and Random Forest. Transformer models such as AraBERT [54] and MARBERT [55] help mitigate overfitting through pretraining on large corpora, contextual representations, and regularization techniques like dropout and early stopping [6,41]. They reduce bias by using diverse pretraining data, fine-tuning on balanced datasets, and offering attention-based interpretability to help identify and adjust biases [42,43]. While transformers are not entirely immune to bias or overfitting, they significantly reduce these issues compared to traditional models, making them more suitable for Arabic mental health NLP tasks.

The imbalance between class distributions is indeed a significant issue in the context of Arabic social media data, where some mental health conditions may be underrepresented, leading to potential biases in classification models. Transformer-based models such as AraBERT and MARBERT provide several advantages for addressing class imbalance in these applications. These models are trained on large and diverse datasets, allowing them to develop an understanding of contextual relationships across various conditions, including rare ones. Fine-tuning strategies like class weighting, data augmentation, oversampling/under-sampling, loss function modifications, and ensemble learning can significantly improve model performance. Class weighting adjusts the loss function to penalize misclassifications of rare conditions [57], while data augmentation techniques like back-translation and synthetic data generation increase underrepresented samples [58]. Oversampling the minority class or undersampling the majority class also help to alleviate imbalance [59]. Loss function modifications such as focal loss [60] or Dice loss focus the model on hard-to-classify examples, while ensemble learning methods [61] enhance performance by combining multiple models. These strategies enable transformer models to effectively handle imbalanced mental health datasets and improve the identification of underrepresented conditions like panic disorder and adjustment disorder.

The comparative analysis of different NLP techniques revealed significant variations in their effectiveness, with some approaches demonstrating superior performance in detecting and predicting mental health issues among Arabic-speaking populations. Traditional machine learning models, such as SVM and RF, were effective in several studies. For instance, Abdulsalam et al. [29] found that SVM and RF models trained on character n-gram features performed well in detecting suicidal thoughts, achieving 86% accuracy and an F1 score of 79%. These models were relatively straightforward to implement and interpret, making them suitable for initial explorations into NLP applications in mental health. However, deep learning models, particularly transformer-based models, consistently outperformed traditional machine learning techniques. AraBERT and MARBERT, for example, significantly enhanced the detection of mental health symptoms in Arabic text. Elmajali and Ahmad [35] reported that AraBERT achieved an accuracy of 99.3%, a precision of 99.1%, a recall of 98.8%, and an F1 score of 98.9% in classifying tweets containing depression symptoms. MARBERT, while slightly less effective, still demonstrated strong performance with an accuracy of 98.3% and F1 score of 98%. These transformer models excelled due to their ability to understand and process the nuanced context of the Arabic language, providing deeper insights and more accurate classifications. The use of RNNs also showed promise, particularly in the work of Alabdulkreem [30], who developed an RNN model to predict depression from tweets. Although specific metrics were not detailed, the model demonstrated its effectiveness with a high accuracy rate. Similarly, the Bi-LSTM model augmented with attention mechanisms used by Almars [36] achieved an impressive accuracy of 83%, indicating its capability to capture and weigh significant features crucial for depression detection effectively.

Bi-LSTM excels at capturing sequential dependencies by processing input text in both forward and backward directions, which is crucial for modeling long-range contextual relationships, especially in Arabic, where morphological variations and syntactic ambiguity are common [62]. This capability allows the Bi-LSTM to effectively capture the local context of tokens, including nuances like diacritics. On the other hand, transformer models such as AraBERT and MARBERT leverage self-attention mechanisms to capture global contextual relationships, enabling them to focus on different parts of a sentence, regardless of their distance [8]. This makes transformers highly effective for understanding long-range dependencies and semantic relationships, which are essential for detecting emotions, sentiment, and mental-health-related signals in Arabic social media text. The combination of these architectures offers a synergistic approach to improving Arabic NLP tasks in mental health.

In contrast, while still effective, traditional models such as Mutational Naïve Bayes and feature extraction methods like TF-IDF generally showed lower performance metrics than deep learning models. Alzoubi et al. [32] demonstrated that the Mutational Naïve Bayes algorithm combined with TF-IDF achieved an accuracy of 86%, which, while notable, did not reach the high performance of transformer models. The comparative analysis underscores that advanced NLP techniques, particularly transformer-based models like AraBERT and MARBERT, appear most promising for mental health applications in Arabic-speaking populations. Their superior performance can be attributed to their advanced language understanding capabilities, which allow them to capture the subtle nuances of mental health expressions in text. Deep learning models, such as RNNs and Bi-LSTMs with attention mechanisms, showed strong potential, particularly when enhanced with innovative architectural features. While useful, traditional machine learning models generally lagged in accuracy and depth of insight, suggesting a clear advantage for more sophisticated NLP approaches in this field.

Implicit expressions of symptoms such as depression, anxiety, or stress often require a sophisticated understanding of context, emotion, and language subtleties, particularly in social media texts, where these symptoms may be conveyed through indirect or subtle language.

Transformer-based models, such as AraBERT and MARBERT, are well -equipped to handle these challenges due to their self-attention mechanism, which enables them to capture contextual relationships between words regardless of their position in the sentence. This allows transformers to effectively understand the subtext of a sentence, discerning hidden sentiment or intent even when symptoms are not explicitly stated [8]. Research has demonstrated the efficacy of transformers for implicit sentiment analysis in social media, particularly for languages like Arabic [63]. These models thus represent a powerful tool for detecting implicit mental health symptoms in Arabic social media text.

Limitations

While this review highlights the significant advancements in NLP techniques for mental health research among Arabic-speaking populations, it is important to acknowledge several limitations. This review may be subject to selection bias, as it relies on the inclusion criteria and databases used to source the studies. Although comprehensive search strategies were employed, it is possible that some relevant studies were not identified or included. Additionally, studies published in languages other than English may have been overlooked, potentially limiting the scope of this review. NLP and mental health research are rapidly evolving, with new techniques and methodologies emerging. As a result, the findings of this review may quickly become outdated. Ongoing research and future reviews will be necessary to keep abreast of the latest developments and to validate this review's findings.

While large language models (LLMs) and retrieval-augmented generation (RAG)-based techniques show promise in mental health applications, several challenges hinder their inclusion in this review. First, the lack of high-quality Arabic-specific datasets for fine-tuning LLMs presents a significant barrier, as most LLM solutions are optimized for widely spoken languages like English. Second, the substantial computational resources required for fine-tuning LLMs can be prohibitive, particularly in research settings with limited resources. Lastly, the novelty of these techniques in the mental health field means there is limited research addressing their use in this specific context. These factors led to the exclusion of LLMs and RAG-based solutions, and we have elaborated on these limitations to clarify their relevance to the research.

5. Conclusions

NLP techniques have demonstrated significant potential in detecting mental health issues among Arabic-speaking populations. Transformer-based models, such as AraBERT and MARBERT, have shown superior accuracy in capturing nuanced Arabic expressions of mental health symptoms, outperforming traditional machine learning and recurrent neural networks. While these earlier models offer valuable insights, the advancements with transformers highlight the importance of leveraging advanced NLP. Given the rapidly evolving nature of this field, continuous research is crucial to validate findings and explore new methodologies. Future efforts should focus on standardizing evaluation metrics, expanding datasets to include diverse populations, and exploring emerging NLP innovations to enhance the accuracy and applicability of mental health interventions. This review highlights the progress in applying NLP to detect mental health conditions, focusing on the effectiveness of transformer models in addressing Arabic's linguistic challenges. We examine various mental health conditions, compare NLP techniques, and offer insights into model performance optimization. Ultimately, we emphasize the need for advanced models and suggest future research should prioritize standardized metrics, diverse datasets, and innovative methodologies.

Funding: The authors extend their appreciation to the Deanship of Research and Graduate Studies at King Khalid University for funding this work through small group research (RGP1/337/45).

Institutional Review Board Statement: Not applicable.

Informed Consent Statement: Not applicable.

Data Availability Statement: The original contributions presented in this study are included in the article. Further inquiries can be directed to the corresponding author.

Conflicts of Interest: The authors declare no conflicts of interest.

References

1. Rehm, J.; Shield, K.D. Global burden of disease and the impact of mental and addictive disorders. *Curr. Psychiatry Rep.* **2019**, *21*, 10. [CrossRef] [PubMed]
2. Santomauro, D.F.; Herrera, A.M.M.; Shadid, J.; Zheng, P.; Ashbaugh, C.; Pigott, D.M.; Abbafati, C.; Adolph, C.; Amlag, J.O.; Aravkin, A.Y.; et al. Global prevalence and burden of depressive and anxiety disorders in 204 countries and territories in 2020 due to the COVID-19 pandemic. *Lancet* **2021**, *398*, 1700–1712. [CrossRef] [PubMed]
3. Alasmari, A.; Zhou, L. Share to Seek: The Effects of Disease Complexity on Health Information–Seeking Behavior. *J. Med. Internet Res.* **2021**, *23*, e21642. [CrossRef] [PubMed]
4. Alasmari, A.; Zhou, L. Quality Measurement of Consumer Health Questions: Content and Language Perspectives. *J. Med. Internet Res.* **2024**, *26*, e48257. [CrossRef]
5. Nadkarni, P.M.; Ohno-Machado, L.; Chapman, W.W. Natural language processing: An introduction. *J. Am. Med. Inform. Assoc.* **2011**, *18*, 544–551. [CrossRef]
6. Tausczik, Y.R.; Pennebaker, J.W. The Psychological Meaning of Words: LIWC and Computerized Text Analysis Methods. *J. Lang. Soc. Psychol.* **2010**, *29*, 24–54. [CrossRef]
7. Cho, K.; van Merrienboer, B.; Bahdanau, D.; Bengio, Y. On the Properties of Neural Machine Translation: Encoder-Decoder Approaches. *arXiv* **2014**, arXiv:1409.1259.
8. Vaswani, A.; Shazeer, N.M.; Parmar, N.; Uszkoreit, J.; Jones, L.; Gomez, A.N.; Kaiser, L.; Polosukhin, I. Attention is All you Need. In Proceedings of the Advances in Neural Information Processing Systems 30: Annual Conference on Neural Information Processing Systems 2017, Long Beach, CA, USA, 4–9 December 2017.
9. Althoff, T.; Clark, K.; Leskovec, J. Large-scale Analysis of Counseling Conversations: An Application of Natural Language Processing to Mental Health. *Trans. Assoc. Comput. Linguist.* **2016**, *4*, 463–476. [CrossRef]
10. Ewbank, M.P.; Cummins, R.; Tablan, V.; Bateup, S.; Catarino, A.; Martin, A.J.; Blackwell, A.D. Quantifying the Association Between Psychotherapy Content and Clinical Outcomes Using Deep Learning. *JAMA Psychiatry* **2020**, *77*, 35–43. [CrossRef]
11. Ewbank, M.P.; Cummins, R.; Tablan, V.; Catarino, A.; Buchholz, S.; Blackwell, A.D. Understanding the relationship between patient language and outcomes in internet-enabled cognitive behavioural therapy: A deep learning approach to automatic coding of session transcripts. *Psychother. Res.* **2021**, *31*, 300–312. [CrossRef]
12. Goldberg, S.B.; Flemotomos, N.; Martinez, V.R.; Tanana, M.J.; Kuo, P.B.; Pace, B.T.; Villatte, J.L.; Georgiou, P.G.; Van Epps, J.; Imel, Z.E.; et al. Machine learning and natural language processing in psychotherapy research: Alliance as example use case. *J. Couns. Psychol.* **2020**, *67*, 438–448. [CrossRef] [PubMed]
13. Niels Bantilan Matteo Malgaroli, B.R.; Hull, T.D. Just in time crisis response: Suicide alert system for telemedicine psychotherapy settings. *Psychother. Res.* **2021**, *31*, 289–299. [CrossRef]

14. Miner, A.S.; Shah, N.; Bullock, K.D.; Arnow, B.A.; Bailenson, J.; Hancock, J. Key Considerations for Incorporating Conversational AI in Psychotherapy. *Front. Psychiatry* **2019**, *10*, 746. [CrossRef]
15. Boudjellal, N.; Zhang, H.; Khan, A.; Ahmad, A.; Naseem, R.; Dai, L. A Silver Standard Biomedical Corpus for Arabic Language. *Complexity* **2020**, *2020*, 8896659. [CrossRef]
16. Alnaghaimshi, N.I.S.; Awadalla, M.S.; Clark, S.R.; Baumert, M. A systematic review of features and content quality of Arabic mental mHealth apps. *Front. Digit. Health* **2024**, *6*, 1472251. [CrossRef]
17. Alhumoud, S.O.; Al Wazrah, A.A. Arabic sentiment analysis using recurrent neural networks: A review. *Artif. Intell. Rev.* **2022**, *55*, 707–748. [CrossRef]
18. Al Katat, S.; Zaki, C.; Hazimeh, H.; Bitar, I.; Angarita, R.; Trojman, L. Natural language processing for arabic sentiment analysis: A systematic literature review. *IEEE Trans. Big Data* **2024**, *10*, 576–594. [CrossRef]
19. Alhazmi, A.; Mahmud, R.; Idris, N.; Abo, M.E.M.; Eke, C. A systematic literature review of hate speech identification on Arabic Twitter data: Research challenges and future directions. *PeerJ Comput. Sci.* **2024**, *10*, e1966. [CrossRef]
20. Malgaroli, M.; Hull, T.D.; Zech, J.M.; Althoff, T. Natural language processing for mental health interventions: A systematic review and research framework. *Transl. Psychiatry* **2023**, *13*, 309. [CrossRef]
21. Zhang, T.; Schoene, A.M.; Ji, S.; Ananiadou, S. Natural language processing applied to mental illness detection: A narrative review. *NPJ Digit. Med.* **2022**, *5*, 46. [CrossRef]
22. Teferra, B.G.; Rueda, A.; Pang, H.; Valenzano, R.; Samavi, R.; Krishnan, S.; Bhat, V. Screening for Depression Using Natural Language Processing: Literature Review. *Interact. J. Med. Res.* **2024**, *13*, e55067. [CrossRef] [PubMed]
23. Lee, M.H.; Kyung, R. Mental health stigma and natural language processing: Two enigmas through the lens of a limited corpus. In Proceedings of the 2022 IEEE World AI IoT Congress (AIIoT), Seattle, WA, USA, 6–9 June 2022; pp. 688–691.
24. Scherbakov, D.A.; Hubig, N.C.; Lenert, L.A.; Alekseyenko, A.V.; Obeid, J.S. Natural Language Processing and Social Determinants of Health in Mental Health Research: AI-Assisted Scoping Review. *JMIR Ment. Health* **2025**, *12*, e67192. [CrossRef] [PubMed]
25. Lamichhane, B. Evaluation of ChatGPT for nlp-based mental health applications. *arXiv* **2023**, arXiv:2303.15727.
26. Guo, Z.; Lai, A.; Thygesen, J.H.; Farrington, J.; Keen, T.; Li, K. Large language model for mental health: A systematic review. *arXiv* **2024**, arXiv:2403.15401.
27. Tricco, A.C.; Lillie, E.; Zarin, W.; O'Brien, K.K.; Colquhoun, H.; Levac, D.; Moher, D.; Peters, M.D.J.; Horsley, T.; Weeks, L.; et al. PRISMA extension for scoping reviews (PRISMA-ScR): Checklist and explanation. *Ann. Intern. Med.* **2018**, *169*, 467–473. [CrossRef]
28. Munn, Z.; Peters, M.D.J.; Stern, C.; Tufanaru, C.; McArthur, A.; Aromataris, E. Systematic review or scoping review? Guidance for authors when choosing between a systematic or scoping review approach. *BMC Med. Res. Methodol.* **2018**, *18*, 143. [CrossRef]
29. Abdulsalam, A.; Alhothali, A.; Al-Ghamdi, S. Detecting suicidality in Arabic tweets using machine learning and deep learning techniques. *Arab. J. Sci. Eng.* **2024**, *49*, 12729–12742. [CrossRef]
30. Alabdulkreem, E. Prediction of depressed Arab women using their tweets. *J. Decis. Syst.* **2021**, *30*, 102–117. [CrossRef]
31. Alghamdi, N.S.; Mahmoud, H.A.H.; Abraham, A.; Alanazi, S.A.; Garcia-Hernández, L. Predicting depression symptoms in an Arabic psychological forum. *IEEE Access* **2020**, *8*, 57317–57334. [CrossRef]
32. Alzoubi, A.; Alaiad, A.; Alkhattib, K.; Alkhatib, A.J.; Aqoulah, A.A.; Hayajnah, O. Detection of depression from Arabic tweets using machine learning. *Sustain. Mach. Intell. J.* **2024**, *6*, 1–7. [CrossRef]
33. Baghdadi, N.A.; Malki, A.; Balaha, H.M.; AbdulAzeem, Y.; Badawy, M.; Elhosseini, M. An optimized deep learning approach for suicide detection through Arabic tweets. *PeerJ Comput. Sci.* **2022**, *8*, e1070. [CrossRef] [PubMed]
34. Duwairi, R.; Halloush, Z. A multi-view learning approach for detecting personality disorders among arab social media users. *ACM Trans. Asian Low-Resource Lang. Inf. Process.* **2023**, *22*, 1–19. [CrossRef]
35. Elmajali, S.; Ahmad, I. Towards early detection of depression: Detecting depression symptoms in Arabic tweets using pretrained transformers. *IEEE Access* **2024**, *12*, 88134–88145. [CrossRef]
36. Almars, A.M. Attention-Based Bi-LSTM Model for Arabic Depression Classification. *Comput. Mater. Contin.* **2022**, *71*, 3091–3106. [CrossRef]
37. Mezzi, R.; Yahyaoui, A.; Krir, M.W.; Boulila, W.; Koubaa, A. Mental health intent recognition for Arabic-speaking patients using the mini international neuropsychiatric interview (MINI) and BERT model. *Sensors* **2022**, *22*, 846. [CrossRef]
38. Sivakumar, M.; Basariya, R.; Rajak, A.; Senthil, M.; Vetriselvi, T.; Raja, G.; Rajavarman, R. Transforming Arabic Text Analysis: Integrating Applied Linguistics with m-Polar Neutrosophic Set Mood Change and Depression on Social Media. *Int. J. Neutrosophic Sci.* **2025**, *25*, 313.
39. Helmy, A.; Nassar, R.; Ramdan, N. Cross-lingual depression detection for twitter users: A comparative sentiment analysis of english and arabic tweets. *Preprint* **2023**. [CrossRef]
40. Saadany, H.; Tantawy, A.; Orasan, C. Cyber Risks of Machine Translation Critical Errors: Arabic Mental Health Tweets as a Case Study. *arXiv* **2024**, arXiv:2405.11668.

41. Alaskar, A.; Ykhlef, M. Depression Detection from Arabic Tweets using machine learning techniques. *J. Comput. Sci. Soft. Devel* **2021**, 1–10. [CrossRef]
42. Rabie, E.M.; Hashem, A.F.; Alsheref, F.K. Recognition model for major depressive disorder in Arabic user-generated content. *Beni-Suef Univ. J. Basic Appl. Sci.* **2025**, *14*, 7. [CrossRef]
43. Alatawi, H.; Abudalfa, S.; Luqman, H. Empirical Analysis for Detecting Arabic Online Suicidal Ideation. *Procedia Comput. Sci.* **2024**, *244*, 143–150. [CrossRef]
44. Alhuzali, H.; Alasmari, A. Evaluating the Effectiveness of the Foundational Models for Q&A Classification in Mental Health care. *arXiv* **2024**, arXiv:2406.15966.
45. El-Ramly, M.; Abu-Elyazid, H.; Mo'men, Y.; Alshaer, G.; Adib, N.; Eldeen, K.A.; El-Shazly, M. CairoDep: Detecting depression in Arabic posts using BERT transformers. In Proceedings of the 2021 Tenth International Conference on Intelligent Computing and Information Systems (ICICIS), Cairo, Egypt, 5–7 December 2021; pp. 207–212.
46. Kumar, A.; Kumari, J.; Pradhan, J. Explainable deep learning for mental health detection from english and arabic social media posts. *ACM Trans. Asian Low-Resource Lang. Inf. Process.* **2023**. [CrossRef]
47. Hassib, M.; Hossam, N.; Sameh, J.; Torki, M. Aradepsu: Detecting depression and suicidal ideation in arabic tweets using transformers. In Proceedings of the Seventh Arabic Natural Language Processing Workshop (WANLP), Abu Dhabi, United Arab Emirates, 7–11 December 2022; pp. 302–311.
48. Bensalah, N.; Ayad, H.; Adib, A.; El Farouk, A.I. MindWave app: Leveraging AI for Mental Health Support in English and Arabic. In Proceedings of the 2024 IEEE 12th International Symposium on Signal, Image, Video and Communications (ISIVC), Marrakech, Morocco, 21–23 May 2024; pp. 1–6.
49. Almouzini, S.; Alageel, A. Detecting arabic depressed users from twitter data. *Procedia Comput. Sci.* **2019**, *163*, 257–265. [CrossRef]
50. Maghraby, A.; Ali, H. Modern Standard Arabic mood changing and depression dataset. *Data Br.* **2022**, *41*, 107999. [CrossRef]
51. Musleh, D.A.; Alkhales, T.A.; Almakki, R.A.; Alnajim, S.E.; Almarshad, S.K.; Alhasaniah, R.S.; Aljameel, S.S.; Almuqhim, A.A. Twitter Arabic Sentiment Analysis to Detect Depression Using Machine Learning. *Comput. Mater. Contin.* **2022**, *71*, 3463–3477. [CrossRef]
52. Al-Musallam, N.; Al-Abdullatif, M. Depression Detection Through Identifying Depressive Arabic Tweets From Saudi Arabia: Machine Learning Approach. In Proceedings of the 2022 Fifth National Conference of Saudi Computers Colleges (NCCC), Makkah, Saudi Arabia, 17–18 December 2022; pp. 11–18.
53. Habash, N.Y. *Introduction to Arabic Natural Language Processing*; Hirst, G., Ed.; University of Toronto: Toronto, ON, Canada; Morgan & Claypool: San Rafael, CA, USA, 2010; Volume 3.
54. Antoun, W.; Baly, F.; Hajj, H. Arabert: Transformer-based Model for Arabic Language Understanding. In Proceedings of the 4th Workshop on Open-Source Arabic Corpora and Processing Tools, with a Shared Task on Offensive Language Detection, Marseille, France, 11–16 May 2020; European Language Resource Association: Marseille, France, 2020; pp. 9–15. Available online: https://aclanthology.org/2020.osact-1.2 (accessed on 1 July 2024).
55. Abdul-Mageed, M.; Elmadany, A.; Nagoudi, E.M.B. ARBERT & MARBERT: Deep Bidirectional Transformers for Arabic. In Proceedings of the 59th Annual Meeting of the Association for Computational Linguistics and the 11th International Joint Conference on Natural Language Processing (Volume 1: Long Papers), Online, August 2021; Association for Computational Linguistics: Stroudsburg, PA, USA, 2021; pp. 7088–7105.
56. Alhuzali, H.; Alasmari, A.; Alsaleh, H. MentalQA: An Annotated Arabic Corpus for Questions and Answers of Mental Healthcare. *IEEE Access* **2024**, *12*, 101155–101165. [CrossRef]
57. Buda, M.; Maki, A.; Mazurowski, M.A. A systematic study of the class imbalance problem in convolutional neural networks. *Neural Netw.* **2018**, *106*, 249–259. [CrossRef]
58. Wei, J.; Zou, K. EDA: Easy Data Augmentation Techniques for Boosting Performance on Text Classification Tasks. *arXiv* **2019**, arXiv:1901.11196.
59. Chawla, N.V.; Bowyer, K.W.; Hall, L.O.; Kegelmeyer, W.P. SMOTE: Synthetic Minority Over-sampling Technique. *J. Artif. Intell. Res.* **2002**, *16*, 321–357. [CrossRef]
60. Lin, T.-Y.; Goyal, P.; Girshick, R.; He, K.; Dollár, P. Focal Loss for Dense Object Detection. *IEEE Trans. Pattern Anal. Mach. Intell.* **2020**, *42*, 318–327. [CrossRef] [PubMed]
61. Haibo, H.; Garcia, E.A. Learning from Imbalanced Data. *IEEE Trans. Knowl. Data Eng.* **2009**, *21*, 1263–1284. [CrossRef]
62. Schuster, M.; Paliwal, K.K. Bidirectional recurrent neural networks. *IEEE Trans. Signal Process.* **1997**, *45*, 2673–2681. [CrossRef]
63. Tabinda Kokab, S.; Asghar, S.; Naz, S. Transformer-based deep learning models for the sentiment analysis of social media data. *Array* **2022**, *14*, 100157. [CrossRef]

healthcare

MDPI

Article

A Comparative Study of Hospitalization Mortality Rates between General and Emergency Hospitalized Patients Using Survival Analysis

Haegak Chang [1], Seiyoung Ryu [2], Ilyoung Choi [3], Angela Eunyoung Kwon [4] and Jaekyeong Kim [1,2,*]

1 School of Management, Kyung Hee University, Seoul 02447, Republic of Korea; hkc@khu.ac.kr
2 Department of Bigdata Analytics, Kyung Hee University, Seoul 02447, Republic of Korea; rsy22@khu.ac.kr
3 Divison of Business Administration, Seo Kyeong University, Seoul 02713, Republic of Korea; iychoi@skuniv.ac.kr
4 Sauder School of Business, University of British Columbia, Vancouver, BC 2053, Canada; angela.kwon@sauder.ubc.ca
* Correspondence: jaek@khu.ac.kr

Abstract: Background/Objectives: In Korea's emergency medical system, when an emergency patient arises, patients receive on-site treatment and care during transport at the pre-hospital stage, followed by inpatient treatment upon hospitalization. From the perspective of emergency patient management, it is critical to identify the high death rate of patients with certain conditions in the emergency room. Therefore, it is necessary to compare and analyze the determinants of the death rate of patients admitted via the emergency room and generally hospitalized patients. In fact, previous studies investigating determinants of survival periods or length of stay (LOS) primarily used multiple or logistic regression analyses as their main research methodology. Although medical data often exhibit censored characteristics, which are crucial for analyzing survival periods, the aforementioned methods of analysis fail to accommodate these characteristics, presenting a significant limitation. Methods:Therefore, in this study, survival analyses were performed to investigate factors affecting the dying risk of general inpatients as well as patients admitted through the emergency room. For this purpose, this study collected and analyzed the sample cohort DB for a total of four years from 2016 to 2019 provided by the Korean National Health Insurance Services (NHIS). After data preprocessing, the survival probability was estimated according to sociodemographic, patient, health checkup records, and institutional features through the Kaplan–Meier survival estimation. Then, the Cox proportional hazards models were additionally utilized for further econometric validation. Results: As a result of the analysis, in terms of the 'city' feature among the sociodemographic characteristics, the small and medium-sized cities exert the most influence on the death rate of general inpatients, whereas the metropolitan cities exert the most influence on the death rate of inpatients admitted through the emergency room. In terms of institution characteristics, it was found that there is a difference in determinants affecting the death rate of the two groups of study, such as the number of doctors per 100 hospital beds, the number of nurses per 100 hospital beds, the number of hospital beds, the number of surgical beds, and the number of emergency beds. Conclusions: Based on the study results, it is expected that an efficient plan for distributing limited medical resources can be established based on inpatients' LOS.

Keywords: survival analysis; Kaplan–Meier survival analysis; cox proportional hazards model; national health insurance services cohort DB; survival period; death rate; medical data

1. Introduction

Despite the higher demand for emergency medical care due to various accidents, many patients could not receive proper emergency treatment, leading to an increase in the death rate. Following the COVID-19 era, there have been disruptions in the management and operation of emergency medical services since many of the medical resources, including medical staff, emergency rooms, and hospital beds, were specifically dedicated to being utilized in the COVID-19 emergency medical centers [1].

In Korea's emergency medical system, upon the emergence of an emergency patient, treatment is administered on-site and during transport at the pre-hospital stage, followed by inpatient care at the hospital stage [2,3]. As such, the role of emergency rooms in this emergency medical system is becoming increasingly important. Generally, under Article 31 of the Emergency Medical Service Act, emergency rooms are designed to provide emergency care and other medical tasks and are staffed 24 h by specialist physicians who provide efficient and prompt treatments. In fact, emergency rooms have confronted the issue of overcrowding due to an influx of visits by both patients who require immediate care and those with non-emergency conditions.

Overcrowding in emergency rooms is a phenomenon resulting from the lack of medical resources and treatments, which are insufficient to meet the demands of emergency care. This phenomenon leads to several negative impacts, including a prolonged waiting time in the emergency room, an increase in the death rate due to ambulance delay, an inability to prepare for major disasters, and a decline in the quality of emergency medical services due to the allocation of resources to non-emergency patients. To address such issues, there have been many studies suggesting causes and solutions of emergency room overcrowding [4–7]. Despite the foundation of such issues stemming from knowing the determinants of patients' death in the emergency room, it is often neglected from the perspective of emergency management and treatment. In fact, the post-traumatic death rate in 2019 in Korea is preventable by 15.7%, which is not significantly different from the rates in other developed countries [8]. It has been reported that the post-traumatic death rate could be reduced to below 10% with an augmented emergency medical system [9]. Therefore, to reduce the preventable post-traumatic death rate, it is vital to identify determinants affecting the surviving period of inpatients admitted through the emergency room. However, if the study observes the time of death for inpatients admitted through the emergency room only, it remains ambiguous whether one survived during the observation period, and, thus, preventing full identification of their exact survival time. Moreover, if an inpatient died due to other factors besides one's post-traumatic conditions, it is impossible to know one's survival time. Therefore, the aforementioned types of records regarding patients' death all correspond to the censored data, which is a significant characteristic to be considered prior to conducting data analyses. In fact, multivariate and logistic regression analyses do not account for the censored nature of data, and, thus, this places a limitation to the investigation of determinants affecting the surviving period of patients admitted through the emergency room. It is necessary to minimize the inappropriate use of emergency room treatments by non-emergency patients because care consists of emergency room treatment and inpatient care at the hospital stage of the emergency medical system. In particular, considering an increase in the death rate within the emergency room department in Korea, it is urgent to carefully identify the determinants of survival time for ER-admitted patients. For this purpose, this study aims to identify factors influencing the survival time of general inpatients and those admitted through the emergency room and to compare the results between the two groups of patients. Since data regarding an individual's death are the censored data, it is important to consider the survival time prior to analyzing its determinants. Therefore, we decided to utilize survival analysis as the main methodological tool for our research. In fact, survival analysis enables us to statistically analyze not only the duration until the death of inpatients admitted in the emergency room but also the determinants of the survival time [10,11]. This study aims to compare the survival probabilities over time for ER-admitted patients and general inpatients using the non-parametric statistical method of the Kaplan–Meier survival estimation. Then, using the semi-parametric statistical method of the Cox proportional hazards model, this study seeks to analyze and compare features influencing death rates between inpatients admitted in the emergency room and general inpatients. The Cox proportional hazards model is expressed by the hazard function. That is, the hazard function can be interpreted as the risk of death at time. Therefore, the measure of effect in the Cox model is the hazard rate, i.e., the risk of death given that the patient survived until a specific time. We use the cohort database of the National Health Insurance Corporation of Korea. The data include information on the date of death of emergency patients and general patients after hospitalization, but there is no information on whether the patient was discharged after full recovery or if transferred to another hospital. Therefore, we assume death as a terminal event and perform survival analysis.

In terms of features utilized in this study, we referred to the extant literature and selected ones from the cohort DB provided by the Korean NHIS. The data analysis was conducted in a virtual environment of NHIS using the R statistical program (version 3.7.6). Since this study identifies the main determinants affecting the dying risk of inpatients, we expect medical institutions to allocate medical resources in an effective manner. We also expect guidelines to be established to address emergency room overcrowding, based on information about patients prioritized for emergency care.

2. Theoretical Background

2.1. Emergency Medical Services (EMS)

The emergency medical services (EMS) encompass actions taken for patients from the onset of an emergency until they recover from life-threatening conditions or are alleviated from physical and psychological harm [12]. As a part of public goods, these services include consultation, rescue, transport, emergency treatment, and medical care [13]. As shown in Figure 1(1), the number of patients using emergency rooms increased from 5.59 million in 2016 and 2017 and 5.79 million in 2018 to 5.94 million in 2019, which then decreased to 4.64 million in 2020. The admission and death rates in the emergency room are shown in Figure 1(2). The death rates gradually increased from 0.6% in 2016, 0.6% in 2017, 0.6% in 2018, 0.5% in 2019, and 0.7% in 2020. The admission rates also increased from 20.4% in 2016, 21.1% in 2017, 21.0% in 2018, 21.1% in 2019, and 23.0% in 2020.

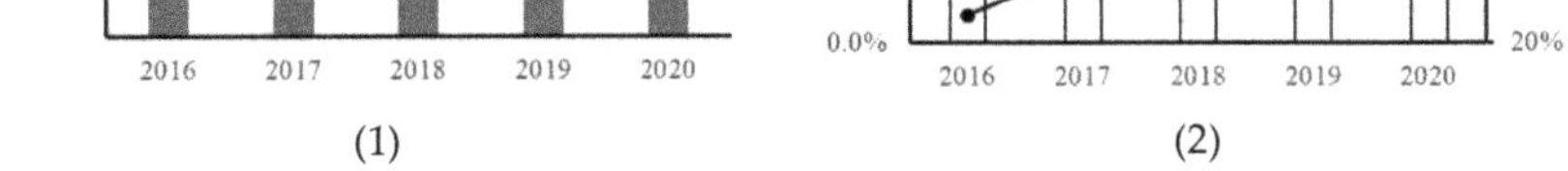

(1) (2)

Figure 1. Current state of EMS in Korea (Source: KOSIS (Korean Statistical Informational Service, Statistics of EMS, 21 November 2022)). The two represent (1) use of emergency room, and (2) admission and death rate in emergency (from left to right).

Despite the increasing trends in death and admission rates of emergency patients, it is difficult to find existing studies examining the relationship of death and admission rates of emergency patients with their survival time. In fact, most existing research related to emergency room is often focused on ER overcrowding; however, it is necessary to analyze the survival time for ER-admitted patients prior to scrutinizing the death and admission rates of these individuals.

2.2. Survival Analysis

Survival analysis is a method widely used in the fields of biology and medicine, which utilizes censored data containing information, such as patients' survival and death, and assesses differences in the elapsed time to an event of interest [11,14–16]. Here, censored data refers to data with unknown occurrence of an event from the beginning of the study to the end. For instance, when observing the time of death among patients as in Figure 2, the characteristics for each data set are as follows. The data for patients 1 and 5 fall under complete data, while patient 2, 3, and 4 correspond to censored data. In particular, the data for patient 4 is considered censored because the cause of death was unrelated to the aggravated disease.

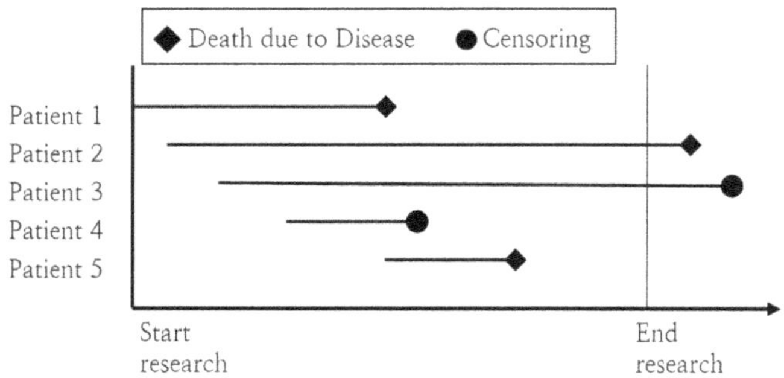

Figure 2. Example of censored data.

Since survival analysis is a statistical approach that estimates the survival time between two events of interest, it is explicitly different from other approaches such as regression and logistic regression, as demonstrated in Table 1. While linear regression considers time as a dependent variable, it is limited by not accounting for the presence of censored data. On the other hand, logistic regression can only include an event, such as whether one has died or has been hospitalized, as a dependent variable, but it cannot consider time in its analysis.

Table 1. Comparison of research methodologies for analyzing survival period.

Category	Characteristics	Limitation
Linear Regression	Dependent variable: time	Cannot consider the presence of censored data
Logistic Regression	Dependent variable: event	Cannot consider time
Survival Analysis	Can consider both time and the presence of censored data	

In fact, survival analysis can be conducted using three types of methods: non-parametric, semi-parametric, and parametric methods. First, a non-parametric method does not require an assumption that the data follow a certain probability distribution. Second, a semi-parametric method still does not require an assumption regarding data distribution yet estimates regression coefficients. Lastly, a parametric method carries an assumption that the data follows a distribution, such as the Weibull distribution, with respect to survival time, t.

Among non-parametric methods, there are the Kaplan–Meier estimation analysis and the log-rank test. The Kaplan–Meier estimation assumes that events are to occur independently of one another and calculates survival probabilities from one interval to the next under the assumption that censoring is independent of the survival time [17]. These probabilities can be illustrated in a survival plot [17]. The log-rank test compares the time-to-event distributions across two or more independent groups, utilizing a chi-squared test of the time occurrence between the observed and expected counts. This test is particularly used to validate the null hypothesis that no significant difference exists in the survival curves between the groups being compared.

Here, Table 2 demonstrates the existing literature that utilized survival analysis for research purposes across various fields of study. In fact, there is one semi-parametric method, which is the Cox proportional hazards model. This model is a multivariate regression method that tests the significance of various predictors relevant to time and processes the censored data, assuming that there is a log-linear relationship between the survival function and the variables [18]. Having acknowledged that the data used in this study do not satisfy a certain distribution over time, such as the Weibull distribution, we decided to utilize the Kaplan–Meier estimation and the Cox proportional hazards model. In other words, this study aims to estimate and compare the survival time of general inpatients and patients admitted through the emergency room using the Korean NHIS cohort DB based on the Kaplan–Meier survival analyses.

Table 2. Extant literature using survival analysis.

Researchers	Research Methodology	Research Subjects	Research Purpose
[19]	Log-rank test Cox proportional hazards model	Resort facilities in Spain	To identify financial and non-financial factors affecting the survival of resort facilities in Spain
[20]	Log-rank test Cox proportional hazards model	Resort facilities in Spain	To investigate factors affecting the survival of resort facilities in Spain
[21]	Cox proportional hazards model	Companies undergoing financial distress	To investigate how restraints to corruptions and financial ratios affect the survival of companies undergoing financial distress
[22]	Cox proportional hazards model	Companies undergoing financial distress	To investigate how factors including corporate governance, financial ratios, and political risk affect the company's survival
[23]	Kaplan–Meier estimation Cox proportional hazards model	Pancreatic cancer patients	To estimate the prognostic effect of the established cancer hallmark genes in various cancer types
[24]	Kaplan–Meier estimation	Playtimes in game	To propose new methods to measure game playtimes

3. Research Methodology

3.1. Research Framework

The purpose of this study is to identify factors affecting the survival time of general inpatients and inpatients admitted through the emergency room, separately, and to compare the results. General inpatients, in this study, refer to those who were hospitalized without the emergency room transport. As demonstrated in Figure 3, we conducted our research in three phases: data collection, data preprocessing, and survival analysis.

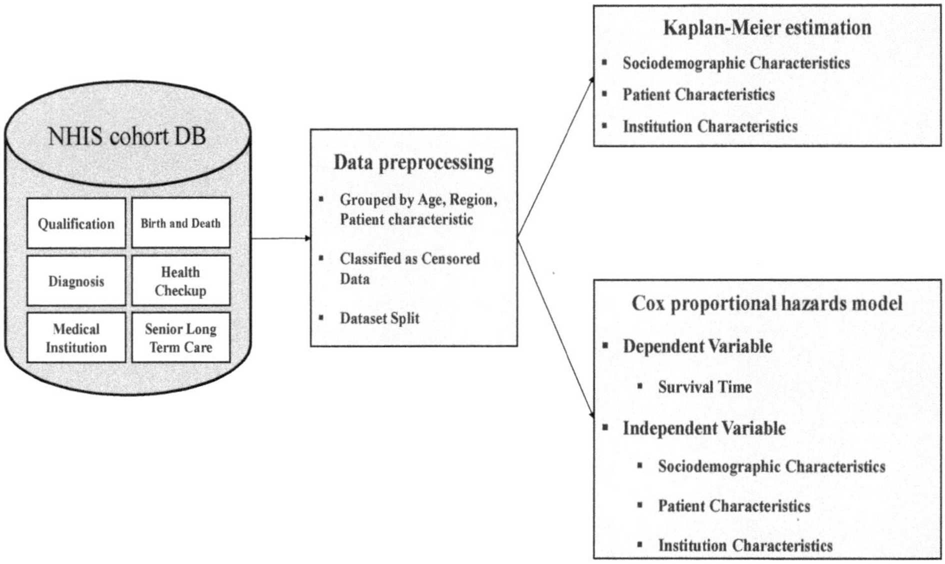

Figure 3. Research framework for investigating determinants of survival time.

During the data collection phase, we collected the Korean National Health Insurance Service (NHIS) cohort DB. For data preprocessing, we grouped the features, classified the censored data, and divided the subjects into general inpatients and those admitted through the emergency room. Lastly, for survival analyses, we investigated the main determinants of survival time for each group of subjects using both the Kaplan–Meier estimation and the Cox proportional hazards model.

3.2. Data Collection

To identify determinants affecting the dying risk of general inpatients and that of inpatients admitted through the emergency room, this study utilized the four-year health checkup cohort DB from the year 2016 to 2019 provided by the Korean National Health Insurance Services. This cohort DB is a sample study DB established in January 2013 based on the health examination records DB, encompassing approximately one million (2% of the total population in Korea) records of patients without violating the privacy terms. This cohort DB is the latest data provided by the Korea Health Insurance Service.

Such DB is largely composed of six different tables as follows: qualification, birth and death, diagnosis, health checkup, medical institution, and senior long-term care (see Table 3).

Referring to prior studies on investigating determinants of survival time, we selected four tables out of the displayed tables in the cohort DB for the purpose of our study: qualification, birth and death, diagnosis, and medical institution. As presented in Table 4, a total of 18 variables were used in this study, where 12 of them were classified into either of the sociodemographic, patient, and institution tables for analyzing the determinants of survival time.

Table 3. Description of health checkup cohort DB.

Table	Description
Qualification	Includes socio-demographic information (gender, age, residential area, income range, insurance type) of a health checkup examinee (excluding foreigners) or information about the matter of death.
Birth and Death	Includes information on subjects whose death has been verified, linked with birth and the cause of death information provided by Statistics Korea.
Diagnosis	Includes medical records (main diagnosis information, prescription history, cost-related information, admission records, the department of treatment, etc.); consists of ten DB partitions.
Health Checkup	Includes checkup records (Lab value, past medical history, hereditary conditions, lifestyle, etc., retrieved from survey questionnaires) of a health checkup examinee.
Medical Institution	Includes information of a medical institution (address, the number of hospital beds) attended by a health checkup examinee.
Senior Long-Term Care	Includes information on subjects' application for long-term care services, usage records, and the status of facilities

Table 4. Features in health checkup cohort DB.

Table	Feature Code *	Feature Description	Purpose of Use
Common	STD_YYYY	Year between 2016 and 2019	Merging between tables
	RN_INDI	A six-digit code for interlinking the tables	
	RN_INST	A six-digit code for interlinking the tables	
Qualification	SEX	1: Male, 2: Female	Sociodemographic feature
	AGE	Patient's age in a corresponding year	
	SIDO	City code	
	GAIBJA_TYPE	A code indicating the type of insurance	Patient feature
	CTRB	Income quantile (1–10)	
	DSB_SVRT_CD	No inclusion, severe, mild level of disability	
Birth and Death	DTH_YYYYMM	The date of one's death	Dependent variable
Diagnosis	HSPTZ_PATH_TYPE	Admission route	Grouping
	MCARE_RSLT_TYPE	Patient's condition on the day of one's final treatment	Censoring
Medical Institution	INST_CLSFC_CD	Type of medical institutions	Institution feature
	CNT_DR_TOT	The number of doctors	
	CNT_NRS_TOT	The number of nurses	
	CNT_BED_INP	The number of hospital beds	
Medical Institution	CNT_BED_OP	The number of surgical beds	Institution feature
	CNT_BED_ER	The number of emergency beds	

* Feature code is directly retrieved from the data provided by NHIS.

First, from the 'qualification' and 'birth and death' tables, we utilized the subjects' sociodemographic and personal information. Among the sociodemographic features, information such as one's gender, age, and region was included. Among the patient features, information such as one's type of health insurance, income quantile, and the severity of disability was included. We used the information regarding one's death from the 'birth and death' table as a dependent variable of our analyses. Second, from the 'Diagnosis' table, we utilized information pertaining to whether one has been hospitalized and also the admission route of hospitalization in order to compare the survival time between general inpatients and those admitted through the emergency room. We also used information regarding the diagnostic results as the censored data. Third, we used various information on institutions from the 'Medical Institution' table. This table includes features, including the types of institutions that one has been admitted, the number of doctors and nurses, and the number of hospital beds.

3.3. Data Preprocessing

This study conducted survival analyses on subjects with hospitalized records between 2016 and 2019 from the sample cohort DB provided by the Korean NHIS. Data preprocessing prior to conducting survival analysis involved eliminating the missing values, merging between tables, and extracting values for each feature followed by identifying the censored data. The details of data preprocessing are presented in Table 5.

Table 5. Preprocessed results by feature (Survival Time Determinant Analysis).

Category	Feature	Preprocessed Results
Sociodemographic Information	Gender Age City	[Grouping] Male/Female [Grouping] 10-year unit [Grouping] Seoul/Metropolitan city/Small and medium-sized city
Patient Information	Insurance status Income quantile Severity of disability	[Grouping] Workplace/Regional/Medical insurees [Grouping] 0/1–3/4–7/8–10 [Grouping] No inclusion, severe, mild
Institution Information	Institution type The number of doctors per 100 hospital beds The number of nurses per 100 hospital beds The number of hospital beds The number of surgical beds The number of emergency beds	[Grouping] top general hospitals/general hospitals [Feature preprocessing] (the number of doctors/the number of hospital beds) × 100 [Grouping] in four quantiles [Feature preprocessing] (the number of nurses/the number of hospital beds) × 100 [Grouping] in four quantiles [Grouping] in four quantiles

First, the process of eliminating missing values was completed using the features corresponding to the income quantile, the severity of disability, diagnostic results, and the date of death. In fact, missing values found within the income quantile and diagnostic results category were eliminated prior to analysis, while ones for the severity of disability were replaced with 'no inclusion (normal)'. Missing values within the date of death feature were instead indicated as 'survived', implying that the patients had not passed away. Second, we only extracted the records for top general hospitals and general hospitals using the codes indicating a type of institution. Next, we utilized common features, such as the standard year code and the code for interlinking the tables to merge the four tables of our research interest. The remaining number of records after merging is 25,722,085. Third, we completed feature preprocessing by, for instance, grouping the variables. In terms of age, since the year of birth was provided by the NHIS data, it was converted to age as of the base year, which was then grouped into ten-year units. For region, we referred to the extant literature [25] to classify the variables into Seoul, metropolitan cities (Busan, Daegu, Daejeon, Incheon, Gwangju, Ulsan), and the others as the small and medium-sized cities. Among the patient characteristics, for insurance status, we regrouped the existing six categories of the feature into three categories: medical insurees, regional insurance, and workplace insurance. For income quantiles, we reclassified the existing ten different quantiles of income into 0 quantile, 1–3 quantiles, 4–7 quantiles, and 8–10 quantiles. For institutional characteristics, considering the size of medical institutions used in this study, we set the number of doctors and nurses by 100 hospital beds, which were then grouped into four separate groups. The same procedure was applied for the number of hospital, surgical, and emergency beds. Fourth, censored data, which are not conventionally considered in other analytical methods, can be utilized in survival analysis. Therefore, this study accounted for subjects who had not died by the last date of treatment—that is, subjects whose current survival status is unknown—to be classified as censored data.

4. Results

This study conducted survival analyses on subjects with hospitalized records between 2016 and 2019 from the sample cohort DB provided by the Korean NHIS. Data preprocessing prior to conducting survival analysis involved eliminating the missing values, the merging between tables, and extracting values for each feature followed by identifying the censored data.

4.1. Determinants of Survival Time among General Inpatients

For the purpose of finding determinants of survival time among general inpatients and those admitted through the emergency room, we first conducted survival analysis on general inpatients. A total of 3,228,933 records was used, and 12 variables were investigated to check which of them affect the risk of death.

4.1.1. Characteristics of General Inpatients

Table 6 presents the characteristics of general inpatients. The gender distribution of the study subjects is 50.13% male and 49.87% female. The age distribution is as follows: 11.66% under 29, 5.62% between 30 and 39, 9.42% between 40 and 49, 17% between 50 and 59, 19.18% between 60 and 69, 21.21% between 70 and 79, 13.86% between 80 and 89, and 2.05% above 90. For region, the result shows 21% in Seoul, 31% in metropolitan cities, and 47% in other small and medium-sized cities. For insurance status, 10% are medical insurees, 29% are those with regional insurance, and 61% are those with workplace insurance. For income quantiles, 10%, 20%, 31%, and 38% are 0, 1–3, 4–7, and 8–10 quantiles, respectively. For the severity of disability, individuals with normal, mild, and severe symptoms are 79%, 11%, and 10%, respectively. There are 70% general hospitals and 30% top general hospitals. For other features, such as the number of doctors per 100 hospital beds, they were previously divided into four groups, and, thus, there is 25% for each category.

Table 6. Characteristics of general inpatients.

Category	Feature		Number of Patients	Number of Dead	Censored Data	
					N	%
Sociodemographic Characteristics	Gender	Male	1,618,558	493,753	1,124,805	69.49
		Female	1,610,375	362,935	1,247,440	77.46
	Age	~29	376,400	8,557	367,843	97.73
		30~39	181,316	11,059	170,257	93.9
		40~49	304,032	38,933	265,099	87.19
		50~59	548,986	97,958	451,028	82.16
		60~69	619,434	155,199	464,235	74.95
		70~79	684,980	261,576	423,404	61.81
		80~89	447,479	236,122	211,357	47.23
		90~	66,306	47,284	19,022	28.69
	City	Seoul	690,213	216,436	473,777	68.64
		Metropolitan city	1,011,287	240,263	771,024	76.24
		Small, medium-sized city	1,527,433	399,989	1,127,444	73.81
Patient Characteristics	Insurance status	Medical insuree	324,647	110,780	213,867	65.88
		Regional insurance	927,937	247,733	680,204	73.30
		Workplace insurance	1,976,349	498,175	1,478,174	74.79
	Income quantile	0 (= Medical aid)	324,647	110,780	213,867	65.88
		1~3	653,717	161,816	491,901	75.25
		4~7	1,014,811	238,137	776,674	76.53
		8~10	1,235,758	345,955	889,803	72.00
	Severity of Disability	Normal	2,543,100	596,918	1,946,182	76.53
		Mild	364,475	129,482	234,993	64.47
		Severe	321,358	130,288	191,070	59.46

Table 6. *Cont.*

Category	Feature		Number of Patients	Number of Dead	Censored Data	
					N	%
Institution Characteristics	Type of medical institution	General hospital	2,256,811	521,261	1,735,550	76.9
		Top general hospital	972,122	335,427	636,695	65.5
	Number of doctors per 100 hospital beds	~13	851,638	164,396	687,242	80.7
		14~30	758,352	173,799	584,553	77.08
		31~46	841,977	271,496	570,481	67.75
		47~	776,966	246,997	529,969	68.21
	Number of nurses per 100 hospital beds	~52	803,234	167,841	635,393	79.1
		53~80	769,585	179,191	590,394	76.72
		81~103	846,852	245,625	601,227	71.00
		104~	809,262	264,031	545,231	67.37
	Number of hospital beds	~280	768,741	144,734	624,007	81.17
		~281~519	844,725	193,682	651,043	77.07
		520~749	806,039	238,870	567,169	70.36
		750~	809,428	279,402	530,026	65.48
	Number of surgical beds	~4	687,623	141,742	545,881	79.39
		5~9	925,752	190,039	735,713	79.47
		10~15	781,024	250,246	530,778	67.96
		16~	834,534	274,661	559,873	67.09
	Number of emergency beds	~15	776,801	146,626	630,175	81.12
		15~22	807,330	190,381	616,949	76.42
		23~35	830,467	250,014	580,453	69.89
		36~	814,335	269,667	544,668	66.89
Total			3,228,933	856,688	2,372,245	

4.1.2. Kaplan–Meier Estimation (General Inpatients)

This study utilizes the Kaplan–Meier estimation to analyze how the sociodemographic, patient, health checkup, and institution features affect LOS for inpatients over time.

First, the estimates for the features responsible for sociodemographic information, including gender, age, and city/province are shown in Figure 4. In the case of gender, the survival rate for men appears to be better than for women up to about 180 days, but after that, the survival rate for women appears to be higher. In terms of age, the survival rate gradually decreases from those in their 30s to those in their 90s or older. Lastly, in the case of regional areas, the survival rate in small and medium-sized cities appears to be high up to about 100 days, but the survival rate decreases rapidly after that. On the other hand, the survival rate in Seoul was the highest from about 100 to 180 days, and the survival rate in metropolitan cities was high after about 180 days.

Second, patient characteristics, such as health insurance subscriber classification, income bracket, and disability severity results, are shown in Figure 5. In the case of health insurance subscriber types, the survival rate of medical benefit recipients was the highest, and the survival rate tended to decrease in that order: local subscribers, and employer subscribers. In terms of income quintile, the 0th quintile showed the highest survival rate, and the survival rate decreased in that order: 8th to 10th quintile, 4th to 7th quintile, and 1st to 3rd quintile. In terms of disability severity, the survival rate was found to be high for severely ill patients, followed by the highest survival rate for mild patients. However, after about 160 days, the survival rate of patients with dysentery is rapidly decreasing, and the survival rate of normal patients (not applicable) appears to be higher.

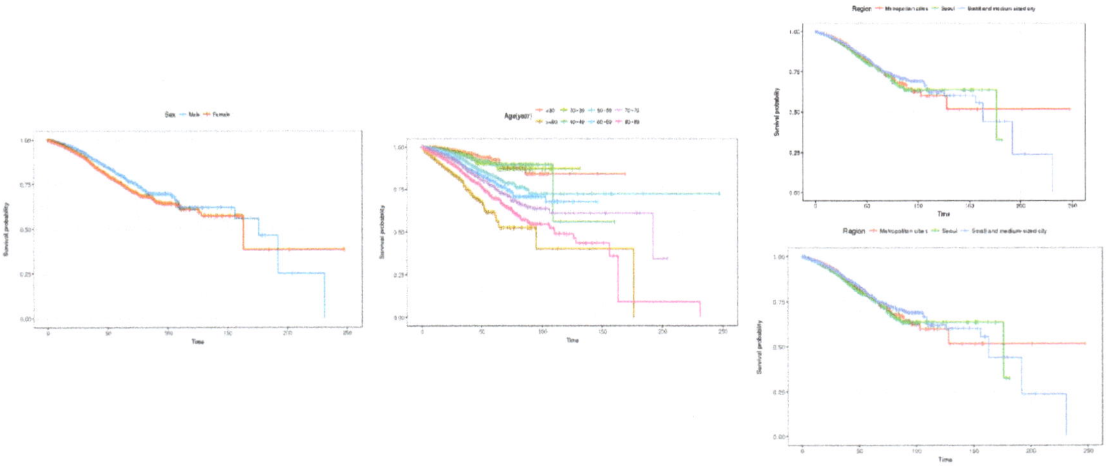

Figure 4. Kaplan–Meier survival curves by socio-demographic characteristics (general inpatients). The three charts represent (1) sex, (2) age, and (3) region (from left to right).

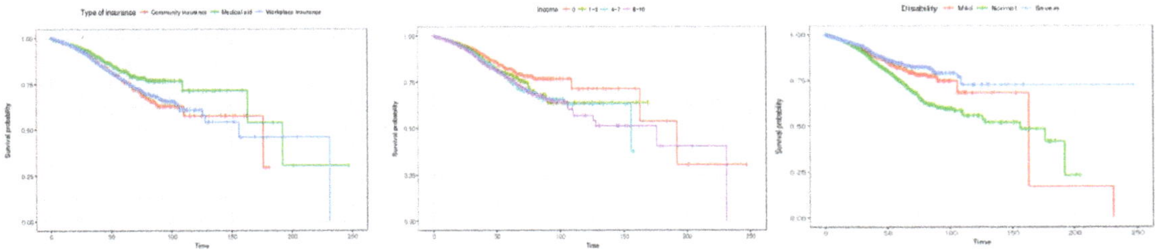

Figure 5. Kaplan–Meier survival curves by patient characteristic (general inpatients). The three charts represent (1) type of insurance, (2) income, and (3) disability (from left to right).

Third, the Kaplan–Meier survival curve by characteristics of medical institutions is shown in Figure 6. Looking at the survival rate by hospital type, it is estimated that the overall survival rate of general hospitals is higher than that of tertiary general hospitals. In terms of the number of doctors per 100 beds, the survival rate is estimated to be lowest in the order of 14 or less in the initial stage of hospitalization, followed by 14 to 30, 47 or more, and 31 to 46. Looking at the number of hospital beds, the survival rate is estimated to be high initially in the order of 281 or less, 281 to 519, 520 to 749, and 750 or more. This shows that, overall, the survival rate is estimated to be lower in larger hospitals. This is believed to be because the period of hospitalization in larger hospitals is limited, meaning there is a lot of censored data.

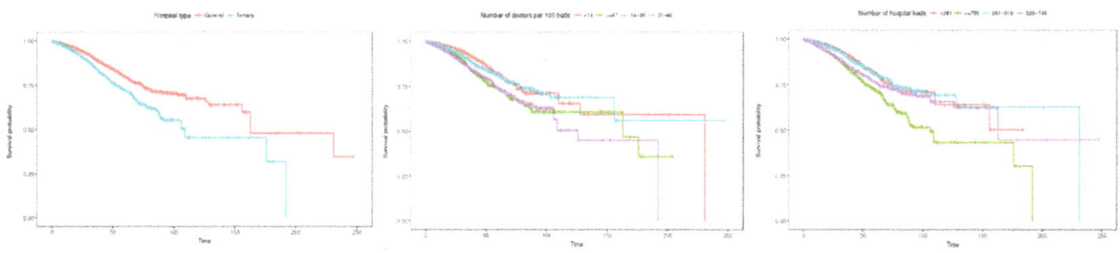

Figure 6. Kaplan–Meier survival curves by institution characteristic (general inpatients). The three charts represent (1) hospital type, (2) number of doctors per 100 beds, and (3) number of hospital beds (from left to right).

4.1.3. Cox Proportional Hazards Model (General Inpatients)

The Cox proportional hazards model results for determinants affecting the dying risk of general inpatients are shown in Figure 7. First, in terms of sociodemographic characteristics, it was found that the death rate for men is 1.54 times higher than for women. The death rate increases from under 30s to the 90s, with those over 90 having a death rate 17.47 times higher than those under 30. For region, compared to the metropolitan cities, the death rate in the small or medium-sized cities increases by 1.07 times, while it decreases by 0.98 times in Seoul. Second, among patient characteristics, the results for the type of insurance showed that the death rate of medical insurees increases by 1.01 times than that of those with regional insurance, while it decreases for those with workplace insurance to 0.96 times, indicating a lesser impact on mortality. In terms of income quantiles, the impact on death rate for patients in the 4–7 quantiles increases by 1.16 times of those in the 0th quantile. For the severity of disability, the impact on the death rate is 1.3 times higher for normal patients compared to those with mild disabilities. Third, the death rate within the top general hospitals is 1.10 times higher than that within the general hospitals. For the number of doctors per 100 hospital beds, the death rates for 31–48, 14–30, and above 47 doctors are 1.32, 1.22, and 1.11 times the death rate below 14 doctors, respectively. For the number of nurses per 100 hospital beds, it was found that compared to a group with fewer than 53 nurses, the death rates are higher in the following order: 1.24 times for the group over 104 nurses, 1.22 times for the group over 81 to 103 nurses, and then for the group between 53 and 80 nurses. In fact, there is no statistically significant difference in the results between different groups of the hospital beds. However, for the number of surgical beds, it was found that hospitals with five to nine beds have a death rate 0.8 times lower than hospitals with fewer than five beds, while there is no statistically significant differences in those with eighteen or more beds and ten to fifteen beds. Lastly, hospitals with the fewest emergency beds, which are less than 15, have the lowest death rate, while those with 23–35, more than 38, and 15–22 beds have the death rates that are 1.54, 1.52, and 1.25 times higher, respectively.

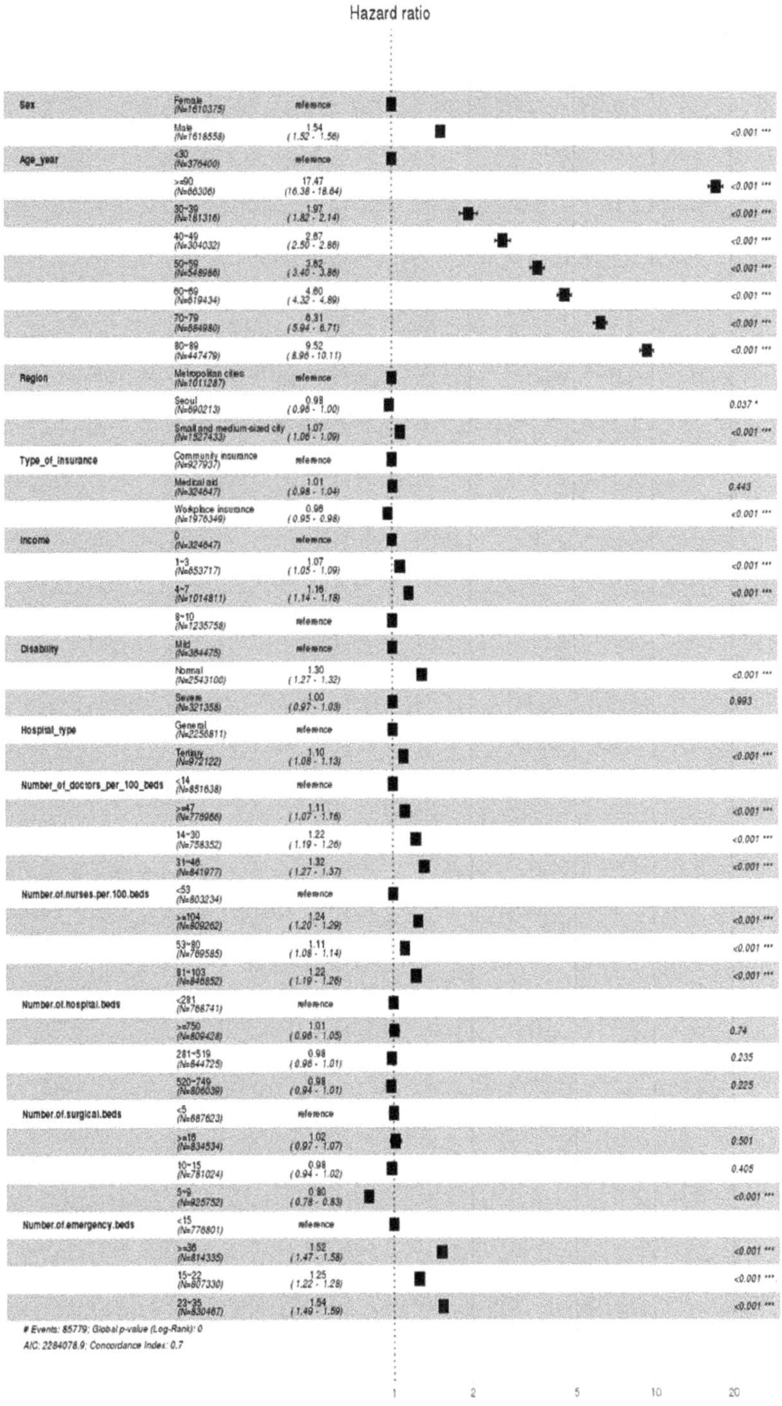

Figure 7. Cox proportional hazards model indicating the hazard ratio of the general inpatients. (* $p < 0.05$, *** $p < 0.001$).

4.2. Determinants of Survival Time among Inpatients Admitted through Emergency Room

4.2.1. Characteristics of Inpatients Admitted through the Emergency Room

Table 7 presents the characteristics of inpatients admitted through emergency room. The gender distribution of the study subjects is 51.26% male and 48.74% female. The age distribution is as follows: 12.88% under 29, 5.72% between 30 and 39, 8.42% between 40 and 49, 14.47% between 50 and 59, 16.76% between 60 and 69, 21.33% between 70 and 79, 17.46% between 80 and 89, and 2.94% above 90. For region, the result shows 23.15% in Seoul, 25.54% in metropolitan cities, and 51.31% in other small and medium-sized cities. For insurance status, 9.88% are medical insurees, 28.78% are those with regional insurance, and 61.34% are those with workplace insurance. For income quantiles, 9.88%, 20.17%, 30.61% and 39.35% are 0, 1–3, 4–7, and 8–10 quantiles, respectively. For the severity of disability, individuals with normal, mild, and severe symptoms are 77.65%, 11.46%, and 10.96%, respectively. There are 61.39% general hospitals and 38.61% top general hospitals. For other features, such as the number of doctors per 100 hospital beds, they were recategorized into four groups during data preprocessing. For the number of doctors per 100 hospital beds, 12.13%, 22.05%, 35.72%, and 30.10% are institutions with below 13, 14–30, 31–46, and above 47 doctors per 100 hospital beds, respectively. For the number of nurses per 100 hospital beds, 12.54%, 20.40%, 35.04%, and 32.02% are institutions with 52, 53–80, 81–103, and above 104 nurses per 100 hospital beds, respectively. For the number of hospital beds, 12.43%, 20.65%, 35.27%, and 31.64% are institutions with below 280, 281–519, 520~749, and above 750 hospital beds, respectively. For the number of surgical beds, 11.71%, 21.86%, 33.41%, and 33.02% are institutions with below 4, 5–9, 10–15, and above 16 surgical beds, respectively. Lastly, for the number of emergency beds, 10.34%, 21.85%, 33.24%, and 34.57% are institutions with below 15, 15–22, 23–35, and above 36 surgical beds, respectively.

Table 7. Characteristics of inpatients admitted through the Emergency Room.

Category	Feature		Number of Patients	Number of Dead	Censored Data	
					N	%
Sociodemographic Characteristics	Gender	Male	571,640	371,216	200,424	35.06
		Female	543,474	388,387	155,087	28.54
	Age	~29	143,679	139,950	3729	2.60
		30~39	63,773	59,087	4686	7.35
		40~49	93,932	81,225	12,707	13.53
		50~59	161,395	127,515	33,880	20.99
		60~69	186,934	129,766	57,168	30.58
		70~79	237,902	132,291	105,611	44.39
		80~89	194,696	81,129	113,567	58.33
		90~	32,803	8640	24,163	73.66
	City	Seoul	258,178	169,368	88,810	34.4
		Metropolitan city	284,779	195,224	89,555	31.45
		Small, medium-sized city	572,157	395,011	177,146	30.96
Patient Characteristics	Insurance status	Medical insuree	110,136	64,425	45,711	41.50
		Regional insurance	320,967	219,090	101,877	31.74
		Workplace insurance	684,011	476,088	207,923	30.4
	Income quantile	0 (=Medical aid)	110,136	64,425	45,711	41.50
		1~3	224,901	158,102	158,102	70.3
		4~7	341,334	247,235	247,235	72.43
		8~10	438,743	289,841	148,902	33.94
	Severity of Disability	Normal	865,904	622,833	242,261	27.98
		Mild	127,769	72,803	54,966	43.02
		Severe	122,251	63,967	58,284	47.68

Table 7. *Cont.*

Category	Feature		Number of Patients	Number of Dead	Censored Data	
					N	%
Institution Characteristics	Type of medical institution	General hospital	684,519	487,287	197,232	28.81
		Top general hospital	430,595	272,316	158,279	36.76
	Number of doctors per 100 hospital beds	~13	135,227	96,104	39,123	28.93
		14~30	245,888	177,896	67,992	27.65
		31~46	398,310	263,256	135,054	33.91
		47~	335,689	222,347	113,342	33.76
	Number of nurses per 100 hospital beds	~52	139,881	97,734	42,147	30.13
		53~80	227,528	163,339	64,189	28.21
		81~103	390,697	267,089	123,608	31.64
		104~	357,008	231,441	125,567	35.17
	Number of hospital beds	~280	138,642	102,709	35,933	25.92
		~281~519	230,297	163,236	67,061	29.12
		520~749	393,323	269,569	123,754	31.46
		750~	352,852	224,089	128,763	36.49
	Number of surgical beds	~4	130,599	94,109	36,940	28.29
		5~9	243,815	179,372	64,443	26.43
		10~15	372,513	248,428	124,085	33.31
		16~	368,187	237,694	130,493	35.44
	Number of emergency beds	~15	115,294	81,769	33,525	29.08
		15~22	243,659	177,732	65,927	27.06
		23~35	370,612	249,681	120,931	32.63
		36~	385,549	250,421	135,128	35.05
Total			1,115,114	759,603	355,511	

4.2.2. Kaplan–Meier Estimation (Inpatients Admitted through the Emergency Room)

To estimate the survival rate for patients admitted to the emergency room over time, Kaplan–Meier estimation was performed by sociodemographic characteristics, patient characteristics, and medical institution characteristics. First, the survival probability estimation results for socio-demographic characteristics, such as gender, age, and region, are shown in Figure 8. In the case of gender, it is estimated that men have a higher survival probability than women in the early days of hospital stay, but after 125 days of hospital stay, the survival rate of men is estimated to be better than that of women.

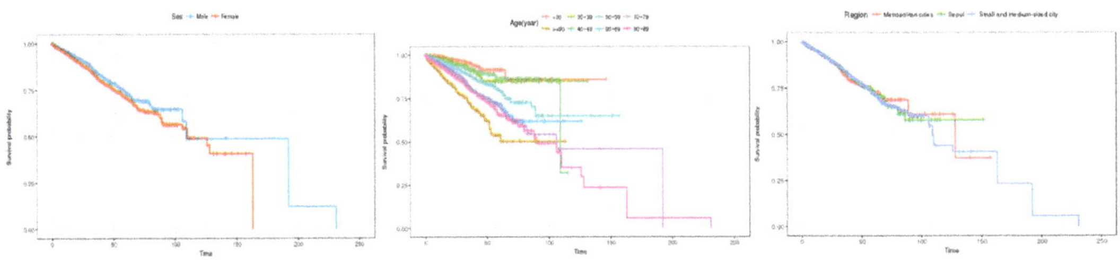

Figure 8. Kaplan–Meier survival curves by socio-demographic characteristics (inpatients admitted through the emergency room). The three charts represent (1) sex, (2) age, and (3) region (from left to right).

In terms of age, the overall survival rate shows a gradual decreasing trend from those in their 30s to those in their 90s, but after the 100th day of hospitalization, the survival rate for those in their 40s is estimated to be lower than that for those in their 90s or older. In the case of regions, there appears to be no difference in the survival rate in the early days of hospitalization, but after 125 days of hospitalization, the survival rate is estimated to be the best in metropolitan cities, followed by Seoul and small and medium-sized cities.

Second, patient characteristics, such as health insurance subscriber type, income bracket, and disability severity, are shown in Figure 9. In the case of health insurance subscriber types, there was no difference in survival rate at the beginning of the length of stay, but after about 50 days, the survival rate was highest for medical benefit recipients, and the survival probability tended to decrease in the order of employer subscribers and local subscribers. In the case of income brackets, it is estimated that there is no difference in survival rate in the early stages of hospital stay. In the 8th to 10th percentiles, the survival rate showed a sharp decline after 100 days of hospitalization. In the case of disability severity, it is estimated that the survival rate is high in the order of severe, mild, and normal patients at the beginning of the length of stay. However, at 125 days, contrary to general hospitalized patients, the survival rate was highest for mild patients, and the survival rate decreased in that order for severe patients and then normal patients. It is estimated that the survival rate of mildly ill patients will decline sharply after 150 days.

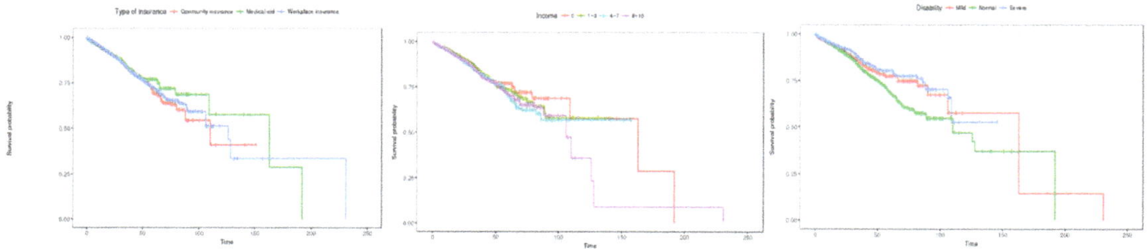

Figure 9. Kaplan–Meier survival curves by patient characteristics (inpatients admitted through the emergency room). The three charts represent (1) type of insurance, (2) incom, and (3) disability (from left to right).

Third, the Kaplan–Meier survival curve by characteristics of medical institutions is shown in Figure 10. Looking at the hospital type, it is estimated that the survival rate is higher in general hospitals than in tertiary general hospitals. In terms of the number of doctors per 100 beds, it was initially estimated that hospitals with less than 14 doctors (the group with the fewest doctors) had the highest survival rate, but the survival rate was found to decline sharply after about 60 days. In terms of the number of hospitalized beds, the survival rate was estimated to be high in the following order: less than 281 beds, 281 to 519, 520 to 749, and more than 750 beds until the length of stay was about 60 days. However, at about 110 days, the survival rate of hospitals with fewer than 281 beds was found to decline sharply.

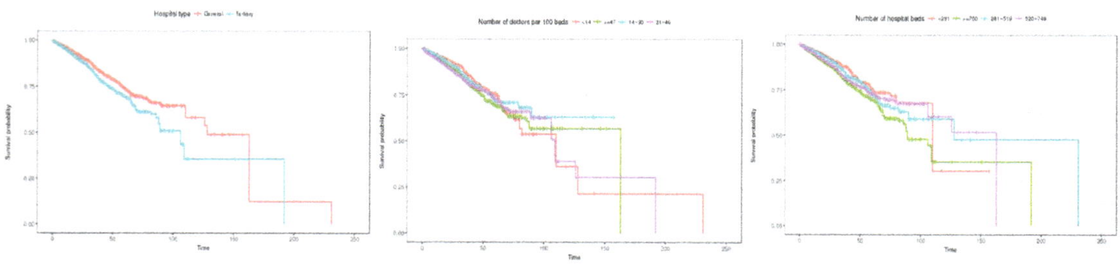

Figure 10. Kaplan–Meier survival curves by institution characteristic (inpatients admitted through the emergency room). The three charts represent (1) hospital type, (2) number of doctors per 100 beds, and (3) number of hospital beds (from left to right).

4.2.3. Cox Proportional Hazards Model (Inpatients Admitted through the Emergency Room)

The Cox proportional hazards model demonstrates the determinants affecting the dying risk of inpatients admitted through the emergency room, as shown in Figure 11.

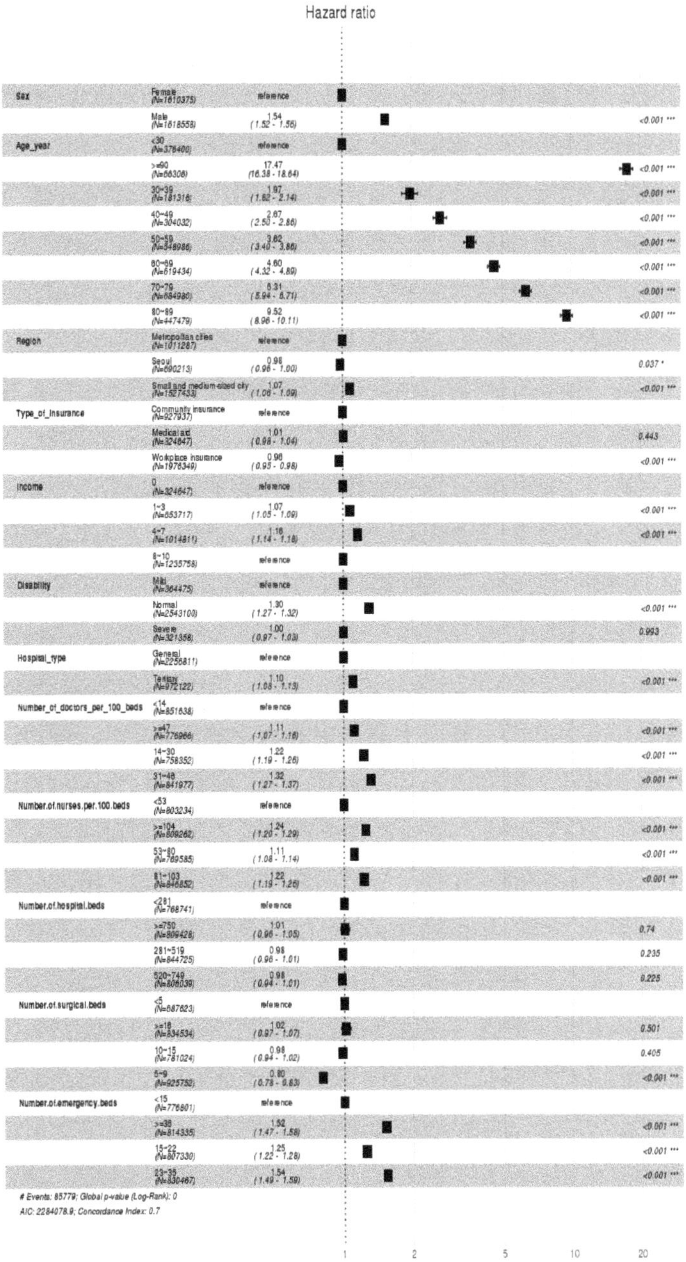

Figure 11. Cox proportional hazards model indicating the hazard ratio of the inpatients admitted through the emergency room. (* $p < 0.05$, *** $p < 0.001$).

First, in terms of sociodemographic characteristics, it was found that the death rate for men is 1.43 times higher than for women. The death rate increases from under 30s to the 90s, with those over 90 having a death rate 12.20 times higher than those under 30. For region, compared to the metropolitan cities, the death rate in the small or medium-sized cities decreases by 0.96 times, while it also decreases by 0.95 times in Seoul. Second, among patient characteristics, the results for the type of insurance showed that the death rate of medical insurees increases by 1.07 times than that of those with regional insurance, while it decreases for those with workplace insurance to 0.93 times, indicating a lesser impact on mortality. In terms of income quantiles, the impact on death rate for patients in the 4–7 quantiles increases by 1.16 times to those in the 0th quantile, while its impact is the same between the 0th quantile and the 8–10 quantiles. Similarly, for the severity of disability, the impact on the death rate is 1.22 times higher for normal patients than for patients with mild disabilities, while the death rate for patients with severe disabilities decreases by 0.94 times than that for patients with mild disabilities. Third, the death rate within the top general hospitals is 1.06 times higher than that within the general hospitals. For the number of doctors per 100 hospital beds, the death rates for 14–30 and 31–46 doctors are 1.21 and 1.19 times the death rate below 14 doctors, respectively. However, there is no statistically significant difference in death rates between the institutions with fewer than 14 doctors and ones with more than 47 doctors. For the number of nurses per 100 hospital beds, the death rates for 281–519 and for more than 750 nurses are 1.10 and 1.07 times the death rate below 53 nurses, respectively. However, there is no statistically significant difference in death rates between the institutions with fewer than 53 nurses and ones with 520–749 nurses.

For the number of hospital beds, institutions with the third highest number of beds (281–519) and those with 750 beds have increased death rates of 1.10 and 1.07 times higher, respectively, than those with the fewest beds (below 281). However, there is no significant difference in the death rates between institutions having lower than 281 beds and those with 520–749 beds. For the number of surgical beds, compared to institutions with the fewest number of surgical beds (below 5), those with the highest number of surgical beds (above 16) and those with 10–15 surgical beds have the death rate of 1.13 and 1.09 times higher, respectively. In contrast, those with 5–9 surgical beds demonstrated the decreased death rate that is 0.80 times than that of those with the fewest number of surgical beds. Lastly, in terms of the number of emergency beds, those with above 36, 23–35, and 15–22 emergency beds have increased death rates of 1.40, 1.34, and 1.16 times higher, respectively, than those with the fewest number of emergency beds (below 15).

4.3. Summarized Results and Implication

Table 8 illustrates the summarized results of this study. In fact, there is no significant difference in determinants of the death rate between the two groups of study. However, in terms of the 'city' feature among the sociodemographic characteristics, the small and medium-sized city exerts the most influence on the death rate of general inpatients, whereas the metropolitan city exerts the most influence on the death rate of inpatients admitted through the emergency room. In terms of institution characteristics, it was found that there is a difference in determinants affecting the death rate of the two groups of study, such as the number of doctors per 100 hospital beds, the number of nurses per 100 hospital beds, the number of hospital beds, the number of surgical beds, and the number of emergency beds.

The theoretical implications of this study are as follows. This study is the pioneering research in analyzing determinants affecting the death rate of general inpatients as well as that of inpatients admitted through the emergency room using survival analyses. Therefore, we first utilized the Kaplan–Meier survival estimation to take a closer look at the change in survival probability of inpatients depending on their sociodemographic, patient, and institutional characteristics. We also incorporated the Cox proportional hazards model to investigate not only the statistically significant features from sociodemographic, patient, and institutional characteristics that influence the death rate of inpatients but also the extent to which each feature affects mortality.

Table 8. Determinants of the death rate (general inpatients vs. inpatients admitted through the ER).

Category	Feature	General inpatient	Inpatients Admitted through ER
Sociodemographic Characteristics	Gender	Male > Female	Male > Female
	Age	Above 90s > 80s > 70s > 60s > 50s > 40s > 30s > below 30s	Above 90s > 80s > 70s > 60s > 50s > 40s > 30s > below 30s
	City	Small and medium-sized city > Seoul > Metropolitan city	Metropolitan city > Small and medium-sized city > Seoul
Patient Characteristics	Insurance status	(Medical insurees = Regional insurance) > Workplace insurance	Medical insurees > Regional insurance > Workplace insurance
	Income quantile	4–7 quantiles > 1–3 quantiles > (0 quantile = 8–10 quantiles)	4–7 quantiles > 1–3 quantiles > (0 quantiles = 8–10 quantiles)
	Severity of disability	Normal > (Severe = Mild)	Normal > Mild > Severe
Institution Characteristics	Type of institution	Top general hospital > General hospital	Top general hospital > General hospital
	Number of doctors per 100 hospital beds	31–48 > 14–30 > above 47 > below 14	14–30 > 31–48 > (above 47 = below 14)
	Number of nurses per 100 hospital beds	Above 104 > 81–103 > 53–80 > below 53	(Below 53 = Above 104) > 53–80 > 81–103
	Number of hospital beds	Below 281 = 281–519 = 520–749 = above 750	281–519 > above 750 > (below 281 = 520–749)
	Number of surgical beds	(Below 5 = 10–15 = above 16) > 5–9	Above 16 > 10–15 > below 5 > 5–9
	Number of emergency beds	23–35 > above 36 > 15–22 > below 15	Above 36 > 23–35 > 15–22 > below 15

The practical implications of this study are as follows. Although Korea has a multiple regional emergency medical centers across the country (Seoul: 27, Incheon: 10, Busan: 8, Daegu: 5, Daejeon: 4, Ulsan: 1, Gwangju: 5, Gyeonggi: 22, Gyeongbuk: 6, Gyeongnam: 6, Chungbuk: 4, Chungnam: 8, Jeonbuk: 8, Jeonnam: 2, Gangwon: 4, Jeju: 4), the survival probability of emergency room patients within the metropolitan cities is found to be the lowest. This is most likely due to the inadequate initial treatment and procedures for critically ill emergency patients at the regional emergency medical centers.

Furthermore, the emergency medical expense system is structured in a way that the more patients visit the emergency room, the more revenue is generated, regardless of the investment towards the emergency room or its quality of care. Therefore, to solve such issues, it is of importance to expand regional emergency centers that specialize in the professional treatment and care of critically ill emergency patients, and to reinforce the expense system that can induce the enhancement in the quality of emergency care. Lastly, it is necessary to secure an intermediary organization that can handle medical accidents that may occur during emergency treatments.

5. Conclusions

5.1. Research Implications

Considering an increase in the death of patients within the emergency room department, it is of necessity to identify the determinants of survival time among inpatients admitted through the emergency room. Therefore, our goal was to conduct a comparative study between general inpatients and those admitted through the emergency room, using survival analyses to identify the determinants of survival time.

In fact, the results reveal that there is not much difference in the death rate between the two groups of interest. However, for the regional variable among sociodemographic features, it was found that the small and medium-sized cities exert the most influence on the death rate among general inpatients, while the metropolitan cities exert the most influence on the death rate among those admitted through the emergency room. Among institutional features, the number of doctors per 100 hospital beds, the number of nurses per 100 hospital beds, the number of hospital beds, the number of surgical beds, and the number of emergency beds were found to affect the death rate of the two groups of study subjects differently.

Many previous studies utilized multiple or logistic regression analyses as their main research methodology. However, multiple regression analysis requires basic assumptions to be met, including linearity, independence, equal variance, normality, and the absence of multicollinearity. Logistic regression analysis, on the other hand, requires assumptions, such as the linearity of the logit, the independence of the error term, and the absence of multicollinearity. Although medical data often exhibit censored characteristics, these two methods fail to accommodate them, both presenting a significant limitation.

Therefore, this study conducted survival analyses to analyze the factors affecting the dying risk of general inpatients and those admitted through the emergency room. For this purpose, we measured the probability of survival as well as that of hospitalization depending on the sociodemographic, patient, health checkup, and institutional features using the Kaplan–Meier estimation. However, the Kaplan–Meier survival estimation has a limitation in that it cannot control for factors outside of those under analysis. Therefore, we also incorporated the Cox proportional hazards models as an additional econometric method to validate the results by controlling for other factors. Since both the Kaplan–Meier survival analysis and the Cox proportional hazards model do not require assumptions regarding the data distribution, these two methods are suitable for analyzing the determinants of survival time using the medical data.

In this study, we conducted survival analyses to compare and analyze the two subject groups: general inpatients and inpatients admitted through the emergency room. It is expected that a plan for the efficient allocation of limited medical resources can be established based on our research findings.

5.2. Limitations and Future Directions

The limitations of this study are as follows. Although there are various features affecting the dying risk of patients, such as sociodemographic and disease-specific features, this study is limited in that we only incorporated the sociodemographic, patient, and institutional features under analyses. Therefore, future studies are to encompass a broader scale of features from various aspects.

This study separately analyzes the two patient populations (general inpatients and inpatients admitted through the ER). An analysis that incorporates both patient populations using the Cox model would enable an assessment of whether the hazard or risk (death rate) differs between the patient populations after adjusting for all the factors considered in this paper.

Moreover, we conducted survival analyses on individuals who were either general inpatients or inpatients who were admitted through the emergency room. However, it is likely that survival time varies depending on a patient's main diagnosis. Therefore, it is highly recommended that future research should rigorously scrutinize and compare the survival times of patients across different diagnoses.

Lastly, this study conducted survival analyses based on the four-year cohort DB provided by the Korean NHIS from the years 2016 to 2019 encompassing tables of qualification, birth and death, diagnosis, health checkup, institution, and senior long-term care characteristics. However, the Korean NHIS further provides key information regarding, for instance, medical treatment (code for drugs, treatment code, main diagnosis code, days of hospitalization, etc.) and prescription details (drug ingredient code, dosage per administration, daily dosage, total days of administration, unit price, total cost, etc.). Therefore, future research should utilize the aforementioned information into their analyses.

Author Contributions: Conceptualization, H.C., and J.K.; methodology, I.C.; formal analysis, S.R.; data curation, A.E.K.; visualization, S.R.; writing—original draft, H.C.; writing—review and editing, J.K. All authors have read and agreed to the published version of the manuscript.

Funding: This research was supported by the BK21 FOUR (Fostering Outstanding Universities for Research) funded by the Ministry of Education (MOE, Korea) and National Research Foundation of Korea (NRF).

Institutional Review Board Statement: The study was conducted in accordance with the Helsinki Declaration and approved by the institutional review board, Kyung Hee University, Seoul, Korea (Protocol No. KHSIRB-22-344), for research involving human subjects.

Informed Consent Statement: Informed consent was obtained from all subjects involved in this study.

Data Availability Statement: Data sharing is not applicable to this article.

Conflicts of Interest: The authors declare no conflicts of interest.

References

1. Yoon, K.J. Infectious diseases and public healthcare through the response to COVID-19. *Health Welf. Issue Focus* **2020**, *377*, 1–11.
2. Oh, Y.H. Problems and policy directions of the emergency medical system in Korea. *Health Welf. Issue Focus* **2011**, *105*, 1–8.
3. Jeon, B.; Kim, K.; Jin, Y. Ontology Design to Improve User Fitness of Emergency Medical Statistics Quality(EMSQ). *J. Korea Acad.-Ind. Coop. Soc.* **2024**, *25*, 208–215.
4. Hwang, H.E.; Kahng, H.; Lee, E.S.; Kim, J.Y.; Yoon, Y.H.; Kim, S.B. Early Prediction of Patient Disposition for Emergency Department Visits Using Machine Learning. *J. Korean Inst. Ind. Eng.* **2021**, *47*, 263–271.
5. Jung, G.H.; Kweon, J. A study on space use analysis at emergency room in local emergency medical center. *J. Digit. Des.* **2017**, *17*, 81–92.
6. Kim, T.Y.; Kang, G.H.; Jang, Y.S.; Kim, W.; Choi, H.Y.; Kim, J.G.; Lee, Y.; Song, H.W. Effect of admission decision by emergency physicians on length of stay of emergency room and prognosis for patients diagnosed with medical diseases. *J. Korean Soc. Emerg. Med.* **2021**, *32*, 189–197.
7. Lee, E.B.; Paek, S.H.; Kwon, J.H.; Park, S.-H.; Kim, M.-J.; Byun, Y.-H. Characteristics of children hospitalized through the pediatric emergency department and effects of pediatric emergency ward hospitalization. *Pediatr. Emerg. Med. J.* **2023**, *10*, 124–131. [CrossRef]
8. Lee, S.D. Preventable Trauma Death Rate Improves over 3 Years: 19.9% → 15.7%. *Medical News*. 2022. Available online: http://www.bosa.co.kr/news/articleView.html?idxno=2169044 (accessed on 21 March 2023).
9. Kim, Y.; Jung, K.Y.; Cho, K.H.; Kim, H.; Ahn, H.C.; Oh, S.H.; Lee, J.B.; Yu, S.J.; Lee, D.I.; Im, T.H.; et al. Preventable trauma deaths rates and management errors in emergency medical system in Korea. *J. Korean Soc. Emerg. Med.* **2006**, *17*, 385–394.
10. Lee, E.J.; Song, Y.S.; Oh, S.H. Survival analysis approach for student departure of freshmen: Focusing on the case of S university. *J. Korean Assoc. Learn.-Centered Curric. Instr.* **2020**, *20*, 235–258. [CrossRef]
11. Shin, W.M.; Kim, J.M.; Park, C.Y.; Shin, E.; Tchoe, B. Analysis of factors influencing the survival of patients with Out-of-Hospital of Cardiac Arrest (OHCA). *Korean Public Health Res.* **2020**, *46*, 93–105.
12. Yoo, I.S. What to do to improve emergency care. *Health Welf. Forum* **2010**, *169*, 45–57.
13. Kim, J.H.; Han, M.S.; Kim, C.-K.; Sun, S.; Kim, G.J.; Bae, S.H.; Kim, Y.K. A Study on the legal definition and the demands of the times of a medical technician according to changes in the medical market. *J. Digit. Converg.* **2021**, *19*, 397–406.
14. Lee, J.R.; Do, N.Y. Effect of brand on survival and closing of stores. *J. Korea Real Estate Anal. Assoc.* **2019**, *25*, 49–62.
15. Jing, B.; Zhang, T.; Wang, Z.; Jin, Y.; Liu, K.; Qiu, W.; Ke, L.; Sun, Y.; He, C.; Hou, D.; et al. A deep survival analysis method based on ranking. *Artif. Intell. Med.* **2019**, *98*, 1–9. [CrossRef] [PubMed]
16. Schober, P.; Vetter, T.R. Survival analysis and interpretation of time-to-event data: The tortoise and the hare. *Anesth. Analg.* **2018**, *127*, 792. [CrossRef] [PubMed]
17. In, J.; Lee, D.K. Survival analysis: Part I-analysis of time-to-event. *Korean J. Anesthesiol.* **2018**, *71*, 182–191. [CrossRef] [PubMed]
18. Ha, S.H.; Yang, J.W.; Min, J.H. Credit prediction based on Kohonen network and survival analysis. *J. Korean Oper. Res. Manag. Sci. Soc.* **2009**, *34*, 35–54.
19. Gémar, G.; Moniche, L.; Morales, A.J. Survival analysis of the Spanish hotel industry. *Tour. Manag.* **2016**, *54*, 428–438. [CrossRef]
20. Gemar, G.; Soler, I.P.; Guzman-Parra, V.F. Predicting bankruptcy in resort hotels: A survival analysis. *Int. J. Contemp. Hosp. Manag.* **2019**, *31*, 1546–1566. [CrossRef]
21. Kristanti, F.T.; Effendi, N. A survival analysis of indonesian distressed company using cox hazard model. *Int. J. Econ. Manag.* **2017**, *11*, 155–167.
22. Kristanti, F.T.; Herwany, A. Corporate governance, financial ratios, political risk and financial distress: A survival analysis. *Account. Financ. Rev.* **2017**, *2*, 26–34. [CrossRef] [PubMed]
23. Nagy, Á.; Munkácsy, G.; Győrffy, B. Pancancer survival analysis of cancer hallmark genes. *Sci. Rep.* **2021**, *11*, 6047. [CrossRef] [PubMed]

24. Viljanen, M.; Airola, A.; Heikkonen, J.; Pahikkala, T. Playtime measurement with survival analysis. *IEEE Trans. Games* **2017**, *10*, 128–138. [CrossRef]
25. Lee, J.B.; Woo, H. Determinants of length of stay in ischemic heart disease patients. *J. Health Inform. Stat.* **2020**, *45*, 52–59. [CrossRef]

healthcare

MDPI

Article

A Data-Driven Approach to Defining Risk-Adjusted Coding Specificity Metrics for a Large U.S. Dementia Patient Cohort

Kaylla Richardson [1,2], Sankari Penumaka [2], Jaleesa Smoot [1,2], Mansi Reddy Panaganti [2], Indu Radha Chinta [2], Devi Priya Guduri [2], Sucharitha Reddy Tiyyagura [2], John Martin [3], Michael Korvink [3] and Laura H. Gunn [1,2,4,*]

1 Department of Public Health Sciences, University of North Carolina at Charlotte (UNC Charlotte), Charlotte, NC 28223, USA; kricha92@charlotte.edu (K.R.); jsmoot3@charlotte.edu (J.S.)
2 School of Data Science, University of North Carolina at Charlotte (UNC Charlotte), Charlotte, NC 28223, USA; ppenumak@charlotte.edu (S.P.); mpanagan@charlotte.edu (M.R.P.); ichinta@charlotte.edu (I.R.C.); dguduri@charlotte.edu (D.P.G.); stiyyagu@charlotte.edu (S.R.T.)
3 ITS Data Science, Premier, Inc., Charlotte, NC 28277, USA; john_martin@premierinc.com (J.M.); michael_korvink@premierinc.com (M.K.)
4 School of Public Health, Faculty of Medicine, Imperial College London, London W6 8RP, UK
* Correspondence: laura.gunn@charlotte.edu

Abstract: Medical coding impacts patient care quality, payor reimbursement, and system reliability through the precision of patient information documentation. Inadequate coding specificity can have significant consequences at administrative and patient levels. Models to identify and/or enhance coding specificity practices are needed. Clinical records are not always available, complete, or homogeneous, and clinically driven metrics to assess medical practices are not logistically feasible at the population level, particularly in non-centralized healthcare delivery systems and/or for those who only have access to claims data. Data-driven approaches that incorporate all available information are needed to explore coding specificity practices. Using N = 487,775 hospitalization records of individuals diagnosed with dementia and discharged in 2022 from a large all-payor administrative claims dataset, we fitted logistic regression models using patient and facility characteristics to explain the coding specificity of principal and secondary diagnoses of dementia. A two-step approach was produced to allow for the flexible clustering of patient-level outcomes. Model outcomes were then used within a Poisson binomial model to identify facilities that over- or under-specify dementia diagnoses against healthcare industry standards across hospitalizations. The results indicate that multiple factors are significantly associated with dementia coding specificity, especially for principal diagnoses of dementia (AUC = 0.727). The practical use of this novel risk-adjusted metric is demonstrated for a sample of facilities and geospatially via a U.S. map. This study's findings provide healthcare facilities with a benchmark for assessing coding specificity practices and developing quality enhancements to align with healthcare industry standards, ultimately contributing to better patient care and healthcare system reliability.

Keywords: coding specificity; ICD-10; dementia

1. Introduction

The precise recording, evaluation, and documentation of patient information through medical coding play a large role in the quality of care delivered, reimbursement from payors, and the reliability of healthcare systems [1]. The process of clinical coding has multiple facets, such as accuracy, completeness, and appropriate levels for the specificity of diagnostic coding. Coding specificity, an important aspect of the coding process, refers to the level of granularity at which a clinical diagnosis is recorded [2].

A widely used medical coding system is the International Classification of Diseases Clinical Modification (or ICD-CM) [3]. ICD-10-CM (herein ICD-10) refers to the 10th revision of the taxonomy and serves to categorize diseases and health conditions at varying degrees of specificity, from coarse or unspecified more general diagnoses to more granular ones representing a deeper level of knowledge of the clinical condition. Medical coding helps standardize documentation across healthcare systems, serves as a tool for medical billing, standardizes risk factors in risk-adjusted quality measures, and helps guide healthcare policy by accurately identifying disease prevalence and supporting national and international decision making [3]. The coding system also helps organize and find medical information easily, impacting how we understand and use medical data, including assessing in real time the spread or prevalence of diseases and the optimization of resource allocations [3–6].

When considering coding practice enhancements, it is important to assess how healthcare professionals in hospitals document the presence of a specific condition or disease. Transcription—potentially including voice transcription for electronic health records (EHRs)—errors, missing information in patient charts, and illegible handwriting all contribute to inadequate specificity in coding [7]. It constitutes a shared responsibility among all parties involved to appropriately code to the highest level of specificity [8]. The move from ICD-9 to ICD-10 on 1 October 2015 led to a fivefold increase in the number of codes, exacerbating the complexity of coders' work and the potential for coding errors following this transition [3]. Clinical specialties have been affected differently, with this ICD-10 transition representing an uneven burden across facilities and patients depending on the diagnosis family and the facility's level of specialization [9,10].

A lower coding specificity is a potential burden for Medicare and other payors, which are billed for potentially under-specified diagnoses when a higher specificity (i.e., enhanced diagnosis quality) could be available [3,8]. Medicare is the health insurance coverage provided by the United States (U.S.) government for individuals 65 years and older. Medicare within the acute care inpatient setting refers to payments reimbursed through the Inpatient Prospective Payment System (IPPS). Through the IPPS, hospitalizations are grouped into medical severity diagnosis-related groups (MS-DRGs) based largely on the presence of principal and secondary ICD-10-CM diagnosis codes, and in some cases, ICD-10-PCS procedure codes. The MS-DRG grouping is associated with a weight that further adjusts the base hospital payment (determined by a set of hospital-level characteristics) to determine the final discharge-level reimbursement. There is a tradeoff between productivity and coding quality, as enhancing the coding specificity can be time intensive in some instances, requiring the coder to explore whether more specific coding is appropriate given the information provided in the patient medical record. At the facility level, the associated costs to the healthcare payor as well as the impact on patients' clinical history, treatment, and resulting health outcomes must also be considered [8]. Coding specificity is especially relevant when a diagnosis is unrelated to the principal cause of hospitalization, or when diagnoses are not made by specialists, as added specification for these codes may not affect the hospital's rate of reimbursement for the hospitalization. Thus, coding specificity is not only important at the administrative level but also has the potential to impact both healthcare facilities and patients.

At the facility level, coding that accurately captures clinical diagnoses ensures that healthcare facilities maintain effective billing operations. Coding specificity has the potential to impact a facility's financial capital and allocation of resources, since facilities, after a short grace period that ended in October 2016, can be denied Medicare-based claims based on insufficient diagnostic specificity [8,11]. ICD-10 codes are the foundation of hospital billing processes, so misdiagnoses or misclassifications of codes can impact hospital reimbursement and insurance eligibility, including Medicare reimbursements [12]. Inaccurate coding further has the potential to affect facilities' reputations and pay-for-performance incentive payments, as such hospital-ranking programs evaluate quality performance using risk-adjusted outcomes that rely on ICD-10 coding [13–18].

From the patient perspective, accurate documentation ensures that the patient is receiving an adequate treatment plan tailored to the specifics of their diagnosis and needs, both during their inpatient stay and after discharge [8]. In addition to individuals who may go undiagnosed, those with an under-specified diagnosis may also suffer worsened clinical outcomes. Among other factors, practitioners' unconscious biases as well as inappropriate facility practices could result in deviations from universal documentation and coding standards, thus potentially exacerbating health disparities [19], which may manifest through specificity gaps across subpopulations. A lack of specificity can lead to patients' clinical histories being affected, thus resulting in potential variations in care and resulting outcomes across social strata [8]. From the standpoint of coding specificity, the literature lacks a wider understanding of how decreased (or increased) levels of specificity may be associated with sociodemographic factors, thus potentially exacerbating the aforementioned healthcare disparities [19].

Not all unspecified diagnoses are inappropriate. In fact, unspecified diagnosis codes are recommended by the United States (U.S.) Centers for Medicare and Medicaid Services (CMS): "*When sufficient clinical information is not known or available about a particular health condition to assign a more specific code, it is acceptable to report the appropriate unspecified code*" [20]. Hence, there is a balance between the necessary level of unspecificity and the unnecessary level of unspecificity that needs to be considered, since a pure minimization of unspecified codes could also lead to incorrectly specified diagnoses. Conversely, achieving a higher level of specificity may require additional clinical tests or interventions, which may be subject to additional considerations regarding cost-effectiveness [21–23], especially when the primary cause of the inpatient stay is not related to nor affected by the unspecified diagnosis. Also, higher levels of specificity may not be warranted by clinical diagnoses. Incorrect levels of both specificity and unspecificity can lead to inappropriate treatment. Thus, when a diagnosis is not confirmed, it is appropriate to provide an initial, temporary unspecified diagnosis [20] until further tests can be performed, if clinically recommended.

While our approach is generalizable and can be applied across clinical strata, our motivating example consists of a large patient cohort across the U.S. of nearly 500,000 unique inpatient individuals who were diagnosed with dementia and discharged in 2022. In 2020, dementia affected the lives of over 55 million people across the world, which is close to 1% of the global population [24]. Projections suggest that this number will experience nearly twofold growth every 20 years, surging to 78 million by 2030 and about 139 million by 2050 [24]. This number is further increased by those providing caregiving and other family members indirectly suffering from this debilitating disease. In the absence of enhanced treatments or preventive measures, adverse outcomes associated with dementia will persistently rise [25]. Many patients are likely to receive unspecified dementia diagnoses when seeing a primary care provider compared to when seeing a specialized provider (like a neurologist or geriatrician) [26,27]. Thus, dementia represents an important disease within an aging population that is likely to be of increased relevance as treatment interventions are developed, and enhanced coding specificity is needed in this area to identify resources properly [25]. In a 2017 study, researchers reviewed the medical records of dementia ICD-10 code cases, and they discovered that many of the cases lacked specific descriptions that would aid in confirming the diagnosis of specific types of dementia [28]. This study revealed that 63% of cases did not provide a specific diagnosis of dementia in the medical records, but instead considered other conditions as the likely explanation of the patient's hospitalization [28]. More generally, mental health conditions have been identified among conditions suffering from higher rates of unspecified diagnoses [8].

Models have been developed for assessing risk-adjusted coding intensity for both diagnoses and procedures, as well as identifying facilities that over- or under-code [29,30]. This area tangentially relates to coding specificity. However, the literature still lacks risk-adjusted approaches that account for factors potentially associated with coding specificity, adjusting for patient and facility characteristics, with only some initial work developed in the area of depression [31], but none, to our knowledge, in the area of dementia or other neurocognitive diseases. The aim of this study is to provide a novel risk-adjusted metric, demonstrated through a population-based dementia patient cohort in the U.S., to estimate dementia ICD-10 coding specificity by facility upon adjusting for a set of commonly available facility- and patient-level characteristics.

While enhancements in coding specificity practices are possible through other means, such as through the clinical identification of potential coding specificity inaccuracies or increased training, such approaches are not cost-effective if they need to be performed at the population level. There is a need for cost-effective approaches that serve to pre-screen and identify facilities which may need such enhancements the most. Clinical assessments may be possible if electronic health records are available, but this is not always the case. In this case, data-driven approaches may provide insights into how coding specificity can vary across patients and facilities and whether these variations occur in ways that may depart from anticipated randomness. Our proposed data-driven metric can serve facilities to self-assess variation in coding specificity compared with their healthcare peers and can provide a benchmark to identify facilities that could benefit from a further analysis of diagnostic coding specificity practices.

2. Materials and Methods

2.1. Data and Variables

De-identified data sourced and provided by Premier, Inc.'s private database serve as the foundation of this analysis [32]. The dataset is composed of N = 487,775 observations containing information on the first inpatient hospitalization for each patient with a principal or secondary diagnosis related to dementia who was discharged in the year 2022 using the F ICD-10 diagnosis codes provided in Supplementary Tables S1 and S2. The ICD-10 codes corresponding to these diagnoses were identified by an expert team of medical coders at Premier, Inc. Patients who were admitted prior to 2022 were also included if they were discharged in 2022.

The data were further categorized into three types of variables: (1) outcome variables; (2) patient characteristics; and (3) facility characteristics. Outcome variables include coding specificity of principal diagnosis of dementia codes and coding specificity of secondary diagnosis of dementia codes. Principal diagnosis specificity denotes whether the ICD-10 dementia-related principal diagnosis code was specified (versus unspecified), and for secondary diagnoses, a specified diagnosis is assumed when at least one secondary diagnosis related to dementia was specified. In addition to masked patient IDs, patient characteristics for this study include the following: age group; sex; race; length of stay; primary payor; point of origin; discharge status; number of procedure codes; ICD-10 coding period (2022 for coding prior to 1 October 2022 and 2023 for codes from 1 October 2022); five Centers for Disease Control and Prevention's Agency for Toxic Substances and Disease Registry's (ATSDR) social vulnerability indices [33]; a COVID-19 indicator; and Medicare Severity Diagnosis Related Group (MS-DRG) type for the inpatient stay. In addition to masked facility IDs, facility characteristics include the following: three facility status variables (teaching, academic, and urban); ownership; size (bed count, grouped); case mix index (CMI); and U.S. state.

2.2. Statistical Analysis

Descriptive statistics were calculated and tabulated. Variables for which certain subgroups had limited representation (e.g., charity and indigent payors) were grouped together. Patients under 45 years old were grouped together due to their low counts. Discharge status codes indicating that the patient expired were collapsed into a single category. A diverse set of categories representing patients' points of origin with low counts were grouped into a single 'other' category.

Univariate and multivariate logistic regression analyses were utilized to identify associations between patient- and facility-level characteristics and each of the two outcomes (specificity of dementia principal and secondary diagnoses per patient hospitalization). Univariate and adjusted odds ratios (ORs), as well as corresponding 95% confidence intervals (CIs) and p-values, were computed and tabulated. Receiver operating characteristic

(ROC) curves were calculated and depicted, and area under the curve (AUC) values were extracted to demonstrate the multivariate models' fitted performances to explain principal and secondary dementia diagnoses.

Clustering of this metric is demonstrated at the facility level, though other clustering factors are possible. Importantly, as opposed to variables used for constructing the patient-specific metric, clustering variables do not need to be observable for the full sample. A facility-specific metric of diagnostic coding specificity was also calculated from the risk-adjusted probabilities of specificity. Let $Y_{i,j}$ be the binary variable denoting coding specificity of the principal or secondary diagnosis for hospitalization i at facility j. This variable follows a Bernoulli (Ber) distribution with estimated probability $\hat{p}_{i,j}$ as shown below:

$$Y_{i,j} \sim Ber\left(\hat{p}_{i,j}\right). \quad (1)$$

The set $\hat{p}_{i,j}$ was estimated from the multivariate logistic regression model which was adjusted for patient and facility characteristics. Assuming that each hospitalization's coding specificity was independently, though not identically, distributed per facility, the total count of facility-specific coding specificity follows a Poisson binomial (PoiBin) distribution with probability vector $\hat{p}_j = \left(\hat{p}_{1,j},\hat{p}_{2,j},\ldots,\hat{p}_{n_j,j}\right)$ for n_j hospitalizations in facility j as shown as follows:

$$\sum_{i=1}^{n_j} Y_{i,j} \sim PoiBin\left(\hat{p}_j\right) \quad (2)$$

Facility-specific 95% CIs were extracted through the Poisson binomial facility-specific cumulative distribution functions (CDFs). These were used to identify facilities which under- ($p < 0.025$) and over- ($p > 0.975$) specified in their coding versus facilities' peers using the estimated CDF for the specificity count.

Error bars were constructed to demonstrate the facility-specific metric for a sample of 20 facilities for both dementia principal and secondary diagnoses. Among these facilities, the coding specificity of dementia diagnosis indicator variable was defined, and an observed count (dots) was plotted for each facility (X-axis). A 95% CI for each facility, built on the basis of the Poisson binomial model, was added to identify these facilities' adjusted levels of coding specificity against peers. Over- and under-coding risk-adjusted specificity practices were then identified by the facility.

Finally, geospatial U.S. maps were created to display adjusted ORs of principal and secondary diagnosis coding specificity by state against the reference of New York, which is the state with the highest per capita healthcare expenditure in the U.S. [34].

3. Results

Table 1 provides a summary of the descriptive statistics for N = 487,775 hospitalization records and patients, since each patient is only observed once due to the cohort definition (the first hospitalization for each patient within the year). The dataset comprised observations from 866 facilities, with an average of 563.25 patients per facility. The distribution of age among this dementia patient cohort is naturally skewed, with 61% of individuals being 80 years and older. Females constituted 58% of the patients, and the majority of the patients identified as White (76%). The median length of stay, which was log-transformed due to its large right skewness, was 5 days, and the most common primary payor was Medicare traditional (53%). The point of origin was predominantly non-healthcare facilities (79%), and the discharge status varied, with 19% of the patients being discharged to home or self-care, while the majority were transferred to other healthcare facilities, often skilled nursing facilities (36%). The average number of procedures during inpatient stays was 2.7, with surgical MS-DRGs representing 15% of hospitalizations. Additionally, 13% were COVID-19-positive patients. Most of the facilities were non-teaching (78%) and non-academic (85%). Urban facilities were more prevalent (86%) than rural ones. Voluntary non-profit private was the most common ownership status (64%). The bed capacity varied, with 1–50 beds (3%) and >400 beds (39%) being the least and most common facility sizes, respectively. The mean case mix index was 1.7. The dataset represented multiple states, with New York (9%) and Florida (12%) being the top states in the number of hospitalizations.

Table 1. Descriptive statistics of the dementia-related principal and secondary diagnosis coding specificity outcomes as well as patient and facility characteristics (counts and means/proportions and corresponding percentages/standard deviations).

Study Variables	Count or Mean/Proportion (% or Standard Deviation (SD))
Outcomes	
Specificity of dementia principal diagnosis (count, proportion)	1788 (17%)
Specificity of dementia secondary diagnoses (count, proportion)	186,300 (39%)
Patient Characteristics	
Age (Years)	
0–44	809 (<1%)
45–54	2735 (1%)
55–59	5492 (1%)
60–64	13,512 (3%)
65–69	27,970 (6%)
70–74	53,037 (11%)
75–79	83,694 (17%)
80–84	103,805 (21%)
85+	196,721 (40%)
Sex	
Female	282,090 (58%)
Male	205,685 (42%)
Race	
Asian	12,539 (3%)
Black	68,784 (14%)
Other	26,675 (5%)
Unable to determine	10,463 (2%)
White	369,314 (76%)
Log(Length of Stay) (Days) (mean, SD)	1.6 (0.85)
Primary Payor	
Charity/Indigent	200 (<1%)
Commercial indemnity	4613 (1%)
Direct employer contract	217 (<1%)
Managed care capitated	417 (<1%)
Managed care non-capitated	9370 (2%)
Medicaid managed care capitated	1028 (<1%)
Medicaid managed care non-capitated	7807 (2%)
Medicaid traditional	5512 (1%)
Medicare managed care capitated	20,202 (4%)
Medicare managed care non-capitated	165,874 (34%)
Medicare traditional	258,584 (53%)
Other	2713 (1%)
Other government payors	9097 (2%)
Self-pay	1950 (<1%)
Workers' compensation	191 (<1%)

Table 1. *Cont.*

Study Variables	Count or Mean/Proportion (% or Standard Deviation (SD))
Patient Characteristics	
Point of Origin	
Clinic	16,400 (3%)
Court/Law enforcement	215 (<1%)
Information not available	3174 (1%)
Non-healthcare facility	385,271 (79%)
Other	425 (<1%)
Transfer from ambulatory surgery center	2767 (1%)
Transfer from dept unit in same hospital, separate claim	302 (<1%)
Transfer from health facility	7337 (2%)
Transfer from hospice and under hospice care	131 (<1%)
Transfer from hospital (different facility)	27,141 (6%)
Transfer from SNF [1] or ICF [2]	44,612 (9%)
Discharge Status	
Acute inpatient readmission	847 (<1%)
Discharged to home health organization	89,392 (18%)
Discharged to home or self-care	91,843 (19%)
Discharged to hospice home	25,625 (5%)
Discharged to hospice medical facility	24,993 (5%)
Discharged/Transferred to another rehab facility	15,425 (3%)
Discharged/Transferred to cancer center/children's hospital	209 (<1%)
Discharged/Transferred to court/law enforcement	247 (<1%)
Discharged/Transferred to critical access hospital	71 (<1%)
Discharged/Transferred to federal hospital	279 (<1%)
Discharged/Transferred to ICF [2]	12,891 (3%)
Discharged/Transferred to long-term care hospital	5448 (1%)
Discharged/Transferred to nursing facility	1732 (<1%)
Discharged/Transferred to other facility	5270 (1%)
Discharged/Transferred to other health institute not in list	1391 (<1%)
Discharged/Transferred to psychiatric hospital	2341 (<1%)
Discharged/Transferred to SNF [1]	177,780 (36%)
Discharged/Transferred to swing bed	1605 (<1%)
Expired	28,217 (6%)
Information not available	232 (<1%)
Left against medical advice	1901 (<1%)
Still a patient—expected to return	36 (<1%)
Count of Procedures (mean, SD)	(2.7) 2.2
CMS [3] Fiscal Year	
2022	359,803 (74%)
2023	127,972 (26%)
Social Vulnerability Indices (mean, SD)	
Household characteristics	0.52% (0.25)
Housing type and transportation	0.62% (0.24)
Overall	0.61% (0.25)
Racial and ethnic minority status	0.71% (0.23)
Socioeconomic status	0.56% (0.26)
COVID-19 Status	
Not identified	425,762 (87%)
Positive	62,013 (13%)
MS-DRG [4] Type	
Medical	412,512 (85%)
Surgical	75,263 (15%)

Table 1. *Cont.*

Study Variables	Count or Mean/Proportion (% or Standard Deviation (SD))
Facility Characteristics	
Teaching Status	
No	378,768 (78%)
Not available	6221 (1%)
Yes	102,786 (21%)
Academic Status	
No	415,274 (85%)
Yes	72,501 (15%)
Rural/Urban Status	
Rural	66,204 (14%)
Urban	421,571 (86%)
Ownership	
Government—federal	1118 (<1%)
Government—hospital district/authority	32,417 (7%)
Government—local	11,798 (2%)
Government—state	3611 (1%)
Not available	2248 (<1%)
Physician	1032 (<1%)
Proprietary	25,459 (5%)
Voluntary non-profit—church	71,085 (15%)
Voluntary non-profit—other	26,015 (5%)
Voluntary non-profit—private	312,992 (64%)
Bed Count	
1–50	12,300 (3%)
51–100	25,881 (5%)
101–150	38,616 (8%)
151–200	32,908 (7%)
201–250	47,519 (10%)
251–300	50,418 (10%)
301–350	53,077 (11%)
351–400	39,018 (8%)
>400	188,038 (39%)
Case Mix Index (mean, SD)	1.76 (0.26)
State Abbreviation	
AK	253 (<1%)
AL	3966 (1%)
AR	3789 (1%)
AZ	12,029 (2%)
CA	27,281 (6%)
CO	3578 (1%)
CT	5982 (1%)
DE	1125 (<1%)
FL	60,713 (12%)
GA	7318 (2%)
HI	6038 (1%)
IA	4759 (1%)
ID	28 (<1%)
IL	18,082 (4%)
IN	6646 (1%)
KS	2856 (1%)
KY	10,899 (2%)
LA	3505 (1%)
MA	4549 (1%)

Table 1. *Cont.*

Study Variables	Count or Mean/Proportion (% or Standard Deviation (SD))
Facility Characteristics	
State Abbreviation	
MD	7131 (1%)
ME	21 (<1%)
MI	22,526 (5%)
MN	3431 (1%)
MO	3382 (1%)
MS	6744 (1%)
MT	1374 (<1%)
NC	27,936 (6%)
ND	676 (<1%)
NE	1965 (<1%)
NH	57 (<1%)
NJ	9184 (2%)
NM	2360 (<1%)
NV	5537 (1%)
NY	45,302 (9%)
OH	22,769 (5%)
OK	7968 (2%)
OR	7750 (2%)
PA	24,500 (5%)
RI	15 (<1%)
SC	10,009 (2%)
SD	1194 (<1%)
TN	16,120 (3%)
TX	32,134 (7%)
UT	38 (<1%)
VA	16,695 (3%)
VT	163 (<1%)
WA	7833 (2%)
WI	9889 (2%)
WV	9472 (2%)
WY	204 (<1%)

[1] SNF: Skilled nursing facility; [2] ICF: Intermediate care facility; [3] CMS: U.S. Centers for Medicare and Medicaid Services; [4] MS-DRG: Medicare Severity Diagnosis Related Group.

Table 2 contains the adjusted ORs, 95% CIs, and p-values for the univariate and multivariate logistic regression analyses for modeling the coding specificity of dementia-related principal diagnoses. Younger patients were generally associated with higher odds of coding specificity than patients in the oldest age group (85+). Males experienced 45% higher odds of dementia-related principal diagnosis coding specificity than females (OR = 1.454; 95% CI: 1.301–1.625). Race was generally non-significant, except for Black patients, who experienced significantly higher odds of principal diagnosis coding specificity than White patients (OR = 1.237; 95% CI: 1.058–1.446). The log-length of stay was significant, with longer stays associated with higher odds of coding specificity (OR = 1.124; 95% CI: 1.060–1.191), but primary payor and point of origin were generally not significant. Patients with certain discharge statuses experienced significantly higher odds of coding specificity than those discharged to home or self-care, namely patients discharged to hospice homes, hospice medical facilities, or psychiatric hospitals (OR $\geq$ 1.354). The number of procedures was also significant, with each additional procedure performed associated with 23% increased odds of coding specificity (OR = 1.230; 95% CI: 1.179–1.283). The CMS fiscal year was highly significant, indicating 73.6% lower odds of specificity for 2023 (discharges occurring between 1 October and 31 December 2022) compared to 2022 (discharges between 1 January and 30 September 2022) (OR = 0.264; 95% CI: 0.224–0.311). Social vulnerability indices were not significant at the multivariate level, though some were significant univariately, indicating that some of the information content may be present in other patient characteristics. COVID-19 status and MS-DRG type were not statistically significant, except for at the univariate level, at which the latter showed surgical MS-DRGs associated with increased odds of specificity. At the facility level, patients in facilities whose teaching status was not available experienced 65.1% lower odds of specificity than those in non-teaching facilities (OR = 0.349; 95% CI: 0.142–0.856). Neither academic nor rural/urban status showed significant variability at the multivariate level. Most ownership categories were not significantly different from the voluntary non-profit private reference, except for other non-profit voluntary (OR = 0.605; 95% CI: 0.442–0.827) and local government (OR = 2.104; 95% CI: 1.401–3.159). Patients from facilities with bed counts lower than the reference category (>400) experienced lower odds of coding specificity, though only three categories were statistically significant. The case mix index was significant, with each unit increase accompanied by 57.9% increased odds of dementia-related principal diagnosis coding specificity (OR = 1.579; 95% CI: 1.188–2.100). Finally, most states demonstrated no statistically significant differences in principal diagnosis coding specificity compared to New York, with the exception of Hawaii, Louisiana, Minnesota, Oregon, Pennsylvania, and Virginia (which had a higher odds) as well as Illinois and Tennessee (which had lower odds of coding specificity).

Table 2. Univariate and multivariate logistic regression results including odds ratios (ORs), corresponding 95% confidence intervals (CIs), and *p*-values for specificity of a dementia-related principal diagnosis.

	Univariate Analysis			Multivariate Analysis		
Variable	OR	95% CI	*p*-Value	OR	95% CI	*p*-Value
Intercept	-	-	-	0.030	0.016–0.057	<0.001
Age (Ref: 85+)						
0–44	5.698	2.111–15.378	0.001	2.599	0.781–8.646	0.119
45–54	5.976	3.679–9.706	<0.001	4.845	2.731–8.596	<0.001
55–59	3.337	2.276–4.894	<0.001	2.427	1.577–3.735	<0.001
60–64	3.281	2.546–4.227	<0.001	2.601	1.930–3.507	<0.001
65–69	2.722	2.254–3.288	<0.001	2.266	1.843–2.786	<0.001
70–74	1.583	1.330–1.884	<0.001	1.483	1.232–1.785	<0.001
75–79	1.726	1.482–2.009	<0.001	1.663	1.414–1.955	<0.001
80–84	1.556	1.338–1.809	<0.001	1.484	1.266–1.740	<0.001
Sex (Ref: Female)						
Male	1.591	1.436–1.763	<0.001	1.454	1.301–1.625	<0.001
Race (Ref: White)						
Asian	1.485	1.084–2.035	0.014	1.308	0.907–1.888	0.151
Black	1.385	1.213–1.581	<0.001	1.237	1.058–1.446	0.008
Other	1.215	0.986–1.498	0.068	0.907	0.713–1.154	0.428
Unable to determine	0.811	0.570–1.154	0.244	0.801	0.551–1.166	0.247
Log(Length of Stay)	1.272	1.212–1.336	<0.001	1.124	1.060–1.191	<0.001
Primary Payor (Ref: Medicare traditional)						
Charity/Indigent	1.305	0.146–11.694	0.812	0.462	0.038–5.576	0.543
Commercial indemnity	1.334	0.914–1.948	0.136	1.054	0.694–1.601	0.805
Direct employer contract	0.000	0.000-Inf	0.943	0.000	0.000-Inf	0.989
Managed care capitated	0.870	0.105–7.238	0.898	0.604	0.062–5.919	0.665
Managed care non-capitated	1.449	1.107–1.898	0.007	1.195	0.887–1.610	0.240
Medicaid managed care capitated	2.901	1.537–5.477	0.001	0.924	0.436–1.956	0.836
Medicaid managed care non-capitated	1.875	1.350–2.604	<0.001	1.083	0.738–1.590	0.684
Medicaid traditional	2.437	1.677–3.541	<0.001	1.236	0.802–1.907	0.337
Medicare managed care capitated	1.096	0.829–1.449	0.521	0.902	0.659–1.235	0.520
Medicare managed care non-capitated	1.091	0.972–1.224	0.140	1.048	0.924–1.190	0.463
Other	1.555	0.852–2.838	0.150	1.311	0.690–2.492	0.409
Other government payors	1.707	1.234–2.362	0.001	1.129	0.779–1.637	0.521
Self-pay	1.093	0.531–2.250	0.809	0.757	0.353–1.624	0.475
Workers' compensation	2.611	0.236–28.827	0.434	1.416	0.105–19.117	0.793

Table 2. *Cont.*

Variable	Univariate Analysis			Multivariate Analysis		
	OR	95% CI	*p*-Value	OR	95% CI	*p*-Value
Point of Origin (Ref: Non-healthcare facility)						
Clinic	1.339	0.996–1.799	0.053	1.375	0.994–1.902	0.055
Court/Law enforcement	1.788	0.569–5.623	0.320	1.394	0.411–4.724	0.594
Information not available	3.659	2.308–5.802	<0.001	3.949	2.321–6.719	<0.001
Other	1.639	0.17–15.769	0.669	1.473	0.141–15.383	0.746
Transfer from ambulatory surgery center	0.819	0.099–6.812	0.854	0.688	0.080–5.930	0.734
Transfer from dept unit in same hospital, separate claim	1.414	0.868–2.306	0.164	1.475	0.858–2.536	0.160
Transfer from health facility	0.922	0.556–1.530	0.753	1.001	0.586–1.709	0.997
Transfer from hospice and under hospice program	0.000	0.000-Inf	0.946	0.000	0.000-Inf	0.984
Transfer from hospital (different facility)	1.302	1.012–1.677	0.040	1.026	0.776–1.357	0.856
Transfer from SNF [1] or ICF [2]	1.097	0.882–1.364	0.404	1.133	0.893–1.437	0.304
Discharge Status (Ref: Discharged to home or self-care)						
Acute inpatient readmission	0.716	0.213–2.404	0.588	0.840	0.238–2.961	0.786
Discharged to home health organization	1.106	0.929–1.316	0.257	1.144	0.948–1.382	0.161
Discharged to hospice home	1.202	0.921–1.568	0.176	1.367	1.023–1.828	0.035
Discharged to hospice medical facility	1.232	0.937–1.620	0.135	1.354	1.006–1.823	0.046
Discharged/Transferred to another rehab facility	1.131	0.785–1.628	0.510	1.250	0.845–1.848	0.264
Discharged/Transferred to court/law enforcement	15.741	1.633–151.780	0.017	3.375	0.293–38.812	0.329
Discharged/Transferred to federal hospital	2.099	0.460–10.862	0.377	2.089	0.368–11.873	0.406
Discharged/Transferred to ICF [2]	1.218	0.913–1.624	0.180	1.142	0.831–1.570	0.414
Discharged/Transferred to long-term care hospital	0.562	0.280–1.129	0.105	0.519	0.244–1.104	0.089
Discharged/Transferred to nursing facility	1.331	0.772–2.295	0.303	1.185	0.636–2.209	0.594
Discharged/Transferred to other facility	1.088	0.637–1.857	0.758	1.132	0.641–2.000	0.669
Discharged/Transferred to other health institute not in list	1.199	0.552–2.608	0.646	1.217	0.531–2.790	0.642
Discharged/Transferred to psychiatric hospital	1.344	1.013–1.785	0.041	1.457	1.069–1.986	0.017
Discharged/Transferred to SNF [1]	1.127	0.979–1.297	0.096	1.144	0.979–1.338	0.091
Discharged/Transferred to swing bed	1.166	0.251–5.420	0.845	1.227	0.234–6.440	0.809
Expired	1.282	0.901–1.824	0.168	0.991	0.672–1.462	0.965
Information not available	0.000	0.000-Inf	0.954	0.000	0.000-Inf	0.986
Left against medical advice	0.777	0.367–1.648	0.511	0.888	0.400–1.969	0.770
Still a patient—expected to return	0.000	0.000-Inf	0.962	0.000	0.000-Inf	0.989
Count of Procedures	1.145	1.109–1.183	<0.001	1.230	1.179–1.283	<0.001
CMS [3] Fiscal Year (Ref: 2022)						
2023	0.336	0.290–0.388	<0.001	0.264	0.224–0.311	<0.001
Social Vulnerability Index						
Household characteristics	1.506	1.238–1.831	<0.001	1.625	0.873–3.025	0.126
Housing type and transportation	1.329	1.080–1.636	0.007	1.362	0.584–3.177	0.474
Overall	1.326	1.085–1.621	0.006	0.361	0.037–3.561	0.383
Racial and ethnic minority status	1.047	0.830–1.321	0.698	0.829	0.491–1.398	0.482
Socioeconomic status	1.265	1.045–1.532	0.016	2.003	0.600–6.685	0.259
COVID-19 Status (Ref: Not identified)						
Positive	1.130	0.927–1.377	0.227	0.978	0.788–1.215	0.842
MS-DRG [4] Type (Ref: Medical)						
Surgical	2.089	1.482–2.943	<0.001	1.195	0.794–1.800	0.393
Teaching Status (Ref: No)						
Not Available	0.545	0.249–1.190	0.127	0.349	0.142–0.856	0.021
Yes	1.349	1.208–1.506	<0.001	1.047	0.839–1.307	0.685
Academic Status (Ref: No)						
Yes	1.270	1.124–1.435	<0.001	0.900	0.701–1.156	0.411
Rural/Urban Status (Ref: Urban)						
Rural	0.910	0.775–1.068	0.249	0.995	0.803–1.232	0.963
Ownership (Ref: Voluntary non-profit—private)						
Government—federal	0.000	0.000-Inf	0.934	0.000	0.000-Inf	0.981
Government—hospital district/authority	0.945	0.763–1.170	0.602	0.847	0.652–1.101	0.214
Government—local	1.591	1.166–2.170	0.003	2.104	1.401–3.159	<0.001
Government—state	0.718	0.389–1.323	0.228	0.641	0.304–1.352	0.243
Not available	1.871	0.774–4.522	0.164	1.758	0.679–4.553	0.245
Physician	2.272	0.206–25.082	0.503	3.229	0.267–39.096	0.357
Proprietary	0.943	0.762–1.166	0.586	0.984	0.752–1.289	0.908

Table 2. *Cont.*

Variable	Univariate Analysis OR	Univariate Analysis 95% CI	Univariate Analysis p-Value	Multivariate Analysis OR	Multivariate Analysis 95% CI	Multivariate Analysis p-Value
Ownership (Ref: Voluntary non-profit—private)						
Voluntary non-profit—church	0.782	0.661–0.925	0.004	0.869	0.711–1.063	0.173
Voluntary non-profit—other	0.723	0.545–0.958	0.024	0.605	0.442–0.827	0.002
Bed Count (Ref: >400)						
1–50	0.605	0.403–0.908	0.015	0.687	0.426–1.107	0.123
51–100	0.592	0.460–0.760	<0.001	0.671	0.492–0.916	0.012
101–150	0.795	0.649–0.975	0.028	0.842	0.652–1.086	0.185
151–200	0.656	0.514–0.838	0.001	0.706	0.530–0.939	0.017
201–250	0.619	0.510–0.751	<0.001	0.818	0.645–1.037	0.097
251–300	0.603	0.501–0.725	<0.001	0.704	0.559–0.886	0.003
301–350	0.727	0.604–0.876	0.001	0.865	0.688–1.086	0.212
351–400	0.754	0.608–0.935	0.010	0.933	0.718–1.211	0.601
Case Mix Index	1.912	1.574–2.322	<0.001	1.579	1.188–2.100	0.002
State Abbreviation (Ref: NY)						
AK	2.708	0.245–29.975	0.417	4.569	0.382–54.824	0.230
AL	1.504	0.836–2.707	0.713	1.187	0.625–2.254	0.600
AR	0.524	0.224–1.224	0.136	0.413	0.163–1.044	0.062
AZ	0.633	0.313–1.279	0.203	0.554	0.265–1.157	0.116
CA	1.216	0.931–1.588	0.152	1.242	0.901–1.714	0.186
CO	0.478	0.146–1.568	0.223	0.470	0.316–1.621	0.232
CT	1.658	0.916–3.002	0.095	1.770	0.934–3.352	0.080
DE	0.000	0.000-Inf	0.952	0.000	0.000-Inf	0.966
FL	0.928	0.748–1.152	0.500	0.860	0.654–1.130	0.279
GA	1.511	0.943–2.422	0.860	0.874	0.492–1.556	0.648
HI	1.884	1.050–3.379	0.034	2.239	1.019–4.920	0.045
IA	1.625	0.944–2.798	0.080	1.256	0.676–2.336	0.471
IL	0.668	0.465–0.960	0.029	0.644	0.428–0.696	0.035
IN	1.236	0.755–2.023	0.399	1.067	0.621–1.835	0.814
KS	1.489	0.754–2.941	0.251	0.879	0.412–1.873	0.738
KY	1.146	0.751–1.749	0.526	1.017	0.621–1.667	0.945
LA	4.431	2.343–8.379	<0.001	2.794	1.358–5.748	0.005
MA	1.389	0.957–2.015	0.084	1.256	0.819–1.928	0.297
MD	0.931	0.581–1.492	0.766	1.103	0.653–1.862	0.714
ME	0.000	0.000-Inf	0.984	0.000	0.000-Inf	0.989
MI	0.947	0.726–1.236	0.690	0.840	0.599–1.178	0.313
MN	1.743	1.115–2.724	0.015	1.842	1.127–3.01	0.015
MO	0.602	0.237–1.531	0.286	0.362	0.128–1.021	0.055
MS	0.733	0.405–1.329	0.307	0.582	0.306–1.109	0.100
MT	0.226	0.030–1.676	0.146	0.148	0.018–1.205	0.074
NC	1.645	1.282–2.111	<0.001	1.101	0.796–1.523	0.561
ND	2.407	0.736–7.875	0.146	3.664	0.972–13.816	0.055
NE	0.492	0.150–1.617	0.243	0.661	0.912–2.277	0.512
NJ	0.961	0.700–1.318	0.805	0.988	0.692–1.413	0.949
NM	1.444	0.753–2.768	0.268	1.513	0.736–3.113	0.260
NV	0.782	0.515–1.187	0.248	0.906	0.542–1.513	0.705
OH	1.287	1.001–1.654	0.049	1.077	0.791–1.467	0.637
OK	1.281	0.910–1.802	0.156	1.044	0.676–1.613	0.845
OR	2.462	1.567–3.868	<0.001	2.552	1.530–4.257	<0.001
PA	2.003	1.623–2.472	<0.001	2.146	1.656–2.782	<0.001
SC	1.044	0.699–1.559	0.833	0.927	0.592–1.450	0.739
SD	0.000	0.000-Inf	0.944	0.000	0.000-Inf	0.962
TN	0.752	0.534–1.059	0.102	0.598	0.399–0.897	0.013
TX	0.974	0.696–1.361	0.876	0.929	0.627–1.374	0.711
UT	0.000	0.000-Inf	0.988	0.000	0.000-Inf	0.992
VA	1.477	1.097–1.989	0.010	1.506	1.052–2.155	0.025
VT	0.000	0.000-Inf	0.977	0.000	0.000-Inf	0.986
WA	0.896	0.554–1.448	0.653	0.965	0.562–1.656	0.897
WI	1.529	1.026–2.276	0.037	1.500	0.952–2.363	0.080
WV	0.921	0.590–1.437	0.717	0.726	0.434–1.216	0.224
WY	0.000	0.000-Inf	0.974	0.000	0.000-Inf	0.982

[1] SNF: Skilled nursing facility; [2] ICF: Intermediate care facility; [3] CMS: U.S. Centers for Medicare and Medicaid Services; [4] MS-DRG: Medicare Severity Diagnosis Related Group.

Table 3 reports the univariate and multivariate logistic regression results (ORs, 95% CIs, and p-values) for the specificity of secondary dementia diagnoses' outcome. For the multivariate results, all age groups experienced higher odds of specificity of dementia secondary diagnoses than the reference group of ages 85+ (OR $\geq$ 1.316; $p < 0.001$). Male patients had significantly higher odds of dementia secondary diagnosis specificity compared to females (OR = 1.224, 95% CI: 1.209–1.239; $p < 0.001$). Individuals identifying as Black were associated with lower odds of dementia secondary diagnosis specificity (OR = 0.955; 95% CI: 0.937–0.973) compared to White patients, while the opposite was found for those identifying as other races (OR = 1.069; 95% CI: 1.040–1.099). For some categories, primary payor, patient origin, and discharge status also showed significant associations with dementia secondary diagnosis coding specificity (see Table 3). Length of stay (in log terms) was also associated with higher odds of dementia secondary diagnosis specificity (OR = 1.017; 95% CI: 1.008–1.025). Those undergoing a larger number of procedures experienced higher odds of dementia secondary diagnosis specificity (OR = 1.039; 95% CI: 1.036–1.042). The CMS fiscal year was not substantially different, with those who were hospitalized in the new 2023 fiscal year experiencing 1.4% higher odds of specificity (OR = 1.014; 95% CI: 1.000–1.028). Patient socioeconomic (OR = 0.829; 95% CI: 0.717–0.958) and racial/ethnic minority (OR = 1.09; 95% CI: 1.03–1.154) statuses within the social vulnerability indices were significantly associated with decreased and increased, respectively, odds of dementia secondary diagnosis specificity. COVID-19-positive patients were associated with lower odds of dementia secondary diagnosis specificity (OR = 0.948; 95% CI: 0.930–0.965). Patients undergoing a surgical MS-DRG experienced 14% lower odds of dementia secondary diagnosis specificity compared to those undergoing a medical MS-DRG (OR = 0.859; 95% CI: 0.844–0.875). Academic facilities demonstrated higher odds of dementia secondary diagnosis specificity (OR = 1.052; 95% CI: 1.020–1.085), whereas those in rural settings experienced lower odds of dementia secondary diagnosis specificity (OR = 0.976; 95% CI: 0.955–0.997). Patients at facilities of different ownership types also experienced differing odds of dementia secondary diagnosis specificity (see Table 3). Lower bed counts were generally associated with lower odds of dementia secondary diagnosis specificity (OR $\leq$ 0.954) than those in the largest cluster of hospitals (>400 beds), with the exception of facilities with 51–100 beds and those with 351–400 beds. Substantial differences in the odds of dementia secondary diagnosis specificity were found by state when compared to the reference state of New York.

Table 3. Univariate and multivariate logistic regression results including odds ratios (ORs), corresponding 95% confidence intervals (CIs), and p-values for specificity of a dementia-related secondary diagnosis.

	Univariate Analysis			Multivariate Analysis		
Variable	**OR**	**95% CI**	**p-Value**	**OR**	**95% CI**	**p-Value**
Intercept	-	-	-	0.351	0.327–0.378	<0.001
Age (Ref: 85+)						
0–44	1.956	1.701–2.248	<0.001	1.934	1.676–2.233	<0.001
45–54	1.736	1.607–1.875	<0.001	1.734	1.601–1.877	<0.001
55–59	1.745	1.652–1.843	<0.001	1.736	1.640–1.838	<0.001
60–64	1.532	1.477–1.588	<0.001	1.526	1.468–1.586	<0.001
65–69	1.459	1.421–1.497	<0.001	1.422	1.384–1.461	<0.001
70–74	1.438	1.409–1.467	<0.001	1.421	1.392–1.451	<0.001
75–79	1.410	1.386–1.435	<0.001	1.402	1.377–1.426	<0.001
80–84	1.316	1.295–1.337	<0.001	1.316	1.295–1.338	<0.001
Sex (Ref: Female)						
Male	1.269	1.254–1.284	<0.001	1.224	1.209–1.239	<0.001
Race (Ref: White)						
Asian	0.977	0.941–1.015	0.230	1.009	0.967–1.053	0.680
Black	0.989	0.972–1.006	0.202	0.955	0.937–0.973	<0.001
Other	1.036	1.009–1.063	0.008	1.069	1.040–1.099	<0.001
Unable to determine	0.969	0.930–1.010	0.139	0.973	0.933–1.015	0.210

Table 3. *Cont.*

Variable	Univariate Analysis			Multivariate Analysis		
	OR	95% CI	*p*-Value	OR	95% CI	*p*-Value
Log(Length of Stay)	1.069	1.062–1.077	<0.001	1.017	1.008–1.025	<0.001
Primary Payor (Ref: Medicare traditional)						
Charity/Indigent	1.204	0.903–1.604	0.206	0.976	0.729–1.308	0.873
Commercial indemnity	1.121	1.055–1.192	<0.001	0.979	0.919–1.042	0.499
Direct employer contract	2.934	2.229–3.861	<0.001	2.449	1.854–3.234	<0.001
Managed care capitated	1.087	0.889–1.328	0.416	0.863	0.703–1.060	0.161
Managed care non-capitated	1.090	1.044–1.139	<0.001	1.011	0.967–1.057	0.639
Medicaid managed care capitated	1.130	0.993–1.285	0.063	0.896	0.785–1.023	0.105
Medicaid managed care non-capitated	1.129	1.077–1.183	<0.001	0.896	0.852–0.942	<0.001
Medicaid traditional	1.050	0.993–1.111	0.087	0.844	0.796–0.896	<0.001
Medicare managed care capitated	1.018	0.987–1.049	0.258	0.979	0.948–1.012	0.214
Medicare managed care non-capitated	0.973	0.961–0.986	<0.001	0.945	0.933–0.958	<0.001
Other	0.963	0.888–1.043	0.354	0.909	0.837–0.986	0.022
Other government payors	1.081	1.034–1.129	0.001	0.915	0.875–0.958	<0.001
Self-pay	0.879	0.798–0.968	0.009	0.819	0.742–0.904	<0.001
Workers' compensation	0.467	0.327–0.667	<0.001	0.495	0.344–0.711	<0.001
Point of Origin (Ref: Non-healthcare facility)						
Clinic	0.923	0.893–0.955	<0.001	0.954	0.921–0.987	0.007
Court/Law enforcement	1.029	0.771–1.372	0.848	0.949	0.698–1.291	0.739
Information not available	1.008	0.936–1.085	0.838	1.045	0.968–1.129	0.256
Other	1.071	0.878–1.306	0.497	1.159	0.946–1.419	0.154
Transfer from ambulatory surgery center	0.769	0.599–0.988	0.040	0.715	0.555–0.921	0.009
Transfer from dept unit in same hospital, separate claim	0.976	0.901–1.057	0.543	0.999	0.921–1.084	0.982
Transfer from health facility	1.003	0.956–1.053	0.896	0.950	0.904–0.999	0.044
Transfer from hospice and under hospice program	1.288	0.904–1.834	0.161	1.248	0.871–1.787	0.227
Transfer from hospital (different facility)	0.950	0.926–0.975	<0.001	0.884	0.860–0.908	<0.001
Transfer from SNF [1] or ICF [2]	1.118	1.096–1.141	<0.001	1.082	1.059–1.106	<0.001
Discharge Status (Ref: Discharged to home or self-care)						
Acute inpatient readmission	0.966	0.835–1.117	0.637	1.033	0.891–1.197	0.666
Discharged to home health organization	1.026	1.006–1.046	0.011	1.064	1.043–1.085	<0.001
Discharged to hospice home	1.239	1.204–1.275	<0.001	1.312	1.274–1.352	<0.001
Discharged to hospice medical facility	1.180	1.146–1.215	<0.001	1.228	1.191–1.265	<0.001
Discharged/Transferred to another rehab facility	1.010	0.974–1.047	0.589	1.019	0.982–1.058	0.321
Discharged/Transferred to cancer ctr/children's hospital	0.938	0.702–1.253	0.666	1.109	0.827–1.488	0.490
Discharged/Transferred to court/law enforcement	1.249	0.965–1.616	0.092	1.128	0.856–1.486	0.392
Discharged/Transferred to critical access hospital	0.612	0.355–1.056	0.078	0.581	0.335–1.008	0.054
Discharged/Transferred to federal hospital	1.027	0.800–1.319	0.833	1.027	0.797–1.322	0.839
Discharged/Transferred to ICF [2]	1.289	1.240–1.339	<0.001	1.249	1.201–1.300	<0.001
Discharged/Transferred to long-term care hospital	1.108	1.046–1.173	<0.001	1.002	0.944–1.063	0.950
Discharged/Transferred to nursing facility	1.532	1.389–1.690	<0.001	1.544	1.396–1.706	<0.001
Discharged/Transferred to other facility	0.978	0.922–1.038	0.463	0.947	0.891–1.005	0.074
Discharged/Transferred to other health institute not in list	1.189	1.064–1.328	0.002	1.196	1.068–1.338	0.002
Discharged/Transferred to psychiatric hospital	1.849	1.694–2.019	<0.001	1.685	1.542–1.842	<0.001
Discharged/Transferred to SNF [1]	1.050	1.032–1.068	<0.001	1.075	1.056–1.095	<0.001
Discharged/Transferred to swing bed	1.084	0.977–1.202	0.127	1.151	1.034–1.280	0.010
Expired	0.936	0.910–0.963	<0.001	0.896	0.870–0.923	<0.001
Information not available	0.691	0.514–0.928	0.014	0.830	0.613–1.124	0.228
Left against medical advice	0.850	0.769–0.940	0.002	0.829	0.749–0.917	<0.001
Still a patient—expected to return	1.204	0.603–2.405	0.598	1.006	0.498–2.034	0.987
Count of Procedures	1.038	1.036–1.041	<0.001	1.039	1.036–1.042	0.001
CMS [3] Fiscal Year (Ref: 2022)						
2023	1.030	1.016–1.044	<0.001	1.014	1.000–1.028	0.049
Social Vulnerability Index						
Household characteristics	0.808	0.790–0.827	<0.001	0.829	0.717–0.958	0.011
Housing type and transportation	0.936	0.914–0.958	<0.001	0.963	0.892–1.040	0.336
Overall	0.912	0.889–0.936	<0.001	1.090	1.030–1.154	0.003
Racial and ethnic minority status	0.911	0.889–0.934	<0.001	0.931	0.844–1.027	0.156
Socioeconomic status	0.836	0.817–0.857	<0.001	1.177	0.895–1.548	0.245
COVID-19 Status (Ref: Not identified)						
Positive	0.960	0.943–0.977	<0.001	0.948	0.930–0.965	<0.001

Table 3. *Cont.*

Variable	Univariate Analysis			Multivariate Analysis		
	OR	95% CI	p-Value	OR	95% CI	p-Value
MS-DRG [4] Type (Ref: Medical)						
Surgical	0.932	0.917–0.947	<0.001	0.859	0.844–0.875	<0.001
Teaching Status (Ref: No)						
Not Available	1.153	1.095–1.215	<0.001	1.130	1.066–1.197	<0.001
Yes	1.067	1.051–1.082	<0.001	0.975	0.949–1.001	0.061
Academic Status (Ref: No)						
Yes	1.078	1.061–1.096	<0.001	1.052	1.020–1.085	<0.001
Rural/Urban Status (Ref: Urban)						
Rural	0.969	0.952–0.986	<0.001	0.976	0.955–0.997	0.025
Ownership (Ref: Voluntary non-profit—private)						
Government—federal	0.952	0.841–1.078	0.437	0.915	0.802–1.042	0.181
Government—hospital district/authority	1.048	1.024–1.074	<0.001	1.033	1.006–1.062	0.017
Government—local	1.102	1.060–1.145	<0.001	1.146	1.097–1.196	<0.001
Government—state	0.898	0.837–0.963	0.003	0.881	0.815–0.951	0.001
Not available	0.905	0.829–0.989	0.028	0.847	0.771–0.930	0.001
Physician	1.364	1.206–1.544	<0.001	1.191	1.045–1.358	0.009
Proprietary	0.837	0.814–0.860	<0.001	0.872	0.845–0.899	<0.001
Voluntary non-profit—church	0.886	0.871–0.902	<0.001	0.904	0.887–0.921	<0.001
Voluntary non-profit—other	0.961	0.935–0.987	0.003	0.890	0.864–0.916	<0.001
Bed Count (Ref: >400)						
1–50	0.940	0.904–0.976	0.002	0.954	0.912–0.997	0.038
51–100	1.035	1.007–1.064	0.001	1.071	1.037–1.105	<0.001
101–150	0.849	0.829–0.869	<0.001	0.878	0.987–1.040	<0.001
151–200	0.952	0.928–0.975	<0.001	0.951	0.854–0.902	<0.001
201–250	0.868	0.849–0.886	<0.001	0.931	0.924–0.978	<0.001
251–300	0.914	0.895–0.933	<0.001	0.945	0.909–0.955	<0.001
301–350	0.908	0.889–0.926	<0.001	0.939	0.922–0.969	<0.001
351–400	0.924	0.903–0.945	<0.001	1.013	0.917–0.961	0.329
Case Mix Index	1.028	1.005–1.052	0.018	0.981	0.951–1.012	0.227
State Abbreviation (Ref: NY)						
AK	1.392	1.081–1.793	0.010	1.335	1.034–1.725	0.027
AL	0.731	0.679–0.787	<0.001	0.723	0.669–0.780	<0.001
AR	0.626	0.579–0.677	<0.001	0.665	0.612–0.722	<0.001
AZ	1.011	0.968–1.055	0.633	1.039	0.992–1.089	0.104
CA	0.946	0.916–0.977	0.001	0.949	0.915–0.984	0.005
CO	0.857	0.795–0.923	<0.001	0.841	0.778–0.909	<0.001
CT	1.240	1.173–1.312	<0.001	1.235	1.166–1.309	<0.001
DE	0.817	0.716–0.932	0.003	0.825	0.720–0.945	0.005
FL	0.912	0.888–0.936	<0.001	0.922	0.894–0.952	<0.001
GA	0.933	0.885–0.984	0.011	0.881	0.829–0.935	<0.001
HI	1.150	1.087–1.217	<0.001	1.219	1.136–1.309	<0.001
IA	1.342	1.261–1.427	<0.001	1.298	1.216–1.386	<0.001
ID	1.307	0.612–2.792	0.489	1.488	0.693–3.197	0.308
IL	1.061	1.023–1.101	0.002	1.087	1.044–1.131	<0.001
IN	1.093	1.035–1.154	0.001	1.095	1.033–1.161	0.002
KS	0.697	0.639–0.760	<0.001	0.685	0.626–0.750	<0.001
KY	1.196	1.144–1.249	<0.001	1.225	1.167–1.287	<0.001
LA	1.330	1.239–1.428	<0.001	1.287	1.194–1.388	<0.001
MA	1.025	0.960–1.095	0.454	0.962	0.899–1.031	0.275
MD	0.969	0.918–1.023	0.254	0.950	0.897–1.007	0.083
ME	1.243	0.515–3.000	0.628	1.372	0.563–3.347	0.487
MI	1.006	0.972–1.041	0.741	1.027	0.987–1.069	0.182
MN	2.162	2.014–2.321	<0.001	2.077	1.930–2.234	<0.001
MO	0.991	0.919–1.068	0.809	0.902	0.833–0.977	0.012
MS	1.005	0.951–1.062	0.861	0.992	0.936–1.052	0.796
MT	0.798	0.708–0.900	<0.001	0.848	0.749–0.960	0.009
NC	1.305	1.265–1.347	<0.001	1.244	1.199–1.290	<0.001
ND	1.495	1.280–1.746	<0.001	1.723	1.469–2.022	<0.001
NE	1.667	1.521–1.827	<0.001	1.808	1.643–1.990	<0.001
NH	0.483	0.250–0.933	0.030	0.514	0.265–0.996	0.049
NJ	0.863	0.821–0.907	<0.001	0.874	0.830–0.921	<0.001
NM	0.880	0.803–0.963	0.006	0.839	0.763–0.921	<0.001

Table 3. *Cont.*

Variable	OR	Univariate Analysis 95% CI	p-Value	OR	Multivariate Analysis 95% CI	p-Value
State Abbreviation (Ref: NY)						
NV	0.793	0.745–0.845	<0.001	0.873	0.815–0.936	<0.001
OH	1.287	1.244–1.331	<0.001	1.356	1.306–1.408	<0.001
OK	1.407	1.339–1.478	<0.001	1.350	1.277–1.426	<0.001
OR	1.756	1.672–1.845	<0.001	1.881	1.784–1.984	<0.001
PA	1.403	1.358–1.450	<0.001	1.439	1.389–1.492	<0.001
RI	3.030	1.078–8.516	0.035	2.763	0.977–7.813	0.055
SC	1.082	1.033–1.133	0.001	1.080	1.028–1.135	0.002
SD	1.409	1.252–1.586	<0.001	1.393	1.233–1.573	<0.001
TN	0.807	0.776–0.840	<0.001	0.826	0.790–0.865	<0.001
TX	1.239	1.203–1.277	<0.001	1.247	1.203–1.292	<0.001
UT	0.855	0.422–1.730	0.663	0.881	0.433–1.789	0.726
VA	1.374	1.324–1.426	<0.001	1.365	1.309–1.422	<0.001
VT	0.797	0.564–1.127	0.199	0.853	0.601–1.211	0.373
WA	1.225	1.165–1.288	<0.001	1.281	1.215–1.352	<0.001
WI	1.509	1.443–1.578	<0.001	1.496	1.426–1.569	<0.001
WV	0.971	0.926–1.019	0.229	0.981	0.930–1.036	0.492
WY	1.416	1.067–1.879	0.016	1.471	1.104–1.960	0.008

[1] SNF: Skilled nursing facility; [2] ICF: Intermediate care facility; [3] CMS: Centers for Medicare and Medicaid Services; [4] MS-DRG: Medicare Severity Diagnosis Related Group.

Figure 1 panel (a) shows the ROC curve for the multivariate model of the coding specificity of a principal diagnosis related to dementia. The estimated AUC was 0.7269, representing the good reliability of the multivariate model in assessing the coding specificity of dementia-related principal diagnoses. Panel (b) shows the ROC curve corresponding to the multivariate logistic regression analysis for assessing the coding specificity of secondary dementia diagnoses. The corresponding AUC was 0.5919, demonstrating a worse model performance when compared to that of the model assessing the coding specificity of primary dementia diagnoses.

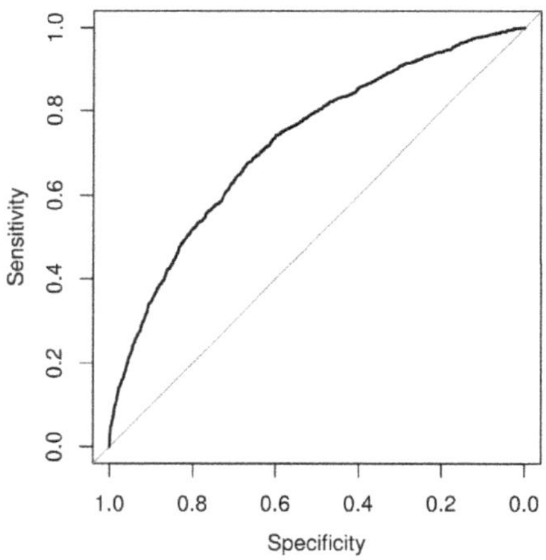

(**a**)

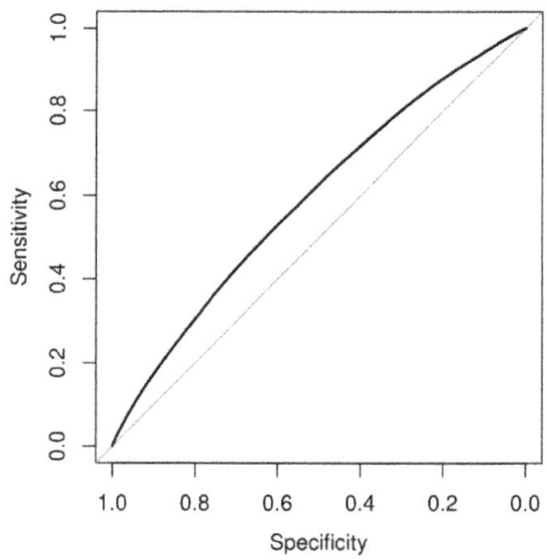

(**b**)

Figure 1. Receiver operating characteristic (ROC) curve of the multivariate logistic regression model for the specificity of a dementia-related principal diagnosis (**a**) and secondary diagnosis (**b**).

Figure 2 represents a subset of the facilities' observed dementia-related principal diagnosis coding specificity (a) and secondary diagnosis coding specificity (b) relative to industry standards. The *p*-values (and the 95% CIs, which are represented as error bars) from the estimated Poisson binomial distribution are used so that under-specificity versus peers ($p < 0.025$) is represented in blue; specificity in line with peers ($0.025 \leq p \leq 0.975$) is represented in black; and over-specificity versus peers ($p > 0.975$) is represented in orange.

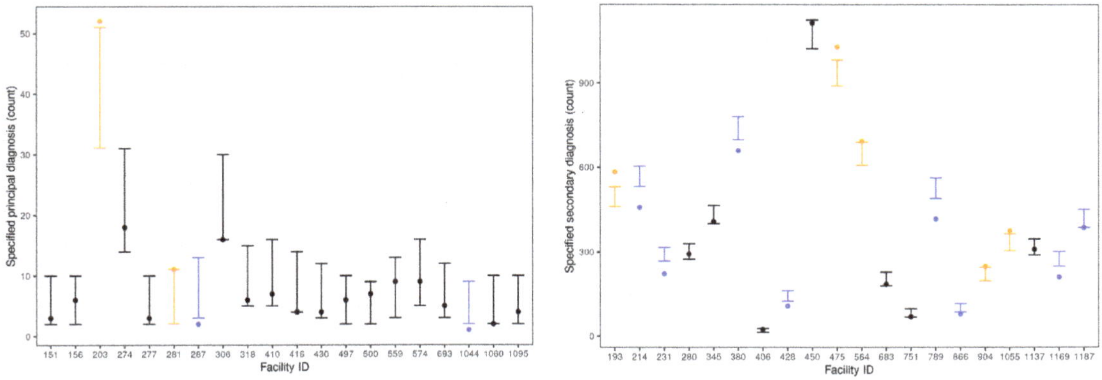

(a) (b)

Figure 2. Observed counts of indicators of principal diagnosis coding specificity (**a**) and secondary diagnosis coding specificity (**b**) for dementia diagnoses by facility (dots) and 95% confidence intervals based on the Poisson binomial metric (error bars), with colors denoting over-specificity (orange), under-specificity (blue), and specificity in line with peers (black).

Figure 3 represents the adjusted ORs for the coding specificity of a dementia-related principal diagnosis (a) and secondary diagnosis (b). All of the adjusted ORs are represented against New York as the reference state. Only a few states demonstrate statistically different adjusted odds of coding specificity of a dementia-related principal diagnosis versus New York, while a larger amount of variability is observed for states' secondary diagnosis coding specificity. The gray states had non-significant adjusted ORs of coding specificity.

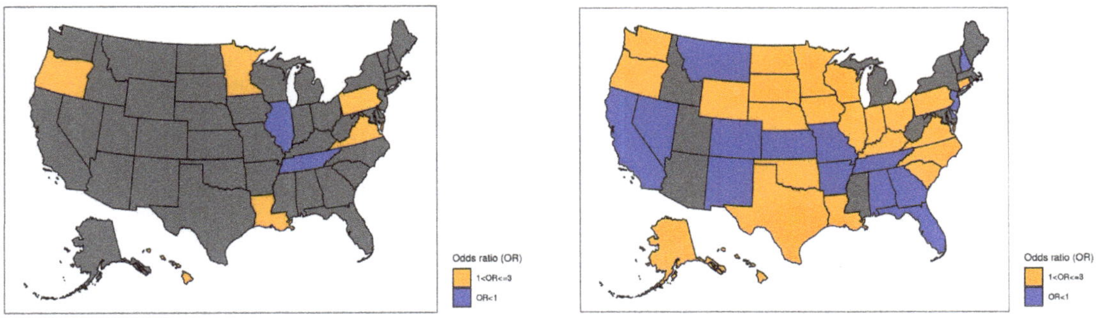

(a) (b)

Figure 3. Geographical U.S. map of adjusted odds ratios (ORs) of coding specificity of dementia-related principal (**a**) and secondary (**b**) diagnoses by state, with a reference state of New York. Odds ratios that were not statistically significant are shown in gray.

4. Discussion

The literature on diagnostic coding specificity remains scarce, with healthcare facilities and practitioners limited in their ability to self-evaluate against healthcare industry standards of practice. It is also unclear whether non-clinical characteristics can explain variability in specificity practices. To address this gap, a novel approach was demonstrated to evaluate facility-specific practices for the dementia-related coding specificity of principal and secondary diagnoses upon making risk adjustments for commonly available patient and facility characteristics. A logistic regression was applied to make risk adjustments to the probability of receiving a specified dementia diagnosis. The statistical output is used in a two-step approach, building on a Poisson binomial model, to evaluate the performance of healthcare facilities in providing specified dementia-related principal, or at least one secondary, diagnoses. This metric can be used to identify facilities that perform differently (under- or over-specifying) compared to their healthcare industry peers and can provide an objective standard against which the coding specificity practices of facilities can be evaluated. These findings offer valuable insights for healthcare stakeholders and quality-control personnel, facilitating the identification of facilities that may benefit from targeted interventions to enhance the levels of specificity of dementia-related diagnosis coding.

Our results indicate that the coding specificity of dementia diagnoses is associated with a range of patient and facility characteristics, particularly for primary diagnoses, as demonstrated through a higher AUC value. Younger patients were generally associated with a higher odds of coding specificity for dementia-related principal and secondary diagnoses. While dementia has been found to be more easily identifiable among older patients [35], our findings indicate that, conditional on a dementia diagnosis, the odds of coding specificity are higher among younger patients. However, it is unclear whether there is a clinical association between the prevalence of specified cases of dementia and age, particularly when comparing age groups with those at least 85 years old.

Prior studies have found that the prevalence of types of dementia is different by sex [36], which could also be due to environmental and behavioral differences according to sex. Males had approximately 22% (secondary) and 45% (principal) higher odds of dementia diagnosis specificity compared to females, though this could be confounded with age. Black patients demonstrated a significantly higher odds of principal diagnosis coding specificity than White patients. However, the reverse is observed for secondary diagnosis specificity. In both cases, there could be confounders due to collinearity with other factors, including social vulnerability indices. Patients have been shown to experience differences in the prevalence of dementia and its associated symptoms and severity by race [37], which could potentially have an association with the ability of doctors to provide a specified dementia diagnosis.

The significant association between longer hospital stays and higher odds of both principal and secondary coding specificity could be due to the additional inpatient time which allows for more comprehensive evaluations, diagnoses, and documentation. Patients discharged to specific destinations, such as hospice homes, hospice medical facilities, or psychiatric hospitals, exhibited significantly higher odds of principal and secondary diagnosis specificity. This could be related to the severity of their case or their prior history, which could, in turn, be associated with a potentially more accurate clinical diagnosis. Patients undergoing more procedures had higher odds of receiving a specified principal or secondary diagnosis. Though the cause of this association is unclear, this could be related to there being more resources allocated for identifying a patient's disease when procedures are necessary during their inpatient stay. While a COVID-19 diagnosis was not associated with differing odds of principal diagnosis specificity, it was associated with lower odds of secondary diagnosis specificity. However, it is unclear whether the association between the severity of patients' COVID-19 symptoms and age could be a confounder [38].

While the differences by CMS fiscal year in secondary diagnosis specificity were minor and are probably clinically irrelevant, the differences were more substantial among those with a dementia primary diagnosis. However, this could be due to seasonal confounders. The new fiscal year, denoted as 2023, was only measured in the October–December 2022 period, which may also be a period with seasonally over-burdened hospitals and less time for healthcare personnel to perform more in-depth diagnoses of patients.

From a payor perspective, none of the payor types were associated with differing odds of principal diagnosis specificity when compared to that of Medicare traditional. This is encouraging, as it indicates that principal diagnosis specificity may not be attributable to healthcare payor type. However, the substantial differences in the univariate results indicate that some complex associations may be embedded, though this is unclear, since the patient mix would not be homogeneous across payor types. For example, age could be acting as a proxy for Medicare status. Also, some differences were found when assessing odds of secondary diagnosis specificity. Some of these differences could be due to other patient characteristics. For example, those receiving Medicare traditional may be in widely different age groups than those for whom the payor comes from a direct employer contract or who receives workers' compensation. Thus, health insurance coverage may be substantially different across patients, leading to the different propensities of patients to seek hospitalization [39].

Additionally, the ownership status of the facilities displayed some significant differences, with local government-owned facilities showing notably higher odds of principal and secondary diagnosis specificity. Again, the non-clinical patient characteristics by facility and facility ownership could differ widely. The case mix index of the hospital was significantly, positively associated with the specificity of principal diagnosis, indicating that the overall complexity of patients' needs in a facility is related to higher degrees of specificity provided during a hospitalization. However, no significant association of specificity and the facility case mix index was found when the dementia diagnosis was secondary during the inpatient stay. Substantial differences were also found by state, particularly for secondary diagnoses. These differences could stem from the population mix or could be related to a substantially larger sample size for this analysis. Differences in health care provision by state across multiple metrics, such as care setting and type of disease/clinical area, have been documented [40]. However, we cannot link the coding specificity with the quality of care directly, since a low quality of care can occur when there are low levels of specificity state-wide but also when there are high levels of specificity and such excessive level of specificity is not clinically warranted.

These variations in coding practices demonstrate the potential influence of organizational characteristics or state-wide standards of practice on coding specificity. State-level variations may be attributed to regional variations in healthcare infrastructure, regulatory frameworks, insurance-related expectations/requirements, or coding practices. Also, there is state clustering of hospitals with a common health system, which may share a coding department and/or coding standards. However, they could also be influenced by the patient mix and other correlated factors in these states, given the socioeconomic, racial, and age differences across states, which may reflect the underlying reasons for non-idiosyncratic specificity disparities [41].

Providing high levels of coding specificity, when possible and appropriate, supports the accuracy and completeness of health records for patients, potentially enhancing their subsequent health outcomes. However, high coding standards require both time and educational/training resources for coders to conduct efficient and consistent coding practices that are current and accurate. Unspecified diagnoses may sometimes be a consequence of insufficient knowledge about all possible ICD-10 codes available related to a condition. Over-specified diagnoses may be a consequence of miscoding. Therefore, there is a tradeoff between the cost of specificity-related accuracy (oftentimes paid by the provider) and the cost of specificity-related inaccuracy (oftentimes a burden for the payor and the patient). Our approach demonstrates that facilities with dementia-related hospitalizations can be compared against a common/industry standard in a risk-adjusted form, so that facilities over- or under-specifying can be identified and their coding standards of practice can be adjusted, when needed.

While the proposed approach is demonstrated with an example of clustering at the facility level, for which full information is available for all patients, clustering by other factors is also possible. For example, clustering by zip code can allow for geospatial analyses of coding specificity. Also, clustering factors do not need to be available for all observations, allowing for more flexible analyses. For example, some hospitals may collect information about patients or systems that other hospitals do not collect. Clustering analyses are possible in such instances, and it is one of the core advantages of the two-step approach of performing patient-level analyses and subsequently clustering by any desired factor.

Our findings emphasize the association of multiple patient and facility characteristics with coding specificity. The relative significance of the evaluated variables in explaining the variability in coding specificity further underscores the importance of risk-adjusted performance metrics when comparing healthcare outcomes and facility performances.

Strengths and Limitations

A large comprehensive dataset with nearly 488,000 patient observations related to dementia was used for this study, which represents, to our knowledge, the largest dementia-related study approaching the topic of diagnostic coding specificity. Developing and utilizing the proposed risk-adjusted metric allows for a fair assessment of coding specificity among healthcare facilities while producing an extrapolatable approach that allows for the incorporation of any available information about patient hospitalizations.

Though the dataset contains the most recently completed year (2022), it only encompasses a single year of discharges, yielding temporal limitations since coding policies and practices can be updated yearly. However, due to these potential dynamics, it is important to have a recent dataset that reflects current practices. The demonstrated method, however, can be applied on a rolling basis, so that facilities can assess their practices over time and evaluate any adjustments made along the way.

While the dataset comprises a large portion of U.S. hospitalizations, there could be data imbalances by state or other factors not considered in the study. This may affect our ability to measure associations with some variables with low counts, such as some of the states. However, this would not affect our results as long as the data imbalances are not directly related to the coding specificity. Also, the cohort definition includes only a subset of dementia-related codes (F ICD-10 diagnosis codes). A more expansive cohort definition is possible, but it would not affect the approach taken, since the cohort definition is common across facilities.

We utilize administrative claims data for explaining a substantial portion of the coding specificity variability in healthcare facilities. While this is insufficient to explain the full variability of diagnostic coding specificity, it is noteworthy that this explanatory power was achieved with minimal access to patients' clinical characteristics, such as those provided in EHRs, many of which are not commonly available in claims data. This indicates that the model provides a baseline from which substantial improvements are possible if additional information is available, such as the granularity and clinical details found in EHRs. However, by making EHRs an optional input, our model gains generalizability, since there is no need for a clinical metric against which to measure the 'correctness' of the degree of coding specificity. Thus, while such clinical metric would be ideal, it is also unfeasible. Therefore, our approach should only be used as a metric to compare against industry standards and averages or against aspirational peer facilities.

Our approach assumes that patients are provided homogeneous treatments within facilities conditional on the set of variables used in the multivariate logistic regression. However, this assumption could be relaxed by introducing additional clustering factors/variables, such as the physicians within facilities, which may explain additional sources of coding specificity variability. The assumption of independence across hospitalizations could also be questionable, since there will be a substantial number of unmeasured factors that could contribute to a lack of independence (e.g., how busy the facilities were during the hospitalizations, who provided treatment, what the commonalities of the unmeasured clinical components across patients were, etc.). However, the model provides an initial metric to flag facilities with the potential for non-standard specificity practices, which can then be investigated more thoroughly by quality-control personnel.

The inclusion of random effects in the model was first considered across a range of facility-level characteristics, particularly the facility identifier. However, for the purpose of this study, we did not include random effects for multiple reasons as follows: (1) Computational complexity—for example, facility-specific random effects added hundreds of random effects in this particular dataset and potentially thousands or tens of thousands for other cohorts, leading to memory limitations. The proposed approach still required nearly 8 Gb RAM. Additionally, if even larger computational resources are needed, then the ability of quality-control personnel to use this approach could be substantially limited; (2) The reduced level of extrapolatability for even more complex or larger datasets, as administrative data may contain few observations or just one observation per facility, particularly if the tool is used for 'live' monitoring purposes; (3) Assumptions behind a random effects approach would be highly questionable, since the random effects would likely be correlated with some of the patient-level characteristics; and (4) While random effects and other modeling enhancements (e.g., different machine learning approaches or semiparametric models with spline components for some of the continuous variables, such as the log-length of stay) could have been considered for variables with lower numbers of categories, the purpose of our approach is not to find the optimal model for a particular cohort/year or set of variables. Instead, this manuscript aims to demonstrate the methodology and utility of administrative information in explaining diagnostic coding specificity variability among patients diagnosed with dementia. The purpose of the two-step approach (first at the patient visit level and then aggregated at any level) is to also provide tools that can be used in different forms, both in a disaggregated form for patient visit monitoring and in an aggregated form for facility monitoring.

The presence of multicollinearity among risk adjustment factors can complicate coefficient interpretation. Alternative approaches that map the information content to smaller sets of uncorrelated factors may be viable to reduce variance inflation, though they would be highly complex to construct due to the mostly categorical structure of the explanatory variable set. Such alternatives could also reduce interpretability. Multicollinearity, however, does not impact the main outcome of this manuscript, which is the estimation of a probability metric for coding specificity at the hospitalization level and a subsequent facility-level aggregation to measure facilities against healthcare industry standards. The goodness of fit or model use for prediction are not affected by collinearity, which allows for wide arrays of explanatory variables to be combined, regardless of potential information overlap in these variables. Thus, the focus of this manuscript is the metrics at the hospitalization and facility levels and their utility in identifying hospitalizations and facilities whose outcomes may substantially differ from industry practices, rather than the specific associations between explanatory variables and outcomes.

Finally, some quantitative data were provided in grouped categories for confidentiality purposes (e.g., age and bed size), and additional variables were not included to maintain the confidentiality of the records. This additional granularity and information could prove to enhance model outcomes within healthcare facility settings.

5. Conclusions

Medical coding is a very important component of healthcare systems, with an extensive impact on patient care quality, reimbursement, and system reliability. An understudied aspect of coding accuracy relates to coding specificity to the highest precision clinically possible. Our study focused on dementia coding specificity in the U.S. and demonstrates that a large number of readily available patient- and facility-level characteristics can be used to make risk adjustments to the odds of coding specificity and thus provide a standardized metric against which facilities can compare their coding specificity practices and standards. This study provides healthcare facilities with a valuable tool to enhance and assess variations in coding specificity, thus contributing to improved healthcare system reliability and financial efficiency as well as improved patient care in an era when accuracy and precision are of the utmost importance. The method demonstrated in this manuscript fills a significant gap in the literature, and its adaptability across patient cohorts, health conditions, and clusters of healthcare provision makes it a valuable tool for quality control and performance assessment. Our results indicate that the variability in the coding specificity of principal diagnoses of dementia can be better explained than the variability in the specificity of secondary diagnoses of dementia. This study addresses a critical need by making risk adjustments for factors that influence coding practices, ultimately contributing to our understanding of coding specificity disparities.

Supplementary Materials: The following supporting information can be downloaded at: https://www.mdpi.com/article/10.3390/healthcare12100983/s1, Table S1: List of specified dementia ICD-10 codes and corresponding descriptions; Table S2: List of unspecified dementia ICD-10 codes and corresponding descriptions.

Author Contributions: Conceptualization, J.M., M.K. and L.H.G.; methodology, L.H.G.; formal analysis, S.P., K.R., J.S., I.R.C., D.P.G., M.R.P., S.R.T. and L.H.G.; data curation, M.K.; writing—original draft preparation, K.R., J.S., S.P., I.R.C., D.P.G., M.R.P., S.R.T. and L.H.G.; writing—review and editing, K.R., J.S., S.P., I.R.C., D.P.G., M.R.P., S.R.T., J.M., M.K. and L.H.G.; visualization, S.P., K.R., J.S., I.R.C., D.P.G., M.R.P., S.R.T. and L.H.G.; supervision, L.H.G. All authors have read and agreed to the published version of the manuscript.

Funding: This research received no external funding.

Institutional Review Board Statement: Ethical review and approval were exempt by the UNC Charlotte Institutional Review Board due to use of existing, de-identified secondary data.

Informed Consent Statement: Data were de-identified and provided by Premier, Inc. No informed consent was needed.

Data Availability Statement: Data were provided by Premier, Inc. and can be requested via https://www.pinc-ai.com/.

Conflicts of Interest: Michael Korvink and John Martin work for Premier, Inc. and own stock in the company. All other authors declare no conflicts of interest.

References

1. Adane, K.; Gizachew, M.; Kendie, S. The role of medical data in efficient patient care delivery: A review. *Risk Manag. Healthc. Policy* **2019**, *12*, 67–73. [CrossRef] [PubMed]
2. Tang, K.L.; Lucyk, K.; Quan, H. Coder perspectives on physician-related barriers to producing high-quality administrative data: A qualitative study. *CMAJ Open* **2017**, *5*, E617–E622. [CrossRef] [PubMed]
3. Centers for Disease Control and Prevention (CDC). International Classification of Diseases, (ICD-10-CM/PCS) Transition—Background. CDC. November 2015. Available online: https://www.cdc.gov/nchs/icd/icd10cm_pcs_background.htm (accessed on 23 October 2023).
4. Asadi, F.; Hosseini, M.A.; Almasi, S. Reliability of trauma coding with ICD-10. *Chin. J. Traumatol.* **2022**, *25*, 102–106. [CrossRef] [PubMed]
5. Wu, J.T.; Leung, K.; Lam, T.T.Y. Nowcasting epidemics of novel pathogens: Lessons from COVID-19. *Nat. Med.* **2021**, *27*, 388–395. [CrossRef] [PubMed]
6. World Health Organization (WHO). International Statistical Classification of Diseases and Related Health Problems, 10th Revision (ICD-10). WHO. September 2012. Available online: https://www.cdc.gov/nchs/data/icd/icdinformationsheet.pdf (accessed on 23 October 2023).
7. Hsia, D.C.; Krushat, W.M.; Fagan, A.B.; Tebbutt, J.A.; Kusserow, R.P. Accuracy of diagnostic coding for Medicare patients under the prospective payment system. *N. Engl. J. Med.* **1988**, *318*, 352–355. [CrossRef] [PubMed]
8. Zegan, J.; Improving Specificity in ICD-10 Diagnosis Coding. American Health Information Management Association. Available online: https://library.ahima.org/doc?oid=302473 (accessed on 23 October 2023).
9. Boyd, A.D.; Li, J.J.; Burton, M.D.; Jonen, M.; Gardeux, V.; Achour, I.; Luo, R.Q.; Zenku, I.; Bahroos, N.; Brown, S.B.; et al. The discriminatory cost of ICD-10-CM transition between clinical specialties: Metrics, case study, and mitigating tools. *J. Am. Med. Inform. Assoc.* **2013**, *20*, 708–717. [CrossRef] [PubMed]
10. Grasso, M.A.; Dezman, Z.D.W.; Jerrard, D.A. Coding disparity and specificity during emergency department visits after transitioning to the tenth version of the International Classification of Diseases. *AMIA Annu. Symp. Proc.* **2022**, *2022*, 495–501. [CrossRef]

11. Centers for Medicare and Medicaid Services, Department of Health and Human Services. ICD-10-CM Official Guidelines for Coding and Reporting FY 2017. Available online: https://www.cms.gov/medicare/coding/icd10/downloads/2017-icd-10-cm-guidelines.pdf (accessed on 23 October 2023).
12. Horsky, J.; Drucker, E.A.; Ramelson, H.Z. Accuracy and completeness of clinical coding using ICD-10 for ambulatory visits. *AMIA Annu. Symp. Proc.* **2017**, *2018*, 912–920.
13. Centers for Medicare and Medicaid Services (CMS). Overall Star Rating for Hospitals. CMS. Available online: https://www.medicare.gov/care-compare/resources/hospital/overall-star-rating (accessed on 23 October 2023).
14. Centers for Medicare and Medicaid Services (CMS). Hospital Value-Based Purchasing Program. Available online: https://www.cms.gov/Medicare/Quality-Initiatives-Patient-Assessment-Instruments/HospitalQualityInits/Hospital-Value-Based-Purchasing (accessed on 30 November 2023).
15. Centers for Medicare and Medicaid Services (CMS). Hospital Readmissions Reduction Program (HRRP). Available online: https://www.cms.gov/Medicare/Medicare-Fee-for-Service-Payment/AcuteInpatientPPS/Readmissions-Reduction-Program (accessed on 30 November 2023).
16. Centers for Medicare and Medicaid Services (CMS). Hospital-Acquired Conditions. Available online: https://www.cms.gov/Medicare/Medicare-Fee-for-Service-Payment/HospitalAcqCond/Hospital-Acquired_Conditions (accessed on 30 November 2023).
17. Austin, J.M.; D'Andrea, G.; Birkmeyer, J.D.; Leape, L.L.; Milstein, A.; Pronovost, P.J.; Romano, P.S.; Singer, S.J.; Vogus, T.J.; Wachter, R.M. Safety in Numbers: The Development of Leapfrog's Composite Patient Safety Score for U.S. Hospitals. *J. Patient Saf.* **2014**, *10*, 64–71. [CrossRef]
18. Fortune and PINC AI. The 2023 Fortune/PINC AI 100 Top Hospitals. Available online: https://fortune.com/article/100-top-hospitals-2023-pinc-ai (accessed on 30 November 2023).
19. Torres, J.M.; Hessler-Jones, D.; Yarbrough, C.; Tapley, A.; Jimenez, R.; Gottlieb, L.M. An online experiment to assess bias in professional medical coding. *BMC Med. Inform. Decis. Mak.* **2019**, *19*, 115. [CrossRef]
20. Department of Health and Human Services. Information and Resources for Submitting Correct ICD-10 Codes to Medicare. MLN Matters 2014. Available online: https://www.hhs.gov/guidance/sites/default/files/hhs-guidance-documents/SE1518.pdf (accessed on 23 October 2023).
21. American Hospital Association (AHA). *Using the X-ray Report for Specificity*; AHA Coding Clinic for ICD-10-CM and ICD-10-PCS (First Quarter 2013), 28; AHA Central Office: Chicago, IL, USA, 2013.
22. American Hospital Association (AHA). *Use of Imaging Reports for Greater Specificity*; AHA Coding Clinic for ICD-10-CM and ICD-10-PCS (Third Quarter 2014), 5; AHA Central Office: Chicago, IL, USA, 2014.
23. American Hospital Association (AHA). *Use of X-ray to Determine Site of Pain*; AHA Coding Clinic for ICD-10-CM and ICD-10-PCS (Fourth Quarter 2016), 143; AHA Central Office: Chicago, IL, USA, 2016.
24. Alzheimer's Disease International. Dementia Statistics. Available online: https://www.alzint.org/about/dementia-facts-figures/dementia-statistics (accessed on 23 October 2023).
25. Arvanitakis, Z.; Shah, R.C.; Bennett, D.A. Diagnosis and management of dementia: Review. *JAMA* **2019**, *322*, 1589–1599. [CrossRef] [PubMed]
26. Butler, D.; Kowall, N.W.; Lawler, E.; Gaziano, J.M.; Driver, J.A. Underuse of diagnostic codes for specific dementias in the Veterans Affairs New England healthcare system. *J. Am. Geriatr. Soc.* **2012**, *60*, 910–915. [CrossRef] [PubMed]
27. Drabo, E.F.; Barthold, D.; Joyce, G.; Ferido, P.; Chang, C.H.; Zissimopoulos, J. Longitudinal analysis of dementia diagnosis and specialty care among racially diverse Medicare beneficiaries. *Alzheimers Dement.* **2019**, *15*, 1402–1411. [CrossRef] [PubMed]
28. Fujiyoshi, A.; Jacobs, D.R., Jr.; Alonso, A.; Luchsinger, J.A.; Rapp, S.R.; Duprez, D.A. Validity of death certificate and hospital discharge ICD codes for dementia diagnosis: The Multi Ethnic Study of Atherosclerosis. *Alzheimer Dis. Assoc. Disord.* **2017**, *31*, 168–172. [CrossRef] [PubMed]
29. Rios, N.G.; Oldiges, P.E.; Lizano, M.S.; Daucet-Wadford, D.S.; Quick, D.L.; Martin, J.; Korvink, M.; Gunn, L.H. Modeling coding intensity of procedures in a U.S. population-based hip/knee arthroplasty inpatient cohort adjusting for patient- and facility-level characteristics. *Healthcare* **2022**, *10*, 1368. [CrossRef] [PubMed]
30. Mishra, R.; Verman, H.; Aynala, V.B.; Arredondo, P.R.; Martin, J.; Korvink, M.; Gunn, L.H. Diagnostic coding intensity among a pneumonia inpatient cohort using a risk-adjustment model and claims data: A U.S. population-based study. *Diagnostics* **2022**, *12*, 1495. [CrossRef] [PubMed]
31. Glass, A.; Melton, N.C.; Moore, C.; Myrick, K.; Thao, K.; Mogaji, S.; Howell, A.; Patton, K.; Martin, J.; Korvink, M.; et al. A novel method for assessing risk-adjusted diagnostic coding specificity for depression using a U.S. cohort of over one million patients. *Diagnostics* **2024**, *14*, 426. [CrossRef] [PubMed]
32. PINC AI Applied Sciences. *PINC AI Healthcare Database White Paper: Data That Informs and Performs*; Premier Inc.: Charlotte, NC, USA, 2023; Available online: https://offers.premierinc.com/rs/381-NBB-525/images/PINC_AI_Healthcare_Data_White_Paper.pdf (accessed on 23 October 2023).
33. Centers for Disease Control and Prevention (CDC), Agency for Toxic Substances and Disease Registry. CDC SVI Documentation 2020. Available online: https://www.atsdr.cdc.gov/placeandhealth/svi/documentation/SVI_documentation_2020.html (accessed on 10 November 2023).

34. Centers for Medicare & Medicaid Services, Office of the Actuary, National Health Statistics Group. National Health Expenditure Data: Health Expenditures by State of Residence, August 2022. Available online: https://www.cms.gov/data-research/statistics-trends-and-reports/national-health-expenditure-data/state-residence (accessed on 10 November 2023).
35. Bradford, A.; Kunik, M.E.; Schulz, P.; Williams, S.P.; Singh, H. Missed and delayed diagnosis of dementia in primary care: Prevalence and contributing factors. *Alzheimer Dis. Assoc. Disord.* **2009**, *23*, 306–314. [CrossRef] [PubMed]
36. Podcasy, J.L.; Epperson, C.N. Considering sex and gender in Alzheimer disease and other dementias. *Dialogues Clin. Neurosci.* **2016**, *18*, 437–446. [CrossRef]
37. Lennon, J.C.; Aita, S.L.; Bene, V.A.D.; Rhoads, T.; Resch, Z.J.; Eloi, J.M.; Walker, K.A. Black and White individuals differ in dementia prevalence, risk factors, and symptomatic presentation. *Alzheimers Dement.* **2022**, *18*, 1461–1471. [CrossRef]
38. Herrera-Esposito, D.; de Los Campos, G. Age-specific rate of severe and critical SARS-CoV-2 infections estimated with multi-country seroprevalence studies. *BMC Infect. Dis.* **2022**, *22*, 311. [CrossRef] [PubMed]
39. Zhao, Y.; Paschalidis, I.C.; Hu, J. The impact of payer status on hospital admissions: Evidence from an academic medical center. *BMC Health Serv. Res.* **2021**, *21*, 930. [CrossRef] [PubMed]
40. Agency for Healthcare Research and Quality. Health Care Quality: How Does Your State Compare? Available online: https://www.ahrq.gov/data/infographics/state-compare-text.html (accessed on 14 November 2023).
41. Aranda, M.P.; Kremer, I.N.; Hinton, L.; Zissimopoulos, J.; Whitmer, R.A.; Hummel, C.H.; Trejo, L.; Fabius, C. Impact of dementia: Health disparities, population trends, care interventions, and economic costs. *J. Am. Geriatr. Soc.* **2021**, *69*, 1774–1783. [CrossRef] [PubMed]

healthcare

MDPI

Article

Modeling Multivariate Distributions of Lipid Panel Biomarkers for Reference Interval Estimation and Comorbidity Analysis

Julian Velev [1,2,*], Luis Velázquez-Sosa [3], Jack Lebien [2], Heeralal Janwa [4] and Abiel Roche-Lima [3]

1. Department of Physics, University of Puerto Rico, Puerto Rico, PR 00925-2537, USA
2. Abartys Health, San Juan, PR 00907-3913, USA; jlebien@abartyshealth.com
3. Center for Collaborative Research in Health Disparities, RCMI Program, Medical Science Campus, University of Puerto Rico, San Juan, PR 00936-5067, USA; luisfernandojavier.velazquez@upr.edu (L.V.-S.); abiel.roche@upr.edu (A.R.-L.)
4. Department of Mathematics, University of Puerto Rico, Puerto Rico, PR 00925-2537, USA; heeralal.janwa@upr.edu

* Correspondence: julian.velev@upr.edu

Abstract

Background/Objectives: Laboratory tests are a cornerstone of modern medicine, and their interpretation depends on reference intervals (RIs) that define expected values in healthy populations. Standard RIs are obtained in cohort studies that are costly and time-consuming and typically do not account for demographic factors such as age, sex, and ethnicity that strongly influence biomarker distributions. This study establishes a data-driven approach for deriving RIs directly from routinely collected laboratory results. **Methods**: Multidimensional joint distributions of lipid biomarkers were estimated from large-scale real-world laboratory data from the Puerto Rican population using a Gaussian Mixture Model (GMM). GMM and additional statistical analyses were used to enable separation of healthy and pathological subpopulations and exclude the influence of comorbidities all without the use of diagnostic codes. Selective mortality patterns were examined to explain counterintuitive age trends in lipid values while comorbidity implication networks were constructed to characterize interdependencies between conditions. **Results**: The approach yielded sex- and age-stratified RIs for lipid panel biomarkers estimated from the inferred distributions (total cholesterol, LDL, HDL, triglycerides). Apparent improvements in biomarker profiles after midlife were explained by selective survival. Comorbidities exerted pronounced effects on the 95% ranges, with their broader influence captured through network analysis. Beyond fixed limits, the method yields full distributions, allowing each individual result to be mapped to a percentile and interpreted as a continuous measure of risk. **Conclusions**: Population-specific and sex- and age-segmented RIs can be derived from real-world laboratory data without recruiting healthy cohorts. Incorporating selective mortality effects and comorbidity networks provides additional insight into population health dynamics.

Keywords: reference intervals; clinical laboratory data; Gaussian mixture models

1. Introduction

Cardiovascular disease (CVD) remains the leading cause of death in the United States, responsible for roughly one in every five deaths, and has held this position since 1950 [1,2]. Among the spectrum of CVDs, coronary artery disease (CAD) is the most prevalent, claiming over 370,000 lives in 2022, and affecting approximately 5% of adults aged 20 and older [2,3]. Established risk factors include non-modifiable traits such as age, sex, race, and genetics, as well as modifiable lifestyle factors—notably hypertension, hyperlipidemia, diabetes, obesity, smoking, poor diet, and physical inactivity [4]. While genetic predisposition remains significant, the growing obesity epidemic and its metabolic consequences—like diabetes and dyslipidemia—have increasingly driven the rise in cardiac conditions, particularly in developed nations.

Because lipid abnormalities are central to the development and progression of cardiovascular disease, the lipid panel (LP) has become the main laboratory tool for monitoring cardiovascular health and assessing risk [5–7]. It includes total cholesterol (CHOL), triglycerides (TRIG), high-density lipoprotein cholesterol (HDL), low-density lipoprotein cholesterol (LDL), and very-low-density lipoprotein (VLDL). These biomarkers represent different classes of lipoproteins—complexes of lipids and proteins that transport cholesterol and triglycerides through the bloodstream. HDL is termed "good cholesterol" because it helps remove excess cholesterol from tissues and plaques, whereas LDL is labeled "bad cholesterol" since elevated levels promote atherosclerosis and increase CVD risk [8]. Triglycerides, the main form of stored fat, are linked to insulin resistance, metabolic syndrome, and higher CVD risk, particularly when HDL is low [9].

Comorbidities have a significant impact on biomarker levels, and understanding their influence is essential for correctly interpreting LP results. In this study, we focus on two highly prevalent conditions—diabetes mellitus (DM) and chronic kidney disease (CKD)—that strongly affect cardiovascular outcomes [7]. Diabetes is a major risk factor for atherosclerotic cardiovascular disease through its effects on insulin resistance, dyslipidemia, and systemic inflammation [10]. CKD is likewise accompanied by dyslipidemia, typically characterized by elevated triglycerides and reduced HDL concentrations [7,11]. Their two key diagnostic markers—glycated hemoglobin (A1C) for diabetes and serum creatinine (CREA) for renal function—are included in the comprehensive metabolic panel (CMP) [5]. Since LP and CMP are often ordered together in routine general health screening, ample data are available for assessing how comorbidities influence lipid biomarkers.

Interpretation of these biomarkers depends on reference intervals (RIs), which define the expected range of values in healthy populations [12–15]. This term is preferred over "normal range" because it emphasizes comparison with a defined reference group rather than implying an absolute standard of health [14,16]. By convention, RIs correspond to the central 95% of the distribution in a healthy population [13]. Their use has been standardized by the International Federation of Clinical Chemistry (IFCC) and the Clinical and Laboratory Standards Institute (CLSI), which have issued detailed guidelines for their estimation and periodic updating [17].

Standard RIs are established through cohort studies, which require at least 120 healthy individuals for each analyte [17]. This approach is time-consuming and costly, making it difficult to update RIs regularly. As a result, many published intervals are outdated and lack stratification by sex, age, or ethnicity—factors known to strongly influence biomarker distributions [18–23]. These limitations can be addressed by indirect methods, which infer RIs from secondary use of data sources not originally collected for this purpose, such as clinical laboratory results [24–26].

Building on these advances, we have previously proposed indirect methods to estimate RIs from real-world clinical laboratory data originally collected for diagnostic purposes [27–29]. These approaches assume that each biomarker distribution consists of a dominant "healthy" component with pathological results superimposed [30]. Using Gaussian mixture models (GMM), we successfully separated these contributions and derived RIs for biomarkers related to CKD [27] and chronic liver disease (CLD) [29] in the Puerto Rican (PR) population.

In the present work, we extend these studies in two important ways. First, methodologically, we advance the GMM framework to multivariate data, using conditional probability distributions with comorbidity markers to better exclude pathological values without relying on diagnostic codes. This approach not only produces RIs that are more representative of the healthy population but also reveals how comorbidities systematically distort biomarker distributions. Second, epidemiologically, we leverage a very large dataset of laboratory results from the PR population to derive age- and sex-specific RIs at single-year resolution for key CVD-related biomarkers, providing the first large-scale characterization of this kind. In doing so, we also identify population-level patterns such as selective mortality, which help explain counterintuitive improvements in biomarker values at older ages, and we construct comorbidity implication networks to capture interdependencies among conditions and their impact on lipid biomarkers.

2. Materials and Methods

2.1. Data

In this study, data were obtained from the clinical results datalake of Abartys Health, a clinical laboratory data processor headquartered in San Juan, PR, which aggregates laboratory test results from hundreds of laboratories across the island. All data were de-identified by removing personally identifiable information (e.g., names, dates of birth, addresses); unique patients were assigned non-descriptive identifiers, with only age and sex retained as demographic information. In accordance with US CFR 46.104(d), analysis of de-identified results does not require patient consent. The study protocol was reviewed and approved by the University of Puerto Rico—Medical Sciences IRB (Ref. 2301072914).

After extracting the data for each measure, results are coarse-grained by month: multiple readings for the same individual within a given month are averaged. Most patients have only a single monthly reading, but a small subset—likely hospitalized patients—show multiple results. In such cases, coarse-graining helps reduce bias toward more severely ill individuals. Finally, the datasets for all measures are merged by patient ID and the corresponding year and month of testing.

The dataset covers LP results [5] from 2019 to 2024. Because LP and CMP are routinely prescribed as screening tests during medical visits, the resulting data for these biomarkers is extensive, as summarized in Table 1.

Table 1. Lipid panel and comorbidity biomarkers: number of test results and unique individuals for the period 2019–2024. The merged ("Joined") dataset refers to the subset of cases where all biomarkers were available in the same time window.

Biomarker	Results	Persons	Male	Female
Total cholesterol (CHOL) Triglycerides (TRIG) Low-density lipoprotein (LDL) High-density lipoprotein (HDL)	4,349,050	1,353,928	574,275	779,653
Hemoglobin A1c (A1C)	2,322,403	842,429	347,790	494,639
Creatinine (CREA)	6,003,119	1,613,033	689,537	923,496
Joined	1,775,134	717,312	296,470	420,842

From 2019 to 2024, the dataset contains over 4.3 million LP results covering more than 1.3 million unique individuals, with a comparable number of records for the renal panel. About two million glycemic tests are available in the data. The sex distribution across these datasets is fairly consistent at approximately 42% male and 58% female. When restricted to lipid biomarkers tests performed within the same time window and alongside contemporary glycemic and renal tests, the joint dataset includes about 1.8 million results representing roughly 0.7 million individuals (Table 1). Additional details on the data collection and processing are given in the Supplementary Materials.

2.2. Methods

As described in our previous work, GMM was used to analyze the data distribution [27,29].

2.2.1. Transformation

The quantitative biomarkers considered in this study are strictly positive, as they represent concentrations, counts, or ratios. Their empirical distributions are typically either approximately normal or lognormal, depending on the underlying physiology. Many biomarkers are subject to homeostatic regulation, which constrains their values within a narrow physiological range around an equilibrium. Deviations from this equilibrium arise due to differences in body size, metabolic rate, and other natural variations. In such cases, a normal distribution provides an adequate description. Conversely, biomarkers such as those in the lipid panel often display multiplicative variability, leading to skewed distributions that are more appropriately modeled as lognormal. To accommodate this, we apply logarithmic transformations to skewed variables prior to further analysis, thereby stabilizing the variance and producing approximately symmetric distributions suitable for multivariate Gaussian modeling.

Each analyte i have an invertible, monotone transform T_i (e.g., $T_i(x) = \log x$ or identity). The model is fit in the transformed space $Z_i = T_i(X_i)$ where $Z \sim \mathcal{N}(\mu, \Sigma)$ are normally distributed. All conditioning values b (and any bounds used elsewhere) are first mapped to Gaussian space via $b_i^{(G)} = T_i(b_i)$. After sampling or computing percentiles/ellipsoids in Gaussian space, results are mapped back analyte-wise by $X_i = T_i^{-1}(Z_i)$.

2.2.2. Joint Distribution

After log-transforming skewed biomarkers, the resulting data can be modeled using Gaussian mixtures. We assume that the observed population consists of a dominant distribution corresponding to physiologically healthy individuals, with pathological results appearing as secondary modes superimposed on this background. GMM provides a natural framework to disentangle these contributions and identify the principal component associated with health [31].

Formally, the probability distribution of an d-dimensional biomarker vector $X = (X_1, X_2, \ldots, X_d) \in R^d$ Gaussian space (after any feature-wise transforms), modeled as a convex combination of multivariate Gaussian densities

$$p(X) = \sum_{k=1}^{K} w_k \mathcal{N}(X \mid \mu_k, \Sigma_k) \tag{1}$$

where w_k are non-negative mixture weights satisfying $\sum_{k=1}^{K} w_k = 1$, and $\mu_k \in R^d$ is the mean vector, and $\Sigma_k \in R^{d \times d} \succ 0$ denote the positive definite covariance matrix of the k-th Gaussian component, respectively.

To estimate these parameters from data, we employ a Bayesian Gaussian Mixture Model (BGMM), which performs variational inference rather than standard maximum likelihood estimation. A key advantage of BGMM is its adaptive treatment of the number of active mixture components: instead of fixing K, a Dirichlet process prior allows redundant components to be suppressed, yielding a parsimonious representation. In practice, we implement this approach using the scikit-learn BGMM algorithm [32,33]. The healthy reference distribution is then defined as the principal Gaussian component, i.e., the mixture element with the largest weight w_k, which captures the central tendency of the majority population.

2.2.3. Marginal and Conditional Distributions

Let $X = (X_1, \ldots, X_d) \sim \mathcal{N}(\mu, \Sigma)$ be a d-dimensional Gaussian random vector.

- Marginals

For a subset of indices $A \subset \{1, \ldots, d\}$, the marginal distribution of the subvector X_A is itself Gaussian, with parameters obtained by restricting the mean and covariance:

$$X_A \sim \mathcal{N}(\mu_A, \Sigma_{AA}) \quad (2)$$

where μ_A and Σ_{AA} denote the sub-vector and sub-matrix of μ and Σ, respectively.

In particular, for a single analyte X_i, the univariate distribution is obtained as the marginal with $A = \{i\}$. Marginals reduce the dimensionality of the distribution by integrating out irrelevant axes ($n < d$) and thus summarize the variability of a subset of analytes. Although they discard explicit dependencies with the remaining variables, they implicitly reflect the influence of the full joint distribution and therefore provide more robust information than univariate fits.

- Conditionals

For two disjoint index sets $A, B \subset \{1, \ldots, d\}$, the conditional distribution of X_A given $X_B = b$ is also Gaussian:

$$p(X_A | X_B = b) \sim \mathcal{N}\left(\mu_{A|B}, \Sigma_{A|B}\right) \quad (3)$$

where the partitioned mean and covariance are written as

$$X = \begin{bmatrix} X_A \\ X_B \end{bmatrix}, \mu = \begin{bmatrix} \mu_A \\ \mu_B \end{bmatrix}, \Sigma = \begin{bmatrix} \Sigma_{AA} & \Sigma_{AB} \\ \Sigma_{BA} & \Sigma_{BB} \end{bmatrix} \quad (4)$$

and the conditional parameters are

$$\begin{aligned} \mu_{A|B} &= \mu_A + \Sigma_{AB} \Sigma_{BB}^{-1} (b - \mu_B) \\ \Sigma_{A|B} &= \Sigma_{AA} - \Sigma_{AB} \Sigma_{BB}^{-1} \Sigma_{BA} \end{aligned} \quad (5)$$

Like marginals, conditional distributions reduce dimensionality by integrating out irrelevant coordinates. But first they restrict the distribution to a subset of axes under fixed values of another disjoint subset ($m < d$).

3. Results

3.1. Joint Distribution

We applied the proposed methodology to the metabolic biomarker dataset described in Section 2.1. As an initial step, we constructed the joint distribution of all lipid panel biomarkers together with relevant comorbidity markers. To normalize the skewed distributions, logarithmic transformations were applied CHOL, TRIG, HDL, LDL, and VLDL, while A1C and CREA were left untransformed. Outliers were generally retained to preserve the natural variability of the population, with the exception of physiologically implausible values, which were excluded using predefined biomarker-specific thresholds. An overview of the data preparation, model fitting, and inference workflows is provided in the Supplementary Materials (Figures S1 and S2).

Subsequently, the BGMM was fitted to the full dataset, yielding the joint seven-dimensional distribution of all biomarkers, $p(X)$. The BGMM incorporates a Dirichlet process prior, which adaptively determines the effective number of active components. In this study, we specified a maximum of K = 7 Gaussian components, ensuring that several components could remain inactive if unsupported by the data.

The weights represent the relative proportion of the population assigned to each component. As shown in Figure 1, only two mixture components consistently carried substantial weight (>10%). The dominant component, corresponding to the healthy subpopulation, accounted for 40–80% of the distribution. Its weight was highest in younger age groups, where pathological conditions are less prevalent and the main distribution remains less distorted. The second major component captured pathological or outlier contributions, with its relative weight increasing in older age groups as comorbidities became more frequent. Together, these weights provide a quantitative view of how the balance between healthy and pathological subpopulations shifts across age and sex.

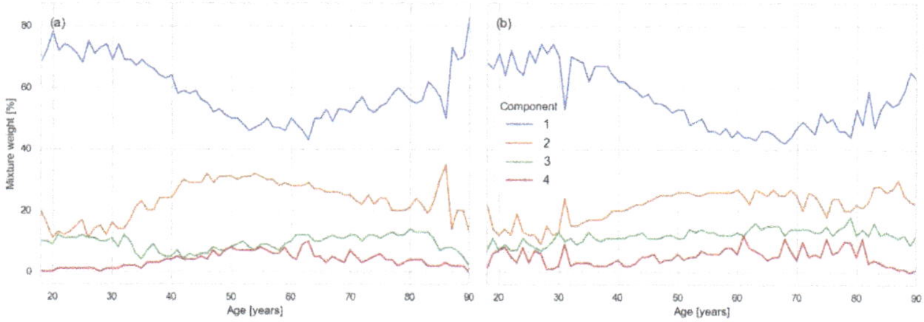

Figure 1. Weights (w_k) of the major mixture components (1–4) of the lipid distributions identified by the BGMM, stratified by sex and age. Panel (**a**) shows results for males and panel (**b**) for females.

We optimized the model hyperparameters to bias the fit toward a dominant "central" Gaussian component representing the healthy population, while still allowing additional components to capture pathological or secondary subpopulations. The prior mean was estimated as the feature-wise median to reduce sensitivity to outliers, and the covariance prior was regularized with diagonal shrinkage to ensure stability and avoid ill-conditioning in higher dimensions. To encourage sparsity, the Dirichlet weight concentration prior was set to a very low value (10^{-6}), thereby limiting the number of active components. Conversely, the mean precision prior was set high (200.0) to constrain the component means more closely around the overall population mean.

The effect of the GMM is twofold: first, it separates multimodal Gaussian structures, and second, it effectively absorbs outliers in the distribution tails by allocating a specific component to them. In one dimension, the healthy and pathological contributions overlap substantially, so pathological values primarily shift the mean and increase the weight of the tail rather than forming distinct modes. In contrast, in the seven-dimensional space, pathological values appear as separate modes that collapse onto each other in the one-dimensional projection. Our results indicate the presence of two to three such satellite modes, each carrying a substantial portion of the total weight (Figure 1). As population segments become less healthy, the weight of these satellite modes increases at the expense of the central distribution, reflecting the growing influence of pathological subgroups.

3.2. Marginal Distributions and Reference Intervals

One-dimensional marginal distributions, $p(X_i)$, for each analyte were obtained from the joint distribution $p(X)$, as described in the Methods. From each marginal distribution, it is possible to calculate the limits corresponding to any quantile q. RIs were defined as the limits (l, h) enclosing the central 95% of the distribution.

First, we estimated RIs for CHOL stratified by sex and age (Figure 2). The gray line represents the marginal distributions of CHOL as described in the Methods. During adolescence, CHOL RIs were similar in males and females. With increasing age, however, both the lower and upper limits rose, with a steeper slope in males. The values peaked around age 45 in males and 55 in females, after which both limits gradually declined. This decline is consistent with the effect of selective mortality, as discussed further in the Discussion.

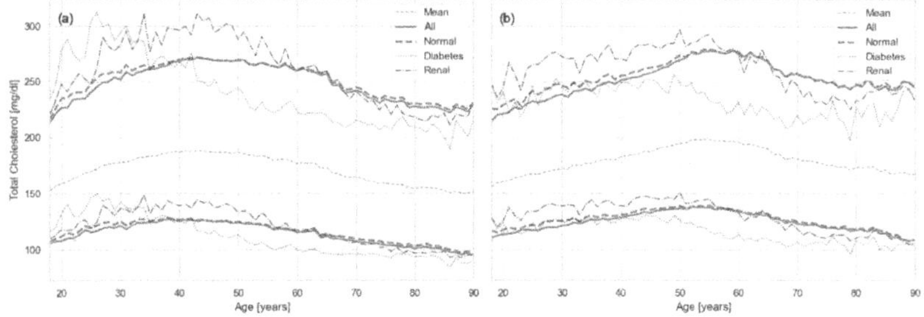

Figure 2. Age- and sex-specific RIs for CHOL: (**a**) males and (**b**) females. Solid gray lines show overall RIs, dashed gray show the mean of the distribution, dashed green show RIs restricted to metabolically normal individuals, while red and blue lines show conditional RIs for individuals with diabetes and renal disease, respectively.

The conditional distributions derived from the joint model provide deeper insight into the structure of RIs. In addition to the overall cohort RIs, we computed 95% intervals for sub-cohorts affected by comorbidities. In Figure 2, the red line corresponds to the diabetic sub-cohort (A1C = 9.0%) and the blue line to the renal disease sub-cohort (CREA = 2.0 mg/dL), where the values in of the diagnostic markers were chosen well in the unhealthy range. The presence of comorbidities markedly altered the lipid profile. Among younger adults with diabetes, the upper limit of CHOL was substantially elevated and the onset of selective mortality occurred earlier. Similarly, renal disease was associated with a pronounced increase in the upper limit of CHOL, although it did not seem to affect the selective mortality.

Conditional modeling also enabled the exclusion of comorbidity effects without requiring explicit diagnostic labels. By constraining analytes to healthy ranges (A1C = 5.7%, CREA = 1.0 mg/dL), the green line in Figure 2 captures the "true" RI for otherwise healthy adults. The near coincidence of the green (constrained) and gray (unconstrained) lines demonstrates that the BGMM successfully isolates the principal healthy distribution from pathological clusters. Nevertheless, along the comorbidity axes the distribution retains the imprint of disease effects, such that conditional probabilities in those directions still reveal how comorbidities distort lipid biomarkers. This illustrates that while the BGMM separates healthy and pathological populations, it also preserves meaningful covariance structure with comorbidity-related variables.

The RIs for the complementary cholesterol biomarkers, HDL and LDL, are shown in Figures 3 and 4, respectively. HDL levels remained relatively stable across the cohort until middle age, after which a modest increase was observed, attributable to selective mortality (Figure 3). More striking, however, was the effect of comorbidities on HDL. In particular, diabetes caused a pronounced reduction in "good" cholesterol, underscoring its role as a strong contributor to cardiovascular risk [10].

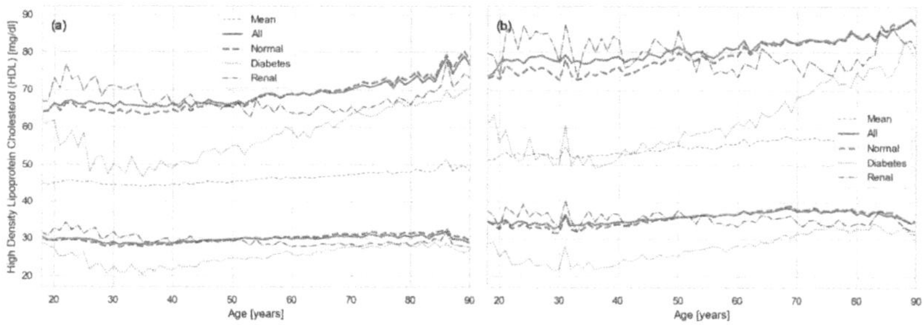

Figure 3. Age- and sex-specific RIs for HDL: (**a**) males and (**b**) females. Solid gray lines show overall RIs, dashed gray show mean of the distribution, dashed green represent RIs constrained to metabolically normal individuals, while red and blue lines indicate conditional RIs for diabetes and renal disease, respectively.

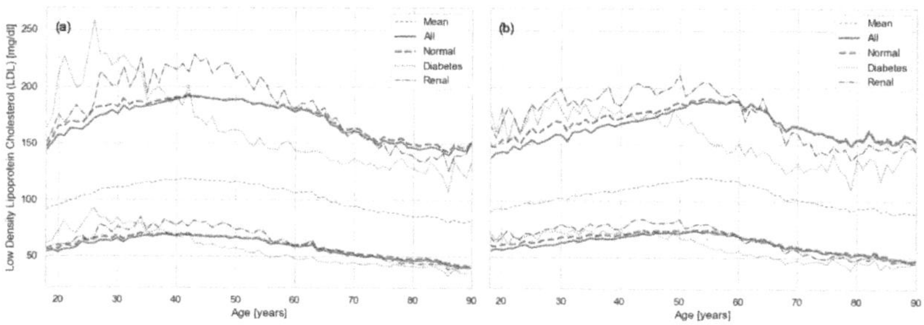

Figure 4. Age- and sex-specific RIs for LDL: (**a**) males and (**b**) females. Solid gray lines show overall RIs, dashed gray show the mean of the distribution, dashed green represent RIs constrained to metabolically normal individuals, while red and blue lines indicate conditional RIs for diabetes and renal disease, respectively.

The RIs for LDL (Figure 4) followed the same pattern as those for CHOL, since LDL values reported in clinical laboratories are typically not measured directly but calculated using the Friedewald formula: $LDL = CHOL - HDL - VLDL$ where VLDL is estimated as $VLDL = TRIG/5$ [34]. As a result, LDL behavior largely mirrored that of total cholesterol. However, the impact of comorbidities was amplified, because LDL incorporates both the elevation of total cholesterol and the reduction in high-density lipoprotein (HDL, "good" cholesterol).

The RIs for TRIG are shown in Figure 5. Their pattern resembled that of CHOL, with values rising until middle age and then declining due to selective mortality. The influence of comorbidities, however, was distinct. Diabetes exerted an even stronger effect on TRIG than on CHOL, consistent with the close metabolic relationship between triglycerides and glucose. Renal disease, in contrast, showed its strongest impact in older individuals, significantly increasing triglyceride levels in the elderly population probably due to less efficient filtration.

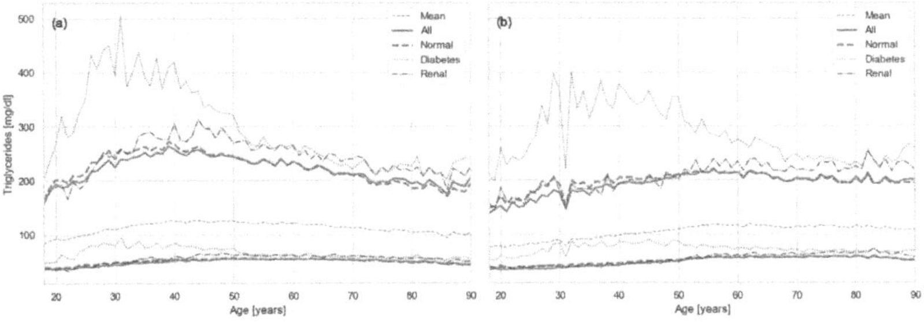

Figure 5. Age- and sex-specific RIs for TRIG: (**a**) males and (**b**) females. Solid green lines show overall RIs, dashed gray show the mean of the distribution, dashed green represent RIs constrained to metabolically normal individuals, while red and blue lines indicate conditional RIs for diabetes and renal disease, respectively.

The uncertainty in RI estimation was quantified using bootstrapping. Specifically, 100 random subsamples were drawn, each comprising 50% of the dataset, and RI limits were recalculated for each iteration. The final RI limits were taken as the mean across bootstrap samples, and the associated error was estimated as the standard deviation. The resulting errors were consistently small—on the order of a fraction of a percent—indicating high robustness of the estimates. Comparable stability was observed in our previous studies [27,29].

4. Discussion

4.1. RI Interpretation

Internationally accepted RIs for lipid biomarkers are largely derived from U.S. and European populations [6,7]. These conventional RIs are typically reported as fixed thresholds and are not stratified by sex, age, or race, despite well-documented physiological differences across demographic groups. In contrast, our approach uses real-world clinical laboratory data to derive population-specific RIs, as demonstrated here for the PR population. The scale and richness of the dataset further allow stratification by age and sex, yielding intervals that more accurately capture biological variation within the population.

A key observation from our results (Figures 2–5) is the strong effect of age on lipid biomarker distributions. Applying a single RI across all ages fails to account for the normal, progressive decline in organ function, effectively treating age as a pathological state. In reality, most metabolic biomarkers—including those beyond the lipid panel—shift inexorably toward less favorable values with age [27,29]. Sex differences are also evident, driven by factors such as body size and hormone-related physiology. Thus, the conventional RIs used in current practice represent little more than population-wide averages, obscuring the biologically meaningful variation attributable to age and sex.

Our results for CHOL indicate that the upper RI limit in the PR population exceeds the widely recommended threshold of 200 mg/dL, even among young adults (Figure 2). Values rise quickly beyond the high-risk cutoff of 240 mg/dL, suggesting an accelerated trajectory toward dyslipidemia. A similar trend is observed for LDL, which largely mirrors total cholesterol, with upper limits exceeding the recommended threshold of 100 mg/dL (Figure 4). Triglycerides show the same pattern (Figure 5), with values generally above the established cutoff of 150 mg/dL. HDL levels are consistent with this unfavorable profile: the lower limit in our results falls below the conventional threshold of 40 mg/dL.

Together, these patterns suggest a population-wide shift toward higher cardiometabolic risk, likely influenced by dietary habits rich in fried foods and by the high prevalence of obesity, which increasingly affects younger age groups. Alternatively, this may suggest that the currently recommended cutoffs underestimate the physiological lipid ranges for the PR population—or perhaps for broader populations as well. It could also be that existing RIs for CHOL and LDL are set conservatively low, in part to encourage pharmacological intervention with statins. This interpretation aligns with recent evidence questioning whether elevated LDL levels are consistently associated with increased all-cause mortality [35].

It can also be argued that the distribution mean, rather than the conventional RI upper limit, is a more informative indicator of population health. The standard 95% interval is directly defined by the mean and standard deviation, $[\mu - 1.96\sigma, \mu + 1.96\sigma]$, and narrower published RIs may simply reflect the limited diversity of the clinical trial cohorts from which they were derived. In contrast, our dataset captures the full PR population, providing a more representative picture. This underscores a broader issue with the way RIs and their associated abnormal flags are applied in practice: RIs define only hard cutoffs and do not convey how values are distributed within those limits. As a result, the laboratory abnormal flag is binary—indicating only whether a value lies inside or outside the interval. By modeling the full distribution, we can assign each individual measurement a percentile, offering a continuous measure of risk rather than a simple threshold. We have previously proposed this percentile-based framework as a more nuanced and clinically meaningful approach [27,29].

Finally, it is also important to emphasize the substantial sex differences in lipid profiles that are obscured by generalized recommendations. Females consistently exhibit lower CHOL and LDL levels, substantially higher HDL, and markedly lower TRIG compared to males—differences that are largely attributable to biological factors such as hormonal regulation and body composition. At the same time, the more rapid deterioration of lipid biomarkers observed in males likely reflects behavioral and lifestyle influences, compounding the biological baseline differences between the sexes.

4.2. Selective Mortality

The gradual rise in CHOL and LDL, coupled with a decline in HDL during early and mid-adulthood, aligns with the expected pattern of metabolic aging and physiological decline. This is consistent with the gradual loss of organ function due to normal wear and tear with age. Similar trajectories were seen in our earlier studies of CKD, where creatinine and urea levels increase steadily with age [27], and of CLD, where platelet counts and albumin concentrations progressively decrease [29].

However, lipid biomarkers display an unexpected pattern after midlife: CHOL and LDL values decline, while HDL rises. Although this could appear to reflect improved cardiovascular health, the paradox is better explained by selective mortality. Younger adults are resilient enough to survive despite adverse biomarker profiles, so their gradual health decline is visible in worsening trends. Beyond midlife, however, physiological reserves diminish, and the body can no longer compensate for chronic dysfunction. As a result, the least healthy individuals are more likely to die earlier, shifting the observed population distribution toward healthier values. The apparent improvement in biomarker profiles therefore reflects differential mortality rather than true physiological recovery. This interpretation is consistent with prior epidemiological studies reporting U-shaped cholesterol–mortality associations, where low cholesterol values in older adults were inversely associated with all-cause mortality and partly attributed to selective survival effects [36,37]. Nevertheless, similar reductions have also been observed longitudinally within individuals, suggesting that additional metabolic factors contribute [38].

The magnitude of selective mortality also varies across conditions. Some chronic dysfunctions, such as CKD, can often be tolerated until later in life and therefore do not substantially alter the overall trajectory of the lipid curves. In contrast, conditions that contribute more directly to early mortality, such as diabetes and cardiovascular disease, shift the onset of selective mortality to earlier ages. This difference is evident in our results (Figures 2–5), where CKD does not substantially change the lipid curves, while DM produces a marked shift toward earlier onset of selective mortality.

For comparison, mortality rates for the PR population were estimated using U.S. Census data for the period 2020–2024, stratified by sex [39]. For each year, we calculated the fraction of individuals of age x who survived to age $x + 1$ in the following year and then averaged these survival rates across years to reduce variability. The annual mortality rate, defined as (1 − survival rate), is shown by age and sex in Figure 6a. Mortality remained relatively stable through early and middle adulthood, though subject to fluctuations likely attributable to migration and other demographic factors. Beginning in midlife, however, mortality rose exponentially, consistent with the Gompertz law, a well-documented demographic pattern of age-dependent mortality rise [40].

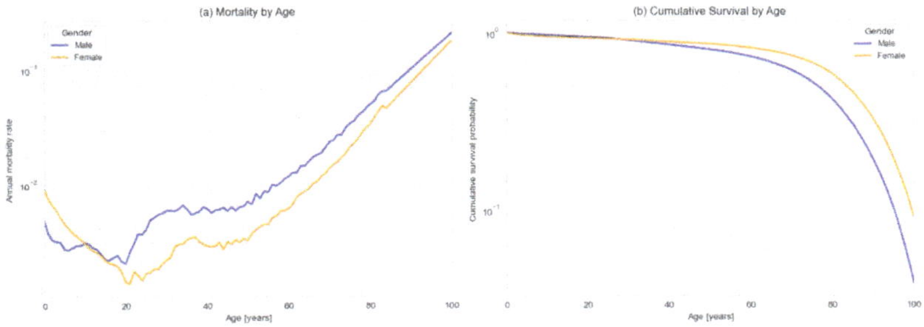

Figure 6. Mortality and survival functions for the PR population (2020–2024), stratified by sex. (**a**) Annual mortality rates by age, shown on a logarithmic scale. (**b**) Corresponding cumulative survival functions.

The corresponding cumulative survival function, $S(x)$, representing the fraction of the population surviving to age x, is shown in Figure 6b. Consistent with the RI curves, survival declines approximately exponentially at advanced ages, with males consistently exhibiting lower survival than females across the entire age range.

Although the survival function aggregates all causes of mortality and cannot be stratified by specific causes using the available census data, it nevertheless explains the patterns observed in the lipid panel RIs. Because male mortality is higher, individuals with adverse lipid profiles are removed from the cohort earlier, producing the earlier decline in elevated CHOL and LDL values in men. Similarly, sub-cohorts affected by specific chronic conditions would be expected to have steeper survival curves than the population average, leading to an earlier onset of mortality and corresponding shifts in their biomarker distributions.

4.3. Implication Network

To better understand how comorbidities influence lipid panel biomarkers, we constructed a comorbidity implication network. For this purpose, a set of diagnostic criteria was developed, as summarized in Table 2, and then joined biomarker data by patient ID and date to apply these rules. This framework allowed us to model disease co-occurrence and explore how multiple conditions interact within individuals. This methodology aligns with contemporary network medicine approaches—where diseases are represented as nodes and statistically derived associations as edges—to uncover patterns of comorbidity and aid in identifying preconditions and complications within patient trajectories [41,42].

Table 2. Diagnostic criteria used to define cardiovascular conditions and comorbidities based on laboratory biomarkers. Thresholds were selected from established clinical guidelines to identify hyperlipidemia, CVD (moderate and high risk), DM, and CKD.

Biomarker	Results
Hypercholesterolemia	cholesterol > 200
Hypertriglyceridemia	triglycerides > 150
CVD (High Risk)	(cholesterol/hdl > 5.0) or (ldl/hdl > 3.5)
CVD (Moderate Risk)	(4.0 < cholesterol/hdl < 5.0) or (2.5 < ldl/hdl < 3.5)
Diabetes Mellitus	hga1c > 6.5
Chronic Kidney Disease	creatinine > 1.3

After assigning diagnoses, we calculated the conditional probability that an individual has condition B given the presence of condition A

$$P(B|A) = \frac{N(A \cap B)}{N(A)} \tag{6}$$

where $N(A \cap B)$ is the number of individuals with both A and B, and $N(A)$ is the number of individuals with A. Together with the complementary probability $P(A|B)$, these values were used to construct the implication matrix, defined as $I[A, B] = P(A|B)$. This matrix serves as the foundation for the comorbidity implication network, where directed edges capture the strength and asymmetry of conditional relationships between diseases. Additional details on the construction of the implication matrix, together with its heatmap representation, are provided in Figure S3.

We then constructed a comorbidity network defined as a directed graph, using the implication matrix I as the adjacency matrix. The resulting network, illustrated in Figure 7, was analyzed with the Hyperlink-Induced Topic Search (HITS) algorithm to identify hub and authority nodes [43]. Conditions with high hub scores act as precursors, pointing toward multiple downstream comorbidities and serving as initiators of disease cascades. In contrast, conditions with high authority scores function as endpoints, receiving links from many hubs and representing common complications or outcomes of diverse pathological pathways.

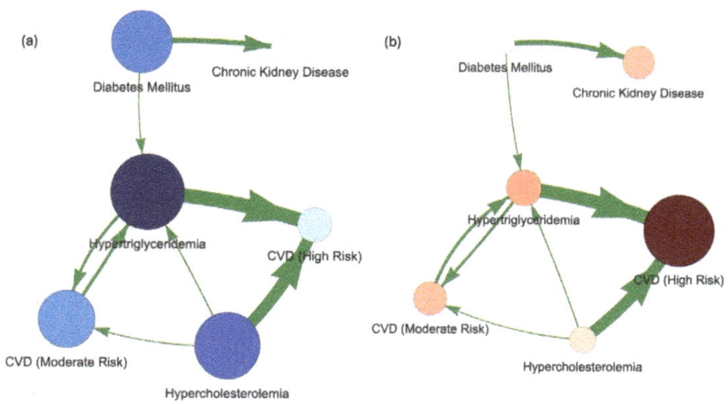

Figure 7. Comorbidity implication network for cardiovascular risk conditions. (**a**) Hub representation, where larger nodes indicate conditions with strong hub scores (precursors leading to multiple downstream comorbidities). (**b**) Authority representation, where larger nodes correspond to conditions with high authority scores (common complications influenced by multiple precursors). Arrow direction and thickness indicate conditional probabilities P(A | B), and only the strongest 75% of edges are displayed for clarity.

The network provides a qualitative view of the relationships among comorbidities. As expected, both hypercholesterolemia and hypertriglyceridemia showed strong implications for CVD, reflected in both edge strengths and high hub scores (Figure 7a). Diabetes also emerged as an important precondition. Conversely, CVD appeared as the most common complication of hyperlipidemia (Figure 7b), while CKD was more closely associated as a complication of diabetes. The strong linkage between hyperlipidemia and CVD is partly tautological, since CVD risk is clinically estimated using cholesterol ratios (Table 2). Nevertheless, the network highlights important nuances: elevated triglycerides were more strongly associated with moderate CVD risk, whereas high cholesterol was more indicative of severe CVD risk. Furthermore, high cholesterol also appeared as a possible precondition for elevated triglycerides.

Even more importantly, the network helps to elucidate how comorbidities directly affect lipid biomarkers. For instance, diabetes appears as a precondition for elevated triglycerides. Impaired glucose metabolism in diabetes promotes hepatic triglyceride synthesis and reduces lipid clearance, leading to hypertriglyceridemia. This, in turn, amplifies cardiovascular risk by contributing to atherogenic dyslipidemia, characterized by high triglycerides, low HDL, and elevated small dense LDL particles.

4.4. Limitations and Future Work

4.4.1. Ground Truth and Laboratory Data Limitations

The principal issue with underrepresented populations, such as PR, is that there are no cohort studies of population that could provide independent validation of the derived RIs. Moreover, chemical laboratory data represents only one side of the health profile of the individual. It lacks important invocators such as vital signs (height, weight, blood pressure, etc.) and other relevant information about the patients' condition such as pregnancy, postpartum, or perimenopause. Better analyses would require linkage with electronic health records (EHRs) to enrich the laboratory data.

4.4.2. Data Standardization and Harmonization

Although Abartys Health's core business involves collecting, cleaning, and standardizing laboratory data across PR, challenges remain due to the lack of standardized and adherence to exchange formats in raw clinical data. Common issues that cannot be easily corrected include—incorrect or ambiguous coding of tests (that cannot distinguish between several closely related tests); lack of detailed metadata on analytical principles, reagents, and platforms that hamper data harmonization; lack of units or incorrect units, etc.

4.4.3. Future Work

The application by this methodology is by no means specific to the PR population. It is fully generalizable provided that routine laboratory test results with demographic information (sex and age) are available. The additional features (e.g., ethnicity) can be easily incorporated to further stratify the RIs. In this case, the PR population serves not only as illustration but also provides valuable epidemiological information of an underrepresented population.

Furthermore, while here we only consider two comorbidities, this is not a limitation of the methodology. This is done to introduce and illustrate the idea of comorbidity networks in a simple form while capturing two of the major comorbidities—DM and CKD—that are highly prevalent in the population. Comorbidity networks construction from laboratory data is only limited by the possibility of diagnosing condition entirely based on laboratory data. There must be sufficient data for the principal biomarkers and the comorbidities available within the same time window.

5. Conclusions

This study demonstrates that Gaussian mixture modeling provides a robust framework for disentangling healthy from pathological distributions in large-scale, real-world laboratory data. By leveraging conditional probability, we were able to estimate definitive RIs for healthy cohorts without relying on diagnostic labels. Conditional modeling further revealed how comorbidities such as diabetes and renal disease systematically alter lipid distributions, while comorbidity implication networks clarified dependencies between conditions and highlighted key precursors and complications.

Unlike traditional RIs, which are reported only as fixed limits, our approach models the entire distribution of biomarker values in the population. This enables each individual result to be placed on a continuous percentile scale of risk, rather than being reduced to a binary abnormal flag. Such distribution-aware reporting provides a more nuanced basis for clinical decision-making.

Finally, our analysis highlights that the narrower RIs in published guidelines likely reflect the limited diversity of the clinical trial cohorts from which they were derived. In contrast, our framework captures the biological and demographic variability of the PR population, underscoring the need for population-specific standards derived from representative real-world data.

Supplementary Materials: The following supporting information can be downloaded at: https://www.mdpi.com/article/10.3390/healthcare13192499/s1, Figure S1: Workflow overview: (a) data preprocessing from raw laboratory results to aligned person–month records, and (b) Bayesian Gaussian mixture model fitting across demographic segments; Figure S2: Inference workflows: (A) construction of reference surfaces (RS) or one-dimensional reference intervals (RI) from the healthy population component, and (B) computation of percentiles for individual biomarker results within the population distribution; Figure S3: Heatmap of the comorbidity implication matrix, showing conditional probabilities $P(B \mid A)$ for all pairs of conditions. Warmer colors indicate stronger directional associations, highlighting asymmetries in comorbidity relationships.

Author Contributions: Conceptualization, J.V., A.R.-L. and H.J.; methodology, J.V. and J.L.; software, J.V.; validation, J.V., J.L. and L.V.-S.; formal analysis, J.V.; investigation, J.V.; resources, J.V.; data curation, J.V.; writing—original draft preparation, J.V.; writing—review and editing, J.V. and A.R.-L.; visualization, J.V.; supervision, A.R.-L.; project administration, A.R.-L.; funding acquisition, A.R.-L. All authors have read and agreed to the published version of the manuscript.

Funding: This research was funded by the Office of the Director, National Institutes of Health Common Fund under award numbers 1OT2OD032581-02-235 and 3OT2OD032581-01S5-826 (Artificial Intelligence/Machine Learning Consortium to Advance Health Equity and Researcher Diversity (AIM-AHEAD)). This research was also supported by the Center for Collaborative Research in Health Disparities (CCRHD), RCMI grant U54 MD007600 (National Institute on Minority Health and Health Disparities) from the National Institutes of Health.

Institutional Review Board Statement: The laboratory test results were retrieved from laboratory information systems serving the clinical laboratories in PR. As stipulated by the US Code of Federal Regulation CFR 46.104(d), the analysis of test results does not require patients' explicit informed consent if the identity of the human subjects cannot readily be ascertained directly or through identifiers linked to the subjects. The use of the datasets has been reviewed and approved by the Institutional Review Board of the office of Human Research Subjects Protection at the University of Puerto Rico—Medical Sciences (reference number 2301072914 on 11 January 2023).

Informed Consent Statement: Informed consent was not required due to data was obtained from the clinical results datalake of Abartys Health. The data is de-identified by removing all personally identifiable information (PII) such as names, dates of birth, and addresses. Unique patients are assigned non-descriptive identifiers and non-PII demographic information, such as age and sex, is also available.

Data Availability Statement: The data that support the findings of this study were licensed from Abartys Health for the purposes of this study alone and are not publicly available. Data access requests can be addressed to the corresponding author who would relay them to Abartys Health. Reasonable requests for access to the original code used to analyze the data can be directed to the corresponding author.

Conflicts of Interest: Julian Velev and Jack LeBien have received compensation and/or own stock in Abartys Health. The company was not involved in the study design, collection, analysis, interpretation of data, the writing of this article or the decision to submit it for publication. The remain authors declare no potential conflict of interest.

Abbreviations

The following abbreviations are used in this manuscript:

PR	Puerto Rico
PII	Personally identifiable information
LP	Lipid panel
CMP	Comprehensive metabolic panel
RI	Reference interval
GMM	Gaussian mixture model
BGMM	Bayesian Gaussian mixture model
CHOL	Total cholesterol
TRIG	Triglycerides
LDL	Low-density lipoprotein
HDL	High-density lipoprotein
A1C	Hemoglobin A1c
CREA	Serum creatinine
DM	Diabetes mellitus
CVD	Cardiovascular disease
CAD	Coronary artery disease
CKD	Chronic kidney disease
CLD	Chronic liver disease

References

1. Tsao, C.W.; Aday, A.W.; Almarzooq, Z.I.; Anderson, C.A.M.; Arora, P.; Avery, C.L.; Baker-Smith, C.M.; Beaton, A.Z.; Boehme, A.K.; Buxton, A.E.; et al. Heart Disease and Stroke Statistics—2023 Update: A Report from the American Heart Association. *Circulation* **2023**, *147*, 8. [CrossRef] [PubMed]
2. Centers for Disease Control and Prevention (CDC) Heart Disease Facts. Available online: https://www.cdc.gov/heart-disease/data-research/facts-stats/ (accessed on 23 August 2025).
3. Centers for Disease Control and Prevention (CDC) Heart Disease Deaths. Available online: https://www.cdc.gov/nchs/hus/topics/heart-disease-deaths.htm (accessed on 23 August 2025).
4. Martin, S.S.; Aday, A.W.; Almarzooq, Z.I.; Anderson, C.A.M.; Arora, P.; Avery, C.L.; Baker-Smith, C.M.; Barone Gibbs, B.; Beaton, A.Z.; Boehme, A.K.; et al. 2024 Heart Disease and Stroke Statistics: A Report of US and Global Data from the American Heart Association. *Circulation* **2024**, *149*, 8. [CrossRef] [PubMed]
5. Van Leeuwen, A.M.; Bladh, M.L. *Davis's Comprehensive Manual of Laboratory and Diagnostic Tests with Nursing Implications*, 9th ed.; F.A. Davis Company: Philadelphia, PA, USA, 2021; ISBN 9781719640589.
6. Arrobas Velilla, T.; Guijarro, C.; Ruiz, R.C.; Piñero, M.R.; Valderrama Marcos, J.F.; Pérez Pérez, A.; Botana López, A.M.; López, A.M.; García Donaire, J.A.; Obaya, J.C.; et al. Consensus Document for Lipid Profile Testing and Reporting in Spanish Clinical Laboratories: What Parameters Should a Basic Lipid Profile Include? *Adv. Lab. Med. Av. Med. Lab.* **2023**, *4*, 138–146. [CrossRef] [PubMed]
7. Davidson, M.H.; Altenburg, M. Dyslipidemia. Available online: https://www.merckmanuals.com/professional/endocrine-and-metabolic-disorders/lipid-disorders/dyslipidemia (accessed on 23 August 2025).

8. Ouimet, M.; Barrett, T.J.; Fisher, E.A. HDL and Reverse Cholesterol Transport. *Circ. Res.* **2019**, *124*, 1505–1518. [CrossRef]
9. Miller, M.; Stone, N.J.; Ballantyne, C.; Bittner, V.; Criqui, M.H.; Ginsberg, H.N.; Goldberg, A.C.; Howard, W.J.; Jacobson, M.S.; Kris-Etherton, P.M.; et al. Triglycerides and Cardiovascular Disease. *Circulation* **2011**, *123*, 2292–2333. [CrossRef]
10. Kosmas, C.E.; Bousvarou, M.D.; Kostara, C.E.; Papakonstantinou, E.J.; Salamou, E.; Guzman, E. Insulin Resistance and Cardiovascular Disease. *J. Int. Med. Res.* **2023**, *51*. [CrossRef]
11. Tonelli, M.; Wanner, C. Kidney Disease: Improving Global Outcomes Lipid Guideline Development Work Group Members Lipid Management in Chronic Kidney Disease: Synopsis of the Kidney Disease: Improving Global Outcomes 2013 Clinical Practice Guideline. *Ann. Intern. Med.* **2014**, *160*, 182. [CrossRef]
12. Geffré, A.; Friedrichs, K.; Harr, K.; Concordet, D.; Trumel, C.; Braun, J.-P. Reference Values: A Review. *Vet. Clin. Pathol.* **2009**, *38*, 288–298. [CrossRef]
13. Ceriotti, F.; Hinzmann, R.; Panteghini, M. Reference Intervals: The Way Forward. *Ann. Clin. Biochem. Int. J. Lab. Med.* **2009**, *46*, 8–17. [CrossRef]
14. Gräsbeck, R. The Evolution of the Reference Value Concept. *Clin. Chem. Lab. Med.* **2004**, *42*, 692–697. [CrossRef]
15. Siest, G.; Henny, J.; Gräsbeck, R.; Wilding, P.; Petitclerc, C.; Queraltó, J.M.; Petersen, P.H. The Theory of Reference Values: An Unfinished Symphony. *Clin. Chem. Lab. Med. (CCLM)* **2013**, *51*, 47–64. [CrossRef]
16. Grasbeck, R.; Saris, N.E. Establishment and Use of Normal Values. *Scand. J. Clin. Lab. Investig.* **1969**, *26*, 62–63.
17. Horowitz, G.L.; Altaie, S.; Boyd, J.C.; Ceriotti, F.; Garg, U.; Horn, P.; Pesce, A.; Sine, H.E.; Zakowski, J. *Defining, Establishing, and Verifying Reference Intervals in the Clinical Laboratory: Approved Guideline*; Clinical and Laboratory Standards Institute: Wayne, PA, USA, 2008; ISBN 1-56238-682-4.
18. Colantonio, D.A.; Kyriakopoulou, L.; Chan, M.K.; Daly, C.H.; Brinc, D.; Venner, A.A.; Pasic, M.D.; Armbruster, D.; Adeli, K. Closing the Gaps in Pediatric Laboratory Reference Intervals: A CALIPER Database of 40 Biochemical Markers in a Healthy and Multiethnic Population of Children. *Clin. Chem.* **2012**, *58*, 854–868. [CrossRef]
19. Yang-Chun, F.; Min, F.; Di, Z.; Yan-Chun, H. Retrospective Study to Determine Diagnostic Utility of 6 Commonly Used Lung Cancer Biomarkers Among Han and Uygur Population in Xinjiang Uygur Autonomous Region of People's Republic of China. *Medicine* **2016**, *95*, e3568. [CrossRef]
20. Schini, M.; Nicklin, P.; Eastell, R. Establishing Race-, Gender- and Age-Specific Reference Intervals for Pyridoxal 5′-Phosphate in the NHANES Population to Better Identify Adult Hypophosphatasia. *Bone* **2020**, *141*, 115577. [CrossRef]
21. Mayr, F.X.; Bertram, A.; Cario, H.; Frühwald, M.C.; Groß, H.-J.; Groening, A.; Grützner, S.; Gscheidmeier, T.; Hoffmann, R.; Krebs, A.; et al. Influence of Turkish Origin on Hematology Reference Intervals in the German Population. *Sci. Rep.* **2021**, *11*, 21074. [CrossRef] [PubMed]
22. Sasamoto, N.; Vitonis, A.F.; Fichorova, R.N.; Yamamoto, H.S.; Terry, K.L.; Cramer, D.W. Racial/Ethnic Differences in Average CA125 and CA15.3 Values and Its Correlates among Postmenopausal Women in the USA. *Cancer Causes Control* **2021**, *32*, 299–309. [CrossRef] [PubMed]
23. Ma, S.; Yu, J.; Qin, X.; Liu, J. Current Status and Challenges in Establishing Reference Intervals Based on Real-World Data. *Crit. Rev. Clin. Lab. Sci.* **2023**, *60*, 427–441. [CrossRef] [PubMed]
24. Sikaris, K.A. Separating Disease and Health for Indirect Reference Intervals. *J. Lab. Med.* **2021**, *45*, 55–68. [CrossRef]
25. Farrell, C.J.L.; Nguyen, L. Indirect Reference Intervals: Harnessing the Power of Stored Laboratory Data. *Clin. Biochem. Rev.* **2019**, *40*, 99–111. [CrossRef]
26. Jones, G.R.D.; Haeckel, R.; Loh, T.P.; Sikaris, K.; Streichert, T.; Katayev, A.; Barth, J.H.; Ozarda, Y. Indirect Methods for Reference Interval Determination-Review and Recommendations. *Clin. Chem. Lab. Med.* **2019**, *57*, 20–29. [CrossRef]
27. Velev, J.; LeBien, J.; Roche-Lima, A. Unsupervised Machine Learning Method for Indirect Estimation of Reference Intervals for Chronic Kidney Disease in the Puerto Rican Population. *Sci. Rep.* **2023**, *13*, 17198. [CrossRef]
28. LeBien, J.; Velev, J.; Roche-Lima, A. Indirect Reference Interval Estimation Using a Convolutional Neural Network with Application to Cancer Antigen 125. *Sci. Rep.* **2024**, *14*, 19332. [CrossRef] [PubMed]
29. Velev, J.; Lebien, J.; Hernandez-Suarez, D.; Roche-Lima, A. Machine Learning Method to Estimate Multivariate Reference Surfaces from Real-World Data Applied to Liver Disease Diagnostics in the Puerto Rican Population. *BMC Med. Inform. Decis. Mak.* 2025, *submitted*.
30. Ammer, T.; Schützenmeister, A.; Prokosch, H.-U.; Zierk, J.; Rank, C.M.; Rauh, M. RIbench: A Proposed Benchmark for the Standardized Evaluation of Indirect Methods for Reference Interval Estimation. *Clin. Chem.* **2022**, *68*, 1410–1424. [CrossRef] [PubMed]
31. Murphy, K.P. *Machine Learning: A Probabilistic Perspective*; MIT Press: Cambridge, MA, USA, 2012; ISBN 9780262018029.
32. Pedregosa, F.; Varoquaux, G.; Gramfort, A.; Michel, V.; Thirion, B.; Grisel, O.; Blondel, M.; Prettenhofer, P. and Weiss, R.; Dubourg, V.; Vanderplas, J.; Passos, A.; et al. Scikit-Learn: Machine Learning in Python. *J. Mach. Learn. Res.* **2011**, *12*, 2825–2830.
33. Scikit-Learn 1.3.0 Bayesian Gaussian Mixture Model. Available online: https://scikit-learn.org/stable/modules/generated/sklearn.mixture.BayesianGaussianMixture.html (accessed on 29 August 2023).

34. Friedewald, W.T.; Levy, R.I.; Fredrickson, D.S. Estimation of the Concentration of Low-Density Lipoprotein Cholesterol in Plasma, without Use of the Preparative Ultracentrifuge. *Clin. Chem.* **1972**, *18*, 499–502. [CrossRef]
35. Ravnskov, U.; Diamond, D.M.; Hama, R.; Hamazaki, T.; Hammarskjöld, B.; Hynes, N.; Kendrick, M.; Langsjoen, P.H.; Malhotra, A.; Mascitelli, L.; et al. Lack of an Association or an Inverse Association between Low-Density-Lipoprotein Cholesterol and Mortality in the Elderly: A Systematic Review. *BMJ Open* **2016**, *6*, e010401. [CrossRef]
36. Jacobs, D.; Blackburn, H.; Higgins, M.; Reed, D.; Iso, H.; McMillan, G.; Neaton, J.; Nelson, J.; Potter, J.; Rifkind, B. Report of the Conference on Low Blood Cholesterol: Mortality Associations. *Circulation* **1992**, *86*, 1046–1060. [CrossRef]
37. Hu, F.; Wang, Z.; Liu, Y.; Gao, Y.; Liu, S.; Xu, C.; Wang, Y.; Cai, Y. Association between Total Cholesterol and All-Cause Mortality in Oldest Old: A National Longitudinal Study. *Front. Endocrinol.* **2024**, *15*. [CrossRef]
38. Ferrara, A.; Barrett-Connor, E.; Shan, J. Total, LDL, and HDL Cholesterol Decrease with Age in Older Men and Women. *Circulation* **1997**, *96*, 37–43. [CrossRef]
39. US Census Bureau Puerto Rico Commonwealth Population by Characteristics: 2020–2024. Available online: https://www.census.gov/data/tables/time-series/demo/popest/2020s-detail-puerto-rico.html (accessed on 23 August 2025).
40. Gompertz, B. XXIV. On the Nature of the Function Expressive of the Law of Human Mortality, and on a New Mode of Determining the Value of Life Contingencies. In a Letter to Francis Baily, Esq. F. R. S. & c. *Philos. Trans. R. Soc. Lond.* **1825**, *115*, 513–583. [CrossRef]
41. Hidalgo, C.A.; Blumm, N.; Barabási, A.-L.; Christakis, N.A. A Dynamic Network Approach for the Study of Human Phenotypes. *PLoS Comput. Biol.* **2009**, *5*, e1000353. [CrossRef]
42. Barabási, A.-L.; Gulbahce, N.; Loscalzo, J. Network Medicine: A Network-Based Approach to Human Disease. *Nat. Rev. Genet.* **2011**, *12*, 56–68. [CrossRef]
43. Kleinberg, J.M. Authoritative Sources in a Hyperlinked Environment. *J. ACM* **1999**, *46*, 604–632. [CrossRef]

healthcare

MDPI

Article

Optimizing Nurse Rostering: A Case Study Using Integer Programming to Enhance Operational Efficiency and Care Quality

Aristeidis Mystakidis [1], Christos Koukaras [2], Paraskevas Koukaras [1], Konstantinos Kaparis [3], Stavros G. Stavrinides [2] and Christos Tjortjis [1,*]

[1] School of Science and Technology, International Hellenic University, 14th km Thessaloniki-Moudania, 57001 Thessaloniki, Greece; a.mystakidis@ihu.edu.gr (A.M.); p.koukaras@ihu.edu.gr (P.K.)
[2] Department of Physics, Democritus University of Thrace, University Campus, St. Lucas, 65404 Kavala, Greece; ckoukara@physics.duth.gr (C.K.); sstavrin@physics.duth.gr (S.G.S.)
[3] School of Business Administration, University of Macedonia, 156 Egnatia Street, 54636 Thessaloniki, Greece; k.kaparis@uom.edu.gr
* Correspondence: c.tjortjis@ihu.edu.gr

Abstract: Background/Objectives: This study addresses the complex challenge of Nurse Rostering (NR) in oncology departments, a critical component of healthcare management affecting operational efficiency and patient care quality. Given the intricate dynamics of healthcare settings, particularly in oncology clinics, where patient needs are acute and unpredictable, optimizing nurse schedules is paramount for enhancing care delivery and staff satisfaction. **Methods:** Employing advanced Integer Programming (IP) techniques, this research develops a comprehensive model to optimise NR. The methodology integrates a variety of constraints, including legal work hours, staff qualifications, and personal preferences, to generate equitable and efficient schedules. Through a case study approach, the model's implementation is explored within a clinical setting, demonstrating its practical application and adaptability to real-world challenges. **Results:** The implementation of the IP model in a clinical setting revealed significant improvements in scheduling efficiency and staff satisfaction. The model successfully balanced workload distribution among nurses, accommodated individual preferences to a high degree, and ensured compliance with work-hour regulations, leading to optimised shift schedules that support both staff well-being and patient care standards. **Conclusions:** The findings underscore the effectiveness of IP in addressing the complexities of NR in oncology clinics. By facilitating a strategic allocation of nursing resources, the proposed model contributes to operational excellence in healthcare settings, underscoring the potential of Operations Research in enhancing healthcare delivery and management practices.

Keywords: nurse rostering; integer programming; healthcare management; operational efficiency; oncology departments; health informatics; healthcare analytics

1. Introduction

Operations Research (OR) applies advanced analytical methods to optimise decision-making in complex organizational contexts. One such challenge is the Nurse Rostering Problem (NRP), where the allocation of nursing staff is vital for both patient care and operational efficiency. In oncology departments, efficient nurse scheduling is essential to ensure continuous, high-quality care [1–4].

To address this, recent OR research integrates mathematical models with healthcare management. Solutions often involve mathematical optimisation, including Integer Programming (IP), which offers a robust framework for improving NR in dynamic clinical settings. However, the use of such models in oncology clinics presents new obstacles and potential. Oncology departments have unpredictable demand patterns and a vital requirement for specialised treatment, which requires a flexible and strong rostering method [5]. Furthermore, the well-being of nursing staff, a vital component of sustainable healthcare delivery, must be included in the optimisation process, guaranteeing schedules that are not only efficient but also equitable and attentive to individual nurses' needs [6].

The method used in this work is mathematical optimisation, focusing on accuracy and simplicity. In order to maximise operational efficiency, the optimal solution under the specified constraints is found, using mathematical formulations, such as linear and IP, whose integration attempts to distribute the work hours among nursing staff in a real case study.

The extension of the current model to incorporate Machine-Learning (ML) techniques offers an innovative approach to decision-making processes traditionally addressed through heuristics. For instance, employing supervised ranking for specific inputs during the subsidiary Mixed-Integer Programming (MIP) phases improves the overall performance of MIP solution mechanisms, aligning with studies indicating the feasibility of such applications [7,8]. Moreover, to improve NR efficiency and decision-making, the conceived approach can benefit from incorporating the modelling of complex information networks [9] to analyse the intricate interactions between nurses, patients, and various clinical factors. Such an approach can use bi-functional ML algorithms tailored to the dynamic nature of healthcare settings.

Finally, using linear regression to predict the annual number of shifts per nurse, coupled with data storage for weekly updates, facilitates adaptive learning by the program, while aiming to correct nurse scheduling over time to balance their workload throughout the year.

1.1. Problem Statement

Oncology departments' NR is a classic operational challenge, driven by the requirement to match healthcare delivery to patient needs. Oncology patients require expert treatment and continuity, making this challenge even greater [3,10]. The traditional scheduling paradigms, often reliant on manual processes and heuristic decision-making, fall short in addressing the multifaceted dimensions of this problem, leading to inefficiencies that impact both patient care and staff welfare [4,11,12]. However, existing methodologies struggle to incorporate real-time data and adapt to sudden changes, resulting in either overstaffing, which strains resources, or understaffing, which compromises care quality and increases stress on the nursing staff [5].

The introduction of IP and other mathematical optimisation techniques offers a viable solution. These models can create flexible scheduling systems that better address the complexities of NR in oncology departments [7]. These advanced models have potential, but applying them in real-world cases is challenging due to the complications of effectively reflecting the nursing workforce's limits and preferences and oncology patient care dynamics.

The contribution of this research lies in revealing how OR challenges are addressed in real healthcare settings. It demonstrates that theoretical models must be adapted and refined to effectively solve operational inefficiencies in healthcare institutions, thereby bridging the gap between theory and practice.

1.2. Integrating OR and Healthcare Management

This paper aims to critically examine the optimisation of rostering processes at a hospital in Greece, addressing the complexities of healthcare staffing. IP coupled with IBM's Cplex program [13], via the Java Iloplex library [14], plays a pivotal role in navigating these challenges. The methodology utilises a dual-strategy approach: applying all constraints initially and subsequently relaxing some to explore alternative solutions. This iterative process highlights the flexibility and adaptability essential in developing efficient rostering systems, emphasizing the importance of stakeholder engagement.

The primary objectives of this work, employing OR in healthcare management, are summarised below:

1. Analyze Existing Rostering Practices: Investigate current NR practices to identify inefficiencies and areas for improvement, creating a foundation for the application of mathematical optimisation techniques to address identified gaps.
2. Integrate IP Models: Explore the use of advanced IP models in NR, aiming to build a system with enhanced flexibility, efficiency, and adaptability. These models will balance the operational demands of oncology care with the preferences and well-being of nursing staff.
3. Enhance Operational Efficiency: Quantify the impact of IP-based rostering systems on operational efficiency, providing evidence through the literature on the practical benefits of optimisation techniques.
4. Promote Staff Satisfaction: Adhering to labour regulations, workload balance, equitable rostering, and personal constraints, the proposed OR solution indirectly aims to create a supportive working environment for nursing staff.
5. Develop a Scalable and Adaptable solution: Create a flexible rostering solution adaptable to various oncology departments, providing a model for systemic improvements in healthcare rostering practices.

2. Background

The origins of OR can be traced back to 1665, when Newton's method for solving differential equations was used. However, OR's major advancements occurred in the 20th century, particularly during World War II, when British and American military forces formed interdisciplinary teams to address wartime operational challenges. This period marked the official recognition of OR and demonstrated the effectiveness of scientific methodologies in solving complex problems [15].

Early efforts to address NRP primarily involved heuristic methods and basic mathematical programming [2,16]. These methods, although foundational, were eventually replaced by more sophisticated optimisation techniques, particularly Mixed Integer Linear Programming (MILP). These approaches facilitated the balancing of strict staffing requirements with nurse preferences, optimizing shift allocations and improving operational efficiency. MILP has been particularly effective in addressing the variable demands of oncology departments, where patient loads can fluctuate unpredictably [17,18].

The development of potent optimisation libraries like CPLEX and Gurobi [19] has accelerated the evolution of OR from theoretical frameworks to computational problem-solving. These tools, integrated into programming environments like Java and Python, have significantly enhanced the ability to apply IP to complex problems such as the NRP. This technological shift has democratised access to advanced methodologies, enabling their application across various healthcare settings.

2.1. *Definition and Challenges of Integer Programming*

LP is a methodological cornerstone in OR that focuses on maximising or minimising a linear objective function under a set of linear constraints [2]. LP's foundational role is pivotal in addressing a wide array of optimisation challenges across diverse fields, from resource allocation to financial planning, providing a structured approach to decision-making [18].

IP emerges as a specialised extension of LP, where decision variables are constrained to integer values, reflecting the discrete nature of many real-world problems. This distinction is crucial in scenarios where fractional solutions are infeasible or lack practical significance, such as scheduling, routing, and allocation tasks [20]. Pure Integer Programming (PIP) and MILP further expand the applicability of IP by accommodating purely integer and mixed (integer and continuous) variables, respectively, thus offering a more versatile toolkit for modelling complex systems [21,22].

Binary decision variables, a subset of IP, introduce the ability to model decisions in a binary format (e.g., yes/no, on/off), enabling the precise representation of choice-based constraints and logical conditions [23]. This binary structure is instrumental in formulating problems where decisions are inherently dichotomous, enhancing IP's utility in designing efficient and effective solutions [18].

Despite IP's rigid framework for addressing optimisation problems, the complexity of solving IP models increases exponentially with problem size, owing to the combinatorial explosion of possible solutions. This complexity necessitates the development of sophisticated solution techniques, such as the Branch and Bound and Branch and Cut algorithms, which systematically explore and prune the solution space to identify optimal or near-optimal solutions [18,24].

Cutting-plane methods are another example of how IP solution strategies are always changing. They provide a strong way to make IP models more specific by repeatedly adding constraints that get rid of parts of the solution space that can not be solved without leaving out any possible integer solutions [25].

2.2. Integer Programming Workforce Problems

The search for more effective scheduling techniques has been a result of the dynamic nature of workforce management, which is characterised by fluctuating employment levels and the need for flexible planning strategies. Innovations such as job rotation and part-time work have emerged as responses to these fluctuating demands, reflecting the evolving landscape of labour arrangements [3,4]. The seminal contributions by [2] introduced IP and MIP into workforce planning, marking a pivotal shift towards more sophisticated and flexible scheduling models.

The subsequent application of IP and MIP to address complex scheduling issues within organizations has been documented by [10,26,27]. These approaches have yielded mathematical models that optimise schedule management and resource allocation, enhancing the adaptability of workforce planning to changing conditions.

Further advancements in this domain, as demonstrated by [28–30], highlight the transformative impact of IP and MIP on improving job satisfaction, minimising employee stress, and boosting overall productivity and service quality. By refining shift scheduling and workload distribution strategies, these models contribute to creating a more equitable and satisfying work environment.

2.3. Mathematical Models of Workforce Planning

Mathematical modeling can address the challenges of workforce scheduling. In nurse scheduling, it can be modelled as a 0–1 shortest path network problem. This model was applied, effectively utilizing IP to optimise the allocation of nursing staff within healthcare settings, ensuring that operational demands were met efficiently and effectively [31].

Building on this foundation, hierarchical workforce scheduling was explored, devising mathematical models to delineate the organisation of staff based on skill levels and operational requirements [26]. These models facilitate the understanding of scheduling dynamics. Here, the flexibility for higher-skilled workers to substitute for lower-skilled ones is crucial, accommodating variable daily workloads and ensuring employees receive mandated days off. The objective function defined by [26] emphasises cost minimisation across the workforce composition (Equation (1)):

$$\min \sum_{k=1}^{m} C_k W_k \tag{1}$$

where W_k = Number of workers of type k, C_k = Cost of type k worker.

Expanding upon Billionnet's framework [26], another model was introduced accommodating diverse shift lengths and work patterns [28]. This adaptation allows for a more granular optimisation of workforce schedules, aligning shift assignments with operational demands and worker preferences. Their revised objective function, incorporating shift-specific costs, showcases the model's flexibility in addressing the scheduling complexities (Equation (2)):

$$\min \sum_{b=1}^{B} \sum_{k=1}^{m} C_{bk} W_{bk} \tag{2}$$

where b = Shift type variable.

b represents the shift type, integrating both cost and workforce considerations into the optimisation process [31]. Workforce scheduling models inherently grapple with the dual objectives of cost minimization and productivity maximisation. The inclusion of the variable C_{bk} in optimisation problems underlines the adaptability of IP in tailoring solutions to specific operational goals. This variable's strategic deployment enables adjustments to scheduling models, reflecting the dynamic interplay between cost efficiency and service quality.

The specific focus of this research on shift balance leverages the previous week's data to inform the scheduling model and stresses the importance of historical patterns in optimizing future workforce allocations. This approach aims to achieve an equitable distribution of morning, afternoon, and night shifts, offering a balanced and sustainable work environment [2].

The exploration of these mathematical models reveals the depth and versatility of IP in solving complex workforce scheduling problems. By incorporating historical data and sophisticated scheduling constraints, these models offer structured pathways towards optimising workforce allocations, proving it as an invaluable tool.

3. Case Study and Problem Definition

3.1. Overview of the Clinic

A specialized Oncology clinic in Greece that provides top-tier care, while representing a critical node in the healthcare landscape. Dedicated to delivering advanced treatments and ensuring optimal patient care through effective staff management and operational practices.

3.2. Description of the NRP

At the heart of the clinic's operational efficiency lies the complex task of NR. The goal is to systematically schedule a diverse and specialised nursing team to maintain continuous, round-the-clock patient care. This section delineates the composition of the nursing staff and the specific constraints that govern their scheduling, reflecting the broader challenges of healthcare workforce management.

3.2.1. Staff Composition and Detailed Scheduling Constraints

The clinic has a team of 13 nurses. Aliases were given to preserve anonymity, as shown in Table 1.

Table 1. Clinic nursing team.

Nurse Identifier	Role
Su	Supervisor (Nursing Supervisor)
De	Deputy (Assistant Nursing Supervisor)
N_0	TE Nurse
N_1	TE Nurse
N_2	TE Nurse
N_3	TE Nurse
N_4	TE Nurse
N_5	TE Nurse
N_6	TE Nurse
N_7	TE Nurse
N_{8S}	SE Nurse
N_{9S}	SE Nurse
N_{10S}	SE Nurse

Both *Su* and *De* are pivotal in ensuring consistent leadership and oversight, working fixed weekday shifts from 07.00 to 15.00. A critical rule is that they cannot be scheduled off on the same day to guarantee managerial continuity.

The roster includes eight Technological Education (TE) nurses and three Secondary Education (SE) nurses. TE nurses and SE nurses are indispensable for providing comprehensive care. A vital scheduling requirement is that SE nurses must always work alongside a TE nurse to ensure a blend of skills and expertise across all shifts, with the rest of the requirements shown in Table 2.

Table 2. Roles and key requirements.

Role/Group	Staff Members	Critical Scheduling Requirements
Leadership	*Su*, *De*	Both cannot be off on the same day. Fixed weekday shifts (07:00–15:00)
TE Nurses	N_0, N_1, N_2, N_3, N_4, N_5, N_6, N_7	TE nurses must work alongside SE nurses on all shifts
SE Nurses	N_{8S}, N_{9S}, N_{10S}.	Must always work with at least one TE nurse

The clinic adheres to a monthly scheduling system aimed at distributing the three eight-hour shifts (07:00–15:00, 15:00–23:00, 23:00–07:00) among the staff in a balanced manner. According to operational regulations, nurses are entitled to a minimum of 11 h of rest between shifts, although in practice, a 16 h rest period is enforced to enhance recovery and well-being. This scheduling paradigm underscores the necessity for a strategic approach to rostering that harmonises regulatory compliance, individual preferences, and clinical demands (Table 3).

Table 3. Basic monthly scheduling.

Shift Timing	Rest Period	Notes
07:00–15:00	Minimum 16 h	Balanced distribution of shifts
15:00–23:00	Minimum 16 h	Ensures adequate recovery
23:00–07:00	Minimum 16 h	Aligns with operational regulations

3.2.2. Problem and Rostering Constraints

The aim of the problem is to establish a fair distribution of morning, afternoon, and night shifts, while avoiding back-to-back shifts and ensuring an equal number of working days among nurses throughout the week (for instance, preventing one nurse from working six shifts while another works only two). It is often noted that nurses are scheduled for successive shifts without a minimum 16 h break between them. Moreover, there are situations where only one nurse is assigned to a shift that requires two due to poor scheduling, and conversely, there are times when four nurses are assigned to a shift that could be handled by fewer staff. During December, the schedule was devised initially with the restrictions applied as shown in Tables 4–6.

Initially, it is evident from the description that the two head nurses are not part of the primary problem since their hours are fixed (i.e., during breakfast) and thus do not need to be considered as parameters in the model. Consequently, the problem focuses on managing 11 nurses (N_0–N_{10S}). The model's objective is to solve the scheduling problem on a weekly basis, leveraging data from the preceding week. As the problem is aimed at minimization without any cost variables (such as labour costs), we incorporate, as additional constraints, the number of shifts worked by each nurse in the prior week and, as a variable, the type of shift assigned (morning, afternoon, or night).

Table 4. Nurse shift and duty scheduling overview.

Time Period	Shift Timing	Staffing Requirements
	Weekdays	
Morning Hours	07:00–15:00	Su, De, and a minimum of 2 nurses
Afternoon Hours	15:00–23:00	2 nurses, at least one must be TE
Evening Hours	23:00–07:00	2 nurses, at least one must be TE
	Public Holidays	
Morning	07:00–15:00	2 nurses, at least one must be TE
Afternoon	15:00–23:00	2 nurses, at least one must be TE
Evening	23:00–07:00	2 nurses, at least one must be TE
Public Holiday Duration	00:00–24:00	Defined from 00:00 to 00:00 the next day
Monthly Shift Coverage	–	62 h each for morning, afternoon, and evening
Night Shift (Extreme Case)	23:00–07:00	1 TE nurse minimum
General On-Call Duty	Various	2 nurses always present
	Additional Scheduling Rules	
Weekly Off-Days	–	If a nurse works on a weekend, they don't work during the week
Max Shifts per Week	–	5 shifts per nurse
Max Afternoon Shifts	–	3 shifts per week
Max Night Shifts	–	2 shifts per week
Public Holidays	–	December 25th, 26th, January 1st
General On-Call Dates	–	1st, 5th, 9th, 13th, 17th, 21st, 25th, 29th December

Table 5. Nurse scheduling requests and constraints.

Nurse	Time Period	Requests and Constraints
Su	07:00–15:00 (Weekdays)	Always works breakfast hours, off on weekends. Public Holidays on 25/12 and 26/12. Leave from 11/12 to 15/12
De	07:00–15:00 (Weekdays)	Works breakfast hours, off on weekends. Public Holiday on 25/12 and 26/12
N_0	23:00–07:00 (4/12)	On-call evening 4/12, can work mornings or take a day off. Parental leave on 7/12. Off on 9/12, 10/12, 23/12, 24/12. Holiday on 25/12 and 26/12
N_1	07:00–15:00 (10/12, 23/12, 25/12, 26/12)	Off on 5/12, 6/12, 7/12. On-call afternoon 11/12. Breakfast shift on 10/12, 23/12, 25/12, 26/12
N_2	07:00–15:00 (Various)	Leave from 4/12 to 8/12. Off on 2/12, 3/12, 9/12, 10/12, 30/12, 31/12. On-call afternoon 20/12
N_3	–	Special schedule adjusted to husband's program (Fixed by herself)
N_4	07:00–15:00 (Various)	Off on 1/12. Collected days off from 14/12 to 20/12 and prefers fewer afternoon shifts.
N_5	07:00–15:00 (Various)	Leave on 1/12 and 4/12. Off on 2/12 and 3/12
N_6	07:00–15:00 (24/12)	Requested to work in the morning on 24/12
N_7	23:00–07:00 (4 shifts)	Contract worker. Can work 4 evening shifts per month and 2 holidays. No afternoon shifts on Thursdays or Fridays
N_{8S}	07:00–15:00, 23:00–07:00 (25/12)	Off on 23/12, 24/12. Works morning and evening on 25/12, and evening on 26/12. Afternoon shift on 31/12
N_{9S}	07:00–15:00 (Mondays, Tuesdays)	Prefers not to work afternoons on Mondays and Tuesdays. Preferably works breakfast hours or takes a day off
N_{10S}	23:00–07:00 (4 shifts)	Contract worker. Can work 4 evening shifts per month and 2 shifts on holidays

Table 6. Additional nurse scheduling information.

Aspect	Details	Notes
Regular Leave Days	25 days	Permanent staff
Solemn Declaration Absence	4 days per year	Permanent staff
Educational Licenses	–	Not specified
Double Shift Rule	07:00–15:00 and 23:00–07:00	Followed by 23:00–07:00 shift or a day off
Night Shift	22:00–06:00	Defined time for night shifts
Public Holidays	00:00–24:00	Duration from midnight to midnight
Regular Leave Days Counting	–	Requires days off before and after the leave (preferable)
First Day After Leave	07:00–15:00 or Double Shift	Must be a morning or double shift
Days Off Per Week	2 days	Not necessarily within the same week
Holiday Work Compensation	–	Entitled to an extra day off
Double Shift After Afternoon	–	No double shift (07:00–15:00 and 23:00–07:00) after the afternoon (15:00–23:00)

Additionally, the general on-call duty may be covered by the two head nurses. The number of on-call shifts they handle is predetermined on a monthly basis. The modeling will proceed in two stages. First, a general model will be constructed, incorporating the weekly constraints, followed by a second stage where the specific constraints for each week will be applied. The data structure results in four distinct weekly scheduling problems, each using the same mathematical framework but subjected to varying limitations. To avoid redundancy, the initial focus will be on solving the problem for the first week. This problem is formulated as an MIP model.

3.3. Objective Function

The objective is to minimise the function $f(x)$, subject to the following constraints (Equation (3)):

$$\forall j \in J: \quad \left(\sum_{i \in I} X_{i,j} = 1\right) \wedge \left(\sum_{i \in I_{T(j)}} X_{i,j} \geq R_{T(j)}\right) \tag{3}$$

The problem for the first week will be solved using the MIP method, considering shift types (morning, afternoon, night) and the number of shifts from the previous week.

4. Methodology and Solution Approach

To address the problem, a combination of optimisation software and a programming language was employed. The software selected was IBM's ILOG CPLEX Optimisation Studio 12.8 (academic license), which is accessible through the library (`IloCplex`) and the jar file (`cplex.jar`, included with the installation of ILOG CPLEX Optimisation Studio). The programming language utilised was Java, though the software also supports Python, C#, and other languages. The Integrated Development Environment chosen for this task was Apache NetBeans 8.2 [32], along with Java version 8 [33]. The mathematical method implemented by the software was the branch-and-cut technique.

Initially, 42 shifts of 8 h each needed to be allocated among 11 employees. We defined $i \rightarrow$ each employee and $j \rightarrow$ each shift, with the first two shifts on the 1st of the month designated as morning shifts (each day comprises 2 morning, 2 afternoon, and 2 night shifts). Additionally, since i, j are indivisible, it follows that $i, j \in \mathbb{Z}$. The distribution of each (s)hift (from s0–s41) is detailed in Table 7.

Table 7. Shift schedule for the first week of December.

	December (1st Week)						
Day	**Fri**	**Sat**	**Sun**	**Mon**	**Tue**	**Wed**	**Thu**
Morning	s_0, s_1	s_6, s_7	s_{12}, s_{13}	s_{18}, s_{19}	s_{24}, s_{25}	s_{30}, s_{31}	s_{36}, s_{37}
Afternoon	s_2, s_3	s_8, s_9	s_{14}, s_{15}	s_{20}, s_{21}	s_{26}, s_{27}	s_{32}, s_{33}	s_{38}, s_{39}
Night	s_4, s_5	s_{10}, s_{11}	s_{16}, s_{17}	s_{22}, s_{23}	s_{28}, s_{29}	s_{34}, s_{35}	s_{40}, s_{41}

The aforementioned number may be adjusted if on-call responsibilities necessitate the presence of an additional nurse during the evening hours of the on-call duty. It is essential to note that, for clarity in code comprehension and for the convenience of programmatic resolution, we assume that the numbering of nurses and shifts commences from 0 rather than 1. Likewise, the same logic applies to shifts. Therefore, we get Equation (4).

$$42 = \sum_{i=0}^{10} \sum_{j=0}^{41} X_{ij} \tag{4}$$

$$X_{ij} \in \{0,1\}, \quad \forall i \in \{0,\ldots,10\}, j \in \{0,\ldots,41\}.$$

Each nurse may be reassigned following the conclusion of their shift, ensuring a minimum of 11 h (inclusive of a 2 h break) prior to commencing the subsequent shift. Also, each nurse cannot be assigned more than 5 consecutive shifts (Equation (5)). If this condition is not met, the schedule is considered invalid, and she will have to take a day off the following day.

$$\sum_{j=0}^{41} X_{ij} \leq 5 \tag{5}$$

Each shift is covered by exactly one nurse (Equation (6)).

$$\sum_{i=0}^{10} X_{ij} = 1 \tag{6}$$

$$X_{ij} \in \{0,1\}, \quad \forall i \in \{0,\ldots,10\}, j \in \{0,\ldots,41\}.$$

Let the morning shifts {0, 1,. . . , 37} belong to set Π and the afternoon shifts {2, 3, . . . , 39} belong to set A, while the night shifts {4, 5, . . . , 41} belong to the set B.

The SE nurses (N_{8S}, N_{9S}, N_{10S}) cannot be scheduled in the same shift without TE nurses. Therefore, two TE nurses cannot be on the same shift together. Thus, the following stands:

$$\begin{aligned} X_{ij} + X_{i(j+1)} &\leq 1, \quad \forall i \in A, j \in B, \\ X_{ij} + X_{k(j+1)} &\leq 1, \quad \forall i,k \in A \cup \{8\}, i \neq k, j \in B, \\ X_{ij} + X_{k(j-1)} &\leq 1, \quad \forall i,k \in A \cup \{8\}, i \neq k, j \in B. \end{aligned}$$

Furthermore, the nurses with limited time contracts, N_7 and N_{10S}, can cover at max 4 night shifts per month with no more than 1 night shift per week. Thus, we get Equation (7):

$$\sum_{j \in B} X_{ij} \leq 1, \quad \forall i \in \{7,10\}. \tag{7}$$

Concerning the remaining nurses, except for N_3, who has her own schedule, each one can cover a maximum of 2 night shifts per week. Thus, we get (Equation (8)):

$$\sum_{j \in B} X_{ij} \leq 2, \quad \forall i \in \{0,1,2,4,5,6,8,9,10\} \tag{8}$$

Additionally, the maximum number of consecutive night shifts that a nurse can work within a scheduling period is three (Equation (9)):

$$\sum_{j\in A} X_{ij} \leq 3, \tag{9}$$

The model will be a minimisation model, aiming to ensure balance in shift allocation among the staff. This is done using the weight index for each employee for each shift, $C_{i\Pi}, C_{iA}, C_{iB}$ (morning, afternoon, night). This estimator-index was determined empirically through trials discussed later and from the feedback provided by the hospital workers.

Making an inquiry for every shift of the upcoming scheduling, it will be shown that the morning, being the most desired and with the largest demand, will not allow a higher shift rate for a nurse to cover the morning shift alone. Consequently, $C_{i\Pi} = 1$.

Similarly, a parallel evaluation is conducted for the night shifts. Considering that the night shift (23:00–07:00) is the hardest to cover, based on the feedback from the nurses, it should carry the highest weight. Initially, with trial values of $C_{iB} = 1.4$, $C_{iB} = 1.3$, or $C_{iB} = 1.2$ for each night shift, it was observed that if a nurse covered many night shifts the previous week, there is a risk that the weight of the night shifts for the upcoming week would become too large, and thus, one night shift would be equivalent to 2 or 3 morning shifts. Consequently, it was determined that for each night shift, $C_{iB} = 1.1$, with the total shift weight from the previous week calculated as (Equation (10)):

$$C_{iB} = 1 + 0.1\left(\sum_{j\in B} X_{ij}\right) \tag{10}$$

Finally, for the afternoon shift, the weight estimator should lie between the weight of the morning shift ($C_{i\Pi} = 1$) and the night shift ($C_{iB} = 1.1$) 8 h period. As with the night shift, through trials ($C_{iA} = 1.04$, $C_{iA} = 1.03$, or $C_{iA} = 1.02$), an attempt is made to find the appropriate estimator so that, in cases where a nurse covers many afternoon shifts, it is not considered that the weight of 3 or 4 afternoon shifts is numerically equivalent to the weight of 1 night shift. Thus, it was estimated that, for each afternoon shift, $C_{iA} = 1.01$, with the total weight of the shifts from the previous week (Equation (11)):

$$C_{iA} = 1 + 0.01\left(\sum_{j\in A} X_{ij}\right) \tag{11}$$

with

$$\min \sum_{i=1}^{11} \sum_{j\in J_i} C_{ij} X_{ij}$$

Note, if N_2 had worked 2 consecutive afternoons and 3 night shifts during the previous week, for the current week, we would get $C_{2A} = 1.02$ and $C_{2B} = 1.3$.

In accordance with the schedule of the last scheduling period—end of November in Table 8. Note that the '+' symbol indicates pairs of nurses on the same shift.

Table 8. ID distribution per shift for November's last week.

Last Week of November							
Day	**Fri**	**Sat**	**Sun**	**Mon**	**Tue**	**Wed**	**Thu**
Morning	$N_2 + N_{8S}$, $N_3 + N_7$	N_2, N_7	N_0, $N_1 + N_7$	$N_0 + N_2$, $N_4 + N_6$	N_2, $N_6 + N_{9S}$	N_1, $N_6 + N_{10}$	$N_0 + N_7$, $N_2 + N_6 + N_{8S}$
Afternoon	N_5, N_{9S}	N_6, N_{9S}	N_{10S}, N_6	N_1, N_7	N_3, N_7	N_3, N_7	N_{10S}, N_4
Night	N_1, N_{10S}	N_2, N_3	N_0, $N_3 + N_{10S}$	N_0, N_4	-, N_4	N_1, N_{9S}	N_{8S}, N_6

We get:

$$C_{i\Gamma} = 1, \quad \forall i \in \{0,1,2,3,4,5,6,7,8,9,10\},$$

$$C_{iA} = \begin{cases} 1 & \text{if } i \in \{0,2,8\}, \\ 1.01 & \text{if } i \in \{1,4,5,10\}, \\ 1.02 & \text{if } i \in \{3,6,9\}, \\ 1.03 & \text{if } i = 7, \end{cases}$$

$$C_{iB} = \begin{cases} 1.2 & \text{if } i \in \{0,1,3,4,10\}, \\ 1.1 & \text{if } i \in \{2,6,9\}, \\ 1 & \text{if } i \in \{5,7,8\}. \end{cases}$$

So, the minimisation model will be (Equation (12)):

$$\min \sum_{i=0}^{10} \sum_{j=0}^{41} C_{ij} X_{ij}, \tag{12}$$

where $X_{ij} \in \{0,1\}$, $i \in \{0,10\}$, and $j \in \{0,41\}$.

This finalises the generic modelization. In the next section, the weekly model is presented.

Weekly Modelling

A minimum number of shifts for each nurse to cover weekly is essential. Since the 11 nurses performing 4 shifts per week cover 44 shifts > 42, we consider that the minimum number of shifts will be 3. However, we will consider that, if a nurse is on call, she will have to work one less shift in the clinic as the same will happen in case of leave. We also believe that if last week someone did less than 5 shifts, the next week they will definitely do 5 (except in cases of leave—on-call duty). Therefore, the minimum number of shifts will be introduced as a final restriction. In addition, in cases such as N_2 or N_0, who has many days off this week, the variables representing the shifts she will cover this week are not eliminated but reset for the sake of flexibility. The model should be flexible in terms of changes each week and able to reflect nurse-specific considerations, such as leave periods, requested off-days, and previously worked shifts. To that end, we incorporate these factors as follows:

Predefined Assignments: Some nurses have fixed assignments based on external factors (e.g., personal requests or coordination with family schedules). For any nurse, i, who must work a specific set of shifts, J_i^{fixed}, we directly set (Equation (13)):

$$X_{i,j} = 1 \quad \forall j \in J_i^{\text{fixed}}. \tag{13}$$

Unavailable Shifts: If nurse i has requested off-days, leave, or cannot be scheduled due to constraints (e.g., adjacency to an on-call night shift), we define J_i^{off} as the set of shifts they cannot cover (Equation (14)):

$$X_{i,j} = 0 \quad \forall j \in J_i^{\text{off}}. \tag{14}$$

Minimum Workload Requirements: After accounting for leaves and on-call duties, each nurse, i, is assigned a minimum required number of shifts, r_i^{min}, for the week (e.g., 3 or 4). We enforce (Equation (15)):

$$\sum_{j=0}^{41} X_{i,j} \geq r_i^{\text{min}}. \tag{15}$$

By encapsulating individualised constraints into sets (J_i^{fixed}, J_i^{off}) and parameters (r_i^{min}), we accommodate personal schedules, leaves, rest requirements, and workload balancing within a single, flexible framework. In line with that, Table 9 presents nurse individualised constraints according to available data.

Table 9. Nurse Individualised Constraints.

Nurse	Constraint Description
N_0	She is scheduled as the on-call nurse on December 4 (23:00–07:00), which prevents her from working 16 h before or after that shift. She also requested parental leave on December 7, making her unavailable for the previous night's shift. As a result, her minimum shifts this week are 3, calculated from 7 days minus 2 off days, 1 on-call day, and 1 leave day.
N_1	She requested days off on December 5 and 6, and Friday, December 7, totalling three days. Therefore, she cannot be assigned a shift on December 5.
N_2	She requested a leave of absence from the 4th to the 8th of the month (the 4th to 7th impacting this week) and days off on the 2nd and 3rd. She also cannot be assigned to the previous night's shift. Therefore, the minimum number of shifts she must work this week is 1, calculated as 7 days minus 2 off days and 4 leave days.
N_3	Sets her schedule based on her husband. She will work on the 1st and 2nd of the month.
N_4	She requested to have December 1 off.
N_5	She requested days off on December 1 and December 4, and additional leave on December 2 and 3. Therefore, she must work 3 shifts this week (7 days–2 off days–2 leave days).
N_6	She does not have any constraints this week.
N_7	She has requested not to be scheduled for the afternoon shift (15:00–23:00) on Thursday and Friday.
N_{8S}	She has no restrictions this week.
N_{9S}	She has requested days off on Monday and Tuesday, meaning she cannot work the night shift on Sunday.
N_{10S}	She worked the 15:00–23:00 shift on Thursday of the previous week (November 3), so she cannot work the morning shift on Friday.
All Nurses except for N_0, N_2 and N_5	Must work at least 4 shifts during the week.

5. Results

The application of a Java-based optimisation algorithm to the nurse scheduling problem at the Clinic of Pathological Oncology has significant improvements. To provide a comprehensive evaluation, Table 10 presents the original, pre-optimisation schedule, which served as the baseline, while Table 11 illustrates the new nurses' schedules, highlighting the optimisation results achieved.

Table 10. Shift schedule for the first week of December with nurse IDs before the solution.

December (First Week)							
Day	**Fri**	**Sat**	**Sun**	**Mon**	**Tue**	**Wed**	**Thu**
Morning	N_1, N_2.N_7	N_{9S}, null	N_4, N_8	N_0.N_{10S}, N_{9S}	N_5, N_6.N_7	N_3.N_{8S}, N_5.N_6	N_4, N_{8S}
Afternoon	N_0, N_{9S}	N_4, N_{10S}	N_6, N_{9S}	N_3, N_{8S}	N_3, N_{8S}	N_4, N_{9S}	N_{9S}, N_5
Night	N_1, N_3.N_{8S}	N_1, N_3	N_4, null	N_0.N_{10S}, N_4	GE, N_7	N_7, N_6	N_3, null

Table 11. Shift schedule for the first week of December with nurse IDs after the solution.

December (First Week)							
Day	**Fri**	**Sat**	**Sun**	**Mon**	**Tue**	**Wed**	**Thu**
Morning	N_1, N_{9S}	N_1, N_7	N_{9S}, N_7	N_{10S}, N_7	N_{10S}, N_5	N_6, N_{10S}	N_6, N_1
Afternoon	N_2, N_0	N_4, N_0	N_1, N_0	N_1, N_3	N_{8S}, N_3	N_4, N_{8S}	N_4, N_{8S}
Night	N_{8S}, N_3	N_6, N_3	N_{8S}, N_4	N_6, N_4	N_7, N_{9S}	N_5, N_{9S}	N_5, N_3

5.1. Key Findings

1. Optimisation Outcome: The process culminated in an optimal solution characterised by an objective function value of 43.69. This denotes a significant enhancement in scheduling efficiency, ensuring an equitable distribution of shifts among nursing staff while meeting all operational and individual constraints. Thus, the optimised schedule demonstrated significant measurable improvements, as shown in Table 12.

Table 12. Quantitative evaluation of optimisation results.

Quantitative Metrics Before and After Optimisation						
Metric	**Rest Violations**	**Skill Mix Compliance**	**Workload Balance**	**Overstaffing**	**Understaffing**	**Objective Function Value**
Before Optimisation	3 violations	85% of shifts	2.3 shifts	2 instances	3 instances	239.5
After Optimisation	0 violations	100% of shifts	0.9 shifts	0 instances	0 instances	43.69

2. Comprehensive Shift Coverage:
    - Morning shifts are adequately staffed with the Su, the De (which are not part of the problem), and at least two additional nurses, guaranteeing leadership oversight and operational readiness.
    - Afternoon and night shifts are consistently staffed with at least one TE nurse each, alongside another nurse, fulfilling the clinic's requirement for specialised care around the clock.
3. Adherence to Constraints: The optimisation algorithm meticulously adhered to a complex set of scheduling constraints, including:

- Prohibiting consecutive shifts for individual nurses to ensure adequate rest.
- Limiting the number of shifts per nurse to a maximum of five per week to prevent overworking.
- Integrating individual availability requests and preferences into the scheduling process without compromising operational integrity.

4. Improvement Over Original Schedule: The optimised schedule presents a stark improvement over the original roster by:
   - Eliminating instances of overstaffing and ensuring that each shift is covered by the exact number of required nurses.
   - Addressing previous scheduling inefficiencies, such as the misallocation of TE nurses or failure to meet skill mix requirements for each shift. The SE do not work together at the same 8-hour shift and are complemented by the TE.
5. Balanced Workload Distribution: The algorithm ensures a fair and balanced distribution of shifts among all nurses, which:
   - Avoids overburdening any single nurse with an excessive number of night or consecutive shifts.
   - Promotes job satisfaction and well-being by respecting individual work–life balance needs and preferences.
   - The contracted nurses can cover at most one night shift per week, while the others can cover a maximum of two night shifts—except for N3 as in Table 13. Furthermore, it is observed that no employee works two consecutive shifts without at least 16 h between the end of one and the start of the next.
   - It is also understood that no nurse works more than 5 shifts or fewer than 4 shifts in a week—except for those on general on-call duty or leave, such as N0, N2, and N5 Table 13.

Table 13. Number of shifts per Nurse.

Nurse	Number of Shifts
N_0	3
N_1	4
N_2	1
N_3	5
N_4	5
N_5	3
N_6	4
N_7	4
N_{8S}	5
N_{9S}	4
N_{10S}	4
Total shifts	42

6. Clinic Feedback: Positive feedback was received from the clinic's staff regarding the optimised scheduling solution. The schedule not only satisfies the clinic's operational and care delivery requirements but also addresses the staff's work–life balance needs, marking it as an effective and sustainable approach to NR. Positive informal feedback was received from the clinic's staff regarding the optimised scheduling solution. While satisfaction was not directly measured, the improvements align with established indicators of staff satisfaction. The optimised schedules achieved compliance with regulatory requirements for rest periods and ensured an equitable distribution of shifts among all nurses—operational enhancements likely contributing to improved staff morale [12,34].
7. Key Observations:

- The solution efficiently covers all nurse shifts, with a total of 42 shifts, ensuring operational continuity without any uncovered periods.
- It strictly adheres to the clinic's nurse-to-shift ratio requirements and, as an indirect result, maintains a high standard of patient care.
- Feedback from the nursing staff indicates a unanimous acceptance of the schedule, highlighting its success in meeting personal preferences and operational demands. To that end, Su's feedback stated that the solution was correct and was unanimously accepted and implemented by the staff, with zero implications.

5.2. Limitations and Threats to Validity

While this study on optimizing nurse rostering shows promising results, several limitations and validity concerns should be flagged.

Data Limitations: The model's success relies on data regarding nurse availability, patient needs, and workload. Data noise can impact the ability to generate optimal schedules, impacting how well the findings reflect real-world conditions.

Real-time Adaptation: The current model does not yet handle real-time scheduling changes. Its effectiveness could be decreased if it cannot promptly respond to changes in staffing needs or in patient demands.

The Human Factor: The model accounts for work-hour constraints and nurse preferences but may not fully capture unexpected human factors like illness or exhaustion. In that sense, it can be less flexible when responding to last-minute changes and potentially impacting the overall staff satisfaction. To address this, structured surveys or interviews could be incorporated to systematically evaluate nurse perceptions of roster fairness, workload distribution, and overall satisfaction. Such feedback mechanisms would complement the operational metrics, providing a more comprehensive understanding of the model's impact on workforce well-being and identifying areas for further improvement.

Specific Context: Conducted in a specific oncology setting, the model was tailored to address high patient care urgency through the optimal organization of the nursing staff. However, the results may not be directly communicable to other healthcare departments where the needs might be different. To do so, further adjustments and testing are required.

Scalability Concerns: Although the developed model showcased potential scalability, the complexity could grow substantially when applied to larger healthcare departments. Something like that can lead to diminishing processing times or even reduced performance in real-time applications, thus confining its use in larger or more fast-paced environments/settings.

Although this study offers a foundation for optimizing nurse schedules in oncology settings, addressing these limitations will be necessary to broaden the applicability prospects and enable real-world use. Thus, Section 6 builds upon these and discusses future directions.

6. Future Research Directions

New methods propose approaches that can improve NR optimisation further. Starting with generic algorithms, a genetic algorithm has been explored to solve the nurse scheduling problem in crisis situations, such as during COVID-19 [35]. The authors in [36] highlight the effectiveness of hybrid approaches combining, for example, IP and Constraint Programming (CP) to address the highly constrained NRP. In other cases, researchers have proposed hybrid approaches for the NRP, combining MIP with deep neural network-assisted heuristics and recurrent neural networks, outperforming other pieces of research in terms of benchmarks [37,38]. The following sections attempt to categorise similar future trends.

6.1. Incorporation of ML Techniques and Others

ML offers promising extensions to traditional NR optimisation, particularly in terms of predictive capabilities and real-time adaptability [39]. For example, using predictive algorithms based on historical data, similar to those in energy forecasting [40–42], might enhance the value of OR in healthcare even more. Such data-driven methods can enhance decision-making, leading to better scheduling and improved patient care. Thus, one direction for future work would be to incorporate supervised learning to predict nurse preferences and availability based on historical data, improving the scheduling system's ability to align nurse shifts with personal preferences. This would enhance both staff satisfaction and operational efficiency by reducing conflicts between organizational requirements and individual nurses' needs [43].

The authors in [44] address the NRP differently, using a two-stage approach. The first stage combines Monte Carlo Tree Search with Hill Climbing to find feasible solutions by satisfying hard constraints. A novel constant C value is proposed to balance search diversification and intensification in MCTS. The second stage improves the solution using Iterated Local Search with Variable Neighbourhood Descent, introducing unique neighbourhood structures and a perturbation strategy to escape local optima. Computational results on the Shift Scheduling dataset report the best new solutions for several instances. In [45], the researchers suggest that partitioning NRP instances into manageable sub-problems and applying sequential optimisation could be further enhanced with ML techniques to adaptively optimise large, complex NRPs. Finally, another work [46], addresses the NRP using a hyper-heuristic approach that combines Reinforcement Learning (RL) with Simulated Annealing (SA) and Reheating. This method improves scheduling by considering multiple constraints such as labour regulations, hospital policies, and nurse availability. The study, conducted in Norwegian hospitals, demonstrates an 82% improvement in solution quality, outperforming other algorithms such as Simple Random-Hill Climbing, Reinforcement Learning-Hill Climbing, and Reinforcement Learning-Simulated Annealing.

6.2. Enhancing Dynamic Capabilities for NR

The enhancement of NR models necessitates additional advancement in dynamic scheduling systems to address the immediate requirements of healthcare settings. The existing frameworks for MIP and ILP, although proficient, exhibit limitations in addressing dynamic constraints, including unexpected nurse absences or varying patient loads. Future research ought to expand these models through the incorporation of stochastic programming, thereby enabling the system to more effectively manage uncertainties by dynamically adjusting schedules in response to real-time feedback regarding nurse availability and patient demand [31]. Another piece of research explored further enhancement of hybrid algorithms, such as combining MIP-based heuristics with metaheuristic methods like SA, to improve solution quality for the NRP [43]. An extended NR model was introduced [47], incorporating unit assignments alongside nurse, day, and shift allocations, addressing the complexities of real-world scenarios where not every nurse can be assigned to every unit due to varying skills and experience. The study also presents a matheuristic solution approach that combines IP for generating initial schedules with Discrete Particle Swarm Optimisation (PSO) for further improvement, ensuring feasibility and near-optimal solutions. In [48], novel strategies for the nurse re-rostering problem are stated, which occurs when unforeseen events disrupt existing schedules and focus on the relaxation of different problem parameters to quickly reconstruct feasible rosters. The integration of accurate optimisation methods can significantly enhance the resilience of scheduling systems, thereby ensuring that optimal solutions maintain stability in the face of variable conditions [43,49].

6.3. Real-Time Scheduling, Adaptive Systems, and Public Perception

The development of real-time scheduling systems is critical for managing the complex and unpredictable nature of NR, particularly in oncology departments where patient demand fluctuates rapidly. Future research should focus on implementing adaptive scheduling models that adjust in real time based on nurse availability, patient admissions, and other external factors. By linking these models to real-time data feeds, such as electronic health records, the system could update schedules automatically, reducing the reliance on manual updates by administrators [10].

Combining systematic IP with adaptive algorithms like SA can improve NR in real time. A systematic two-phase approach for NR was developed, which first determines the workload distribution for each nurse and day, followed by the assignment of specific shifts using IP [45]. The approach was applied in the context of the First International Nurse Rostering Competition (INRC2010), where the problem instances were partitioned into sub-problems and solved sequentially. The method's success was demonstrated by achieving the best results in the competition. In [50], the authors applied SA to a multi-level NRP in hemodialysis services, where nurses with different qualifications must be assigned to various roles, such as in-charge nurse, dispensing nurse, and treatment nurse. The research formulated a 0-1 IP model and used a heuristic algorithm to satisfy both the demand for nurses and their preferences regarding shifts and roles. This adaptive approach successfully addressed the complexity of the problem, ensuring better nurse allocation in a critical healthcare environment.

Another aspect under consideration to enhance NR in oncology departments could be to recognize the impact of social media on public health perceptions and patient engagement [51]. This dynamic can influence staffing decisions, as improved communication with patients through social media may help create schedules that better align with their needs and preferences. Additionally, sentiment analysis from social media discussions on various topics [52] can offer valuable insights into patient concerns, enabling more responsive and effective scheduling strategies for nursing staff.

Future work can also deal with the aspect of cost improvements. The authors in [53] introduce a novel methodology for cyclic preference scheduling using a branch-and-price algorithm to balance individual nurse preferences with cost minimization. The research highlights the growing trend toward cyclic schedules, which are easier to manage, more stable, and generally perceived as equitable in comparison to generating new rosters each period. The proposed approach, which solves instances with up to 200 nurses within minutes, suggests that future research should explore cyclic scheduling models further to enhance stability and manageability in dynamic healthcare environments. Similarly, a cyclic scheduling general IP model which can directly or indirectly support cost minimization is proposed in [54]. More specifically, this work proposes a general IP model for cyclic staff scheduling, which is adaptable to various real-world settings, including a glass plant and a continuous care unit, focusing on the sequence constraints and workload balance through cyclic scheduling.

6.4. Broader Application to Various Healthcare Departments and Combined Metrics

While the current focus is on optimising NR in oncology clinics, future research could expand these optimisation models to other healthcare departments on a larger scale and also include other metrics. To that end, insights from prescriptive maintenance [55] could be utilised to automate the identification of suboptimal schedules. Each department within a hospital, such as emergency services, surgical units, and outpatient care, has unique operational requirements and constraints. Developing customisable modules that can adapt the existing MIP model to fit the specific needs of different departments would allow for a more holistic and integrated scheduling solution across healthcare facilities [56]. The authors in [57] address the challenge of constructing nurse duty schedules for large hospitals, balancing staff availability with individual preferences and fairness. Using a tabu search approach, the study developed a decision support system (NuRoDSS) for Stikland Hospital, a large psychiatric facility, demonstrating the scalability of optimisation methods in nurse scheduling. Similarly, another work [58], describes a hybrid approach to nurse scheduling that combines modern heuristic methods with classical IP models, specifically knapsacks, network flow models, and tabu search, to solve a real-world NRP at a major UK hospital.

Combined with the above, metrics concerning patient outcomes or satisfaction scores from both patients and staff could also be included in future research to further strengthen the validity and value of the proposed solutions.

7. Conclusions

This study has addressed the complex challenge of optimizing NR in oncology clinics through the application of mathematical optimisation techniques. By employing MIP models, the research demonstrated improvements in operational efficiency, nurse satisfaction, and resource allocation. The results show the importance of using precise mathematical tools to navigate the complexities of healthcare staffing, particularly in settings where patient needs are highly variable.

Building on this, the research investigates the application of ILP and hybrid techniques to adjust to both small- and large-scale rostering challenges. While focused on oncology clinics, the methodology may be extended to broader healthcare contexts, offering versatile solutions for staff allocation in uncertain environments. Dynamic scheduling systems incorporating ML and RL offer the potential for real-time adaptability and data-driven decision-making. Hybrid models, such as those combining ILP with metaheuristic algorithms like Variable Neighbourhood Search (VNS), optimise flexibility and computational efficiency [17,59,60]. Stochastic optimisation further strengthens the ability to respond in a dynamic way to changes in nurse availability and patient needs, paving the way for fair, efficient, and patient-focused staffing systems.

Author Contributions: Conceptualization, A.M. and K.K.; methodology, A.M., C.K. and P.K.; validation, A.M., P.K., K.K. and S.G.S.; formal analysis, A.M., C.K., P.K. and C.T.; investigation, A.M. and C.K.; resources, P.K.; data curation, A.M. and K.K.; writing—original draft preparation, A.M. and C.K.; writing—review and editing, C.K., P.K. and C.T.; visualization, C.K.; supervision, K.K.; project administration, P.K., S.G.S. and C.T.; funding acquisition, C.T. All authors have read and agreed to the published version of the manuscript.

Funding: This research received no external funding.

Institutional Review Board Statement: Not applicable. This study did not involve patients nor animals. It does not contain personal health information, thus ethical approval was not required.

Informed Consent Statement: Not applicable. This study did not involve patients nor contains personal health information.

Data Availability Statement: The data supporting the reported results are available upon reasonable request from the corresponding author. The data are not publicly available to preserve anonymity.

Conflicts of Interest: The authors declare no conflicts of interest.

Abbreviations

The following abbreviations were used in this manuscript:

CP	Constraint Programming
CPLEX	IBM's ILOG CPLEX Optimisation Studio
De	Deputy
ILP	Integer Linear Programming
IP	Integer Programming
LP	Linear Programming
MCTS	Monte Carlo Tree Search
MIP	Mixed-Integer Programming
MILP	Mixed-Integer Linear Programming
ML	Machine Learning
NRP	Nurse Rostering Problem
NR	Nurse Rostering
OR	Operations Research
PIP	Pure Integer Programming

RL	Reinforcement Learning
SA	Simulated Annealing
SE	Secondary Education (Nurse)
Su	Supervisor
TE	Technological Education (Nurse)
VNS	Variable Neighbourhood Search

Nomenclature

The following nomenclature was used in this manuscript:

X_{ij}	Binary variable indicating if nurse i is assigned to shift j
i	Nurse index
j	Shift index
I	Set of all nurses
J	Set of all shifts
Π	Set of morning shifts
A	Set of afternoon shifts
B	Set of night shifts
$C_{i\Pi}$	Weight for nurse i assigned to morning shifts
C_{iA}	Weight for nurse i assigned to afternoon shifts
C_{iB}	Weight for nurse i assigned to night shifts
$I_{T(j)} \subseteq I$	Subset of nurses qualified for shift type $T(j)$
$R_{T(j)}$	Required minimum number of qualified nurses for shift type $T(j)$
$T(j)$	Type of shift j (morning, afternoon, or night)
$\sum X_{ij}$	Total shifts assigned to nurse i
$\sum X_{i\Pi}$	Total morning shifts assigned to nurse i
$\sum X_{iA}$	Total afternoon shifts assigned to nurse i
$\sum X_{iB}$	Total night shifts assigned to nurse i
Su	Supervisor nurse
De	Deputy nurse
TE	Technological Education nurse
SE	Secondary Education nurse
$\min \sum C_{ij} X_{ij}$	Objective function to minimize weighted shifts across all nurses

References

1. Tien, J.M.; Kamiyama, A. On Manpower Scheduling Algorithms. *SIAM Rev.* **1982**, *24*, 275–287. [CrossRef]
2. Dantzig, G.; Fulkerson, R.; Johnson, S. Solution of a Large-Scale Traveling-Salesman Problem. *J. Oper. Res. Soc. Am.* **1954**, *2*, 393–410. [CrossRef]
3. Ernst, A.T.; Jiang, H.; Krishnamoorthy, M.; Sier, D. Staff scheduling and rostering: A review of applications, methods and models. *Eur. J. Oper. Res.* **2004**, *153*, 3–27. [CrossRef]
4. Cheang, B.; Li, H.; Lim, A.; Rodrigues, B. Nurse rostering problems–a bibliographic survey. *Eur. J. Oper. Res.* **2003**, *151*, 447–460. [CrossRef]
5. Maenhout, B.; Vanhoucke, M. Analyzing the nursing organizational structure and process from a scheduling perspective. *Health Care Manag. Sci.* **2013**, *16*, 177–196. [CrossRef] [PubMed]
6. Mankins, M.; Steele, R. Turning great strategy into great performance. *Harv. Bus. Rev.* **2005**, *83*, 64–72, 191. [PubMed]
7. Khalil, E.B. Machine Learning for Integer Programming. In Proceedings of the Machine Learning for Integer Programming, New York, NY, USA, 9–15 July 2016; pp. 4004–4005. [CrossRef]
8. Boedvarsdottir, E.B.; Bagger, N.C.F.; Hoffner, L.E.; Stidsen, T.J.R. A flexible mixed integer programming-based system for real-world nurse rostering. *J. Sched.* **2022**, *25*, 59–88. [CrossRef]
9. Koukaras, P.; Berberidis, C.; Tjortjis, C. A Semi-supervised Learning Approach for Complex Information Networks. In *Intelligent Data Communication Technologies and Internet of Things*; Hemanth, J., Bestak, R., Chen, J.I.Z., Eds.; Springer: Singapore, 2021; pp. 1–13.
10. Azmat, C.S.; Hürlimann, T.; Widmer, M. Mixed Integer Programming to Schedule a Single-Shift Workforce under Annualized Hours. *Ann. Oper. Res.* **2004**, *128*, 199–215. [CrossRef]
11. Burke, E.K.; Causmaecker, P.D.; Berghe, G.V.; Landeghem, H.V. The state of the art of nurse rostering. *J. Sched.* **2004**, *7*, 441–499. [CrossRef]
12. Yasmine, A.; Yassine, O.; Farouk, Y.; Hicham, C. Workload balancing for the nurse scheduling problem: A real-world case study from a French hospital. *Socio-Econ. Plan. Sci.* **2024**, *95*, 102046. [CrossRef]

13. IBM ILOG CPLEX Optimization Studio—ibm.com. Available online: https://www.ibm.com/products/ilog-cplex-optimization-studio (accessed on 15 October 2024).
14. IloCplex (CPLEX Java API Reference Manual)—ibm.com. Available online: https://www.ibm.com/docs/en/icos/22.1.1?topic=c-ilocplex-3 (accessed on 15 October 2024).
15. McCloskey, J.F. U. S. operations research in world war II. *Oper. Res.* **1987**, *35*, 910–925. [CrossRef]
16. Miller, H.E.; Pierskalla, W.P.; Rath, G.J. Nurse Scheduling Using Mathematical Programming. *Oper. Res.* **1976**, *24*, 857–870. [CrossRef]
17. Burke, E.K.; Li, J.; Qu, R. A hybrid model of integer programming and variable neighbourhood search for highly-constrained nurse rostering problems. *Eur. J. Oper. Res.* **2010**, *203*, 484–493. [CrossRef]
18. Padberg, M.W.; Rinaldi, G. A Branch-and-Cut Algorithm for the Resolution of Large-Scale Symmetric Traveling Salesman Problems. *SIAM Rev.* **1991**, *33*, 60–100. [CrossRef]
19. The Leader in Decision Intelligence Technology—Gurobi Optimization—gurobi.com. Available online: https://www.gurobi.com/ (accessed on 15 October 2024).
20. Schrijver, A. Theory of Linear and Integer Programming. *J. Oper. Res. Soc.* **2000**, *51*, 892–893. [CrossRef]
21. Grötschel, M.; Nemhauser, G.L. George Dantzig's contributions to integer programming. *Discret. Optim.* **2008**, *5*, 168–173. [CrossRef]
22. Chen, P.S.; Zeng, Z.Y. Developing two heuristic algorithms with metaheuristic algorithms to improve solutions of optimization problems with soft and hard constraints: An application to nurse rostering problems. *Appl. Soft Comput. J.* **2020**, *93*, 106336. [CrossRef]
23. Burke, E.K.; Curtois, T.; Post, G.; Qu, R.; Veltman, B. A hybrid heuristic ordering and variable neighbourhood search for the nurse rostering problem. *Eur. J. Oper. Res.* **2008**, *188*, 330–341. [CrossRef]
24. Land, A.H.; Doig, A.G. An Automatic Method of Solving Discrete Programming Problems. *Econometrica* **1960**, *28*, 497. [CrossRef]
25. Balas, E.; Ceria, S.; Cornuéjols, G.; Natraj, N. Gomory cuts revisited. *Oper. Res. Lett.* **1996**, *19*, 1–9. [CrossRef]
26. Billionnet, A. Integer programming to schedule a hierarchical workforce with variable demands. *Eur. J. Oper. Res.* **1999**, *114*, 105–114. [CrossRef]
27. Corominas, A.; García, A.; Pastor, R. Planning production and working time within an annualised hours scheme framework. *Ann. Oper. Res.* **2007**, *155*, 5–23. [CrossRef]
28. Ulusam Seçkiner, S.; Gökçen, H.; Kurt, M. An integer programming model for hierarchical workforce scheduling problem. *Eur. J. Oper. Res.* **2007**, *183*, 694–699. [CrossRef]
29. Ouda, E.; Sleptchenko, A.; Simsekler, M.C.E. Nurse Rostering via Mixed-Integer Programming. *Adv. Transdiscipl. Eng.* **2023**, *35*, 815–823. [CrossRef]
30. Burke, E.K.; Curtois, T. New approaches to nurse rostering benchmark instances. *Eur. J. Oper. Res.* **2014**, *237*, 71–81. [CrossRef]
31. Jaumard, B.; Semet, F.; Vovor, T. A generalized linear programming model for nurse scheduling. *Eur. J. Oper. Res.* **1998**, *107*, 1–18. [CrossRef]
32. Foundation, A.S. Apache NetBeans Archive. Available online: https://netbeans.apache.org/front/main/download/archive/ (accessed on 28 September 2024).
33. Corporation, O. Java | Oracle. Available online: https://www.java.com/en/ (accessed on 28 September 2024).
34. Hassani, M.R.; Behnamian, J. A scenario-based robust optimization with a pessimistic approach for nurse rostering problem. *J. Comb. Optim.* **2021**, *41*, 143–169. [CrossRef]
35. Heiniger, N.; Massaro, G.; Hanne, T.; Dornberger, R. Solving the Nurse Scheduling Problem in Crisis Situations Applying a Genetic Algorithm. In Proceedings of the 2023 10th International Conference on Soft Computing and Machine Intelligence, ISCMI 2023, Mexico City, Mexico, 25–26 November 2023; pp. 65–71. [CrossRef]
36. Rahimian, E.; Akartunali, K.; Levine, J. A hybrid integer and constraint programming approach to solve nurse rostering problems. *Comput. Oper. Res.* **2017**, *82*, 83–94. [CrossRef]
37. Chen, Z.; Dou, Y.; De Causmaecker, P. Neural networked-assisted method for the nurse rostering problem. *Comput. Ind. Eng.* **2022**, *171*, 108430. [CrossRef]
38. Chen, Z.; De Causmaecker, P.; Dou, Y. A combined mixed integer programming and deep neural network-assisted heuristics algorithm for the nurse rostering problem. *Appl. Soft Comput.* **2023**, *136*, 109919. [CrossRef]
39. Shi, J.; Wei, S.; Gao, Y.; Mei, F.; Tian, J.; Zhao, Y.; Li, Z. Global output on artificial intelligence in the field of nursing: A bibliometric analysis and science mapping. *J. Nurs. Scholarsh.* **2023**, *55*, 853–863. [CrossRef]
40. Mystakidis, A.; Koukaras, P.; Tsalikidis, N.; Ioannidis, D.; Tjortjis, C. Energy Forecasting: A Comprehensive Review of Techniques and Technologies. *Energies* **2024**, *17*, 1662. [CrossRef]
41. Tsalikidis, N.; Mystakidis, A.; Tjortjis, C.; Koukaras, P.; Ioannidis, D. Energy load forecasting: One-step ahead hybrid model utilizing ensembling. *Computing* **2024**, *106*, 241–273. [CrossRef]
42. Mystakidis, A.; Ntozi, E.; Afentoulis, K.; Koukaras, P.; Giannopoulos, G.; Bezas, N.; Gkaidatzis, P.A.; Ioannidis, D.; Tjortjis, C.; Tzovaras, D. One Step Ahead Energy Load Forecasting: A Multi-model approach utilizing Machine and Deep Learning. In Proceedings of the 2022 57th International Universities Power Engineering Conference (UPEC), Istanbul, Turkey, 30 August–2 September 2022; pp. 1–6. [CrossRef]

43. Turhan, A.M.; Bilgen, B. A hybrid fix-and-optimize and simulated annealing approaches for nurse rostering problem. *Comput. Ind. Eng.* **2020**, *145*, 106531. [CrossRef]
44. Goh, S.L.; Sze, S.N.; Sabar, N.R.; Abdullah, S.; Kendall, G. A 2-Stage Approach for the Nurse Rostering Problem. *IEEE Access* **2022**, *10*, 69591–69604. [CrossRef]
45. Valouxis, C.; Gogos, C.; Goulas, G.; Alefragis, P.; Housos, E. A systematic two phase approach for the nurse rostering problem. *Eur. J. Oper. Res.* **2012**, *219*, 425–433. [CrossRef]
46. Muklason, A.; Kusuma, S.D.R.; Riksakomara, E.; Premananda, I.G.A.; Anggraeni, W.; Mahananto, F.; Tyasnurita, R. Solving Nurse Rostering Optimization Problem using Reinforcement Learning - Simulated Annealing with Reheating Hyper-heuristics Algorithm. *Procedia Comput. Sci.* **2024**, *234*, 486–493. [CrossRef]
47. Turhan, A.M.; Bilgen, B. A mat-heuristic based solution approach for an extended nurse rostering problem with skills and units. *Socio-Econ. Plan. Sci.* **2022**, *82*, 101300. [CrossRef]
48. Wickert, T.I.; Smet, P.; Vanden Berghe, G. The nurse rerostering problem: Strategies for reconstructing disrupted schedules. *Comput. Oper. Res.* **2019**, *104*, 319–337. [CrossRef]
49. Strandmark, P.; Qu, Y.; Curtois, T. First-order linear programming in a column generation-based heuristic approach to the nurse rostering problem. *Comput. Oper. Res.* **2020**, *120*, 104945. [CrossRef]
50. Liu, Z.; Liu, Z.; Zhu, Z.; Shen, Y.; Dong, J. Simulated annealing for a multi-level nurse rostering problem in hemodialysis service. *Appl. Soft Comput.* **2018**, *64*, 148–160. [CrossRef]
51. Koukaras, P.; Rousidis, D.; Tjortjis, C. Forecasting and Prevention Mechanisms Using Social Media in Health Care. In *Advanced Computational Intelligence in Healthcare-7: Biomedical Informatics*; Maglogiannis, I., Brahnam, S., Jain, L.C., Eds.; Springer: Berlin/Heidelberg, Germany, 2020; pp. 121–137. [CrossRef]
52. Kapoteli, E.; Koukaras, P.; Tjortjis, C. Social Media Sentiment Analysis Related to COVID-19 Vaccines: Case Studies in English and Greek Language. In *Artificial Intelligence Applications and Innovations*; Maglogiannis, I., Iliadis, L., Macintyre, J., Cortez, P., Eds.; Springer International Publishing: Cham, Switzerland, 2022; pp. 360–372.
53. Purnomo, H.W.; Bard, J.F. Cyclic preference scheduling for nurses using branch and price. *Nav. Res. Logist.* **2007**, *54*, 200–220. [CrossRef]
54. Rocha, M.; Oliveira, J.F.; Carravilla, M.A. Cyclic staff scheduling: Optimization models for some real-life problems. *J. Sched.* **2013**, *16*, 231–242. [CrossRef]
55. Koukaras, P.; Dimara, A.; Herrera, S.; Zangrando, N.; Krinidis, S.; Ioannidis, D.; Fraternali, P.; Tjortjis, C.; Anagnostopoulos, C.N.; Tzovaras, D. Proactive Buildings: A Prescriptive Maintenance Approach. In *Artificial Intelligence Applications and Innovations*; AIAI 2022 IFIP WG 12.5 International Workshops; Maglogiannis, I., Iliadis, L., Macintyre, J., Cortez, P., Eds.; Springer International Publishing: Cham, Switzerland, 2022; pp. 289–300.
56. Smet, P.; Causmaecker, P.D.; Bilgin, B.; Berghe, G.V. Nurse rostering: A complex example of personnel scheduling with perspectives. *Stud. Comput. Intell.* **2013**, *505*, 129–153. [CrossRef]
57. Bester, M.J.; Nieuwoudt, I.; Van Vuuren, J.H. Finding good nurse duty schedules: A case study. *J. Sched.* **2007**, *10*, 387–405. [CrossRef]
58. Dowsland, K.; Thompson, J. Solving a nurse scheduling problem with knapsacks, networks and tabu search. *J. Oper. Res. Soc.* **2000**, *51*, 825–833. [CrossRef]
59. Rahimian, E.; Akartunali, K.; Levine, J. A hybrid Integer Programming and Variable Neighbourhood Search algorithm to solve Nurse Rostering Problems. *Eur. J. Oper. Res.* **2017**, *258*, 411–423. [CrossRef]
60. Della Croce, F.; Salassa, F. A variable neighborhood search based matheuristic for nurse rostering problems. *Ann. Oper. Res.* **2014**, *218*, 185–199. [CrossRef]

healthcare

MDPI

Article

Team Size and Composition in Home Healthcare: Quantitative Insights and Six Model-Based Principles

Yoram Clapper [1], Witek ten Hove [2], René Bekker [1] and Dennis Moeke [2,*]

[1] Department of Mathematics, Vrije Universiteit Amsterdam, 1081 HV Amsterdam, The Netherlands; y.clapper@vu.nl (Y.C.); r.bekker@vu.nl (R.B.)
[2] Academy of Organization and Development, HAN University of Applied Sciences, 6826 CC Arnhem, The Netherlands; witek.tenhove@han.nl
* Correspondence: dennis.moeke@han.nl

Abstract: The aim of this constructive study was to develop model-based principles to provide guidance to managers and policy makers when making decisions about team size and composition in the context of home healthcare. Six model-based principles were developed based on extensive data analysis and in close interaction with practice. In particular, the principles involve insights in capacity planning, travel time, available effective capacity, contract types, and team manageability. The principles are formalized in terms of elementary mathematical models that capture the essence of decision-making. Numerical results based on real-life scenarios reveal that efficiency improves with team size, albeit more prominently for smaller teams due to diminishing returns. Moreover, it is demonstrated that the complexity of managing and coordinating a team becomes increasingly more difficult as team size grows. An estimate for travel time is provided given the size and territory of a team, as well as an upper bound for the fraction of full-time contracts, if split shifts are to be avoided. Overall, it can be concluded that an ideally sized team should serve (at least) around a few hundreds care hours per week.

Keywords: home care; work force; resource allocation; efficiency

1. Introduction

As in many other Western European countries, the long-term sustainability of Dutch home healthcare (HHC) system (here, we define home healthcare as an array of health and social support services provided to clients in their own residence [1]) is under serious pressure. On the one hand, we see an increase in demand due to an aging population, and a shift from care provided in an institutional setting to providing care closer to the care user's own home environment. By 2040, it is projected that one in four Dutch people will be aged 65 or over, and the number of persons older than 80 years is expected to almost double from 0.9 million in 2021 to over 1.6 million in 2040 [2]. This will raise the pressure on the Dutch HHC system because the prevalence of physical or mental disability increases with age [3]. When it comes to the shift of institutional care towards the home environment, it is mainly triggered by two developments: extramuralisation and medical care at home. In this context, extramuralisation can be described as government policy that aims to shift from providing care in a nursing home setting to care at home. Medical care at home is an alternative to (more expensive) inpatient hospital admission, enabling patients to receive hospital-level care at or closer to home.

On the other hand, looking at the supply side we see that the availability of healthcare professionals is under increasing pressure due to labor market tightness and high absenteeism rates. The Dutch healthcare and welfare forecast model shows that the shortage of healthcare workers will increase from 55,000 people in 2023 to about 155,000 people in 2032, with the largest shortages expected in nursing home and home healthcare [4]. Due to the increasing staff shortages, the healthcare sector risks falling into a vicious circle: staff shortages create an increased workload, which leads to more absenteeism, thereby creating an even greater shortage, etc. For example, that this vicious circle is lurking becomes evident from the increasing absenteeism rates. In 2022, the average absenteeism rate in the healthcare sector reached about 8.3% [5]. This is the highest absence rate ever measured and represents an increase of 15% compared to the year 2021.

Because of these challenges, many Dutch HHC providers are searching for ways to improve the balance between the available workforce capacity (i.e., supply) and the needs and preferences of their clients (i.e., demand). In collaboration with our partner HHC organization, we encountered (at least) two fundamental problems in obtaining the appropriate balance. The first problem is the lack of insight into the current demand. Although demand prospects exist for both individual clients, as well as some occasional handcrafted estimates at a more aggregate level, structural monitoring of the total demand requirements of the complete client base is yet uncommon in HHC. The second problem relates to the appropriate dimensioning of teams. In fact, the elementary initial question of our partner HHC organization was 'What is the ideal team size?'. Obviously, this question can be addressed from multiple angles; our aim is to provide some generic rules of thumb for determining the scale at which teams should be organized. In other words, our key research question is as follows: To what extent is it beneficial to utilize the potential of economies of scale in HHC?

1.1. Background: Existing Literature

The problems faced by HHC providers have triggered a body of research over the past decade. In the relatively early study of Matta et al., a framework to model HHC organization from an operations management perspective is proposed, whereas a taxonomic classification is provided by Hulshof et al. [6,7]. From those papers, it is evident that the number of studies focusing on strategic and/or tactical decisions in HHC, from an operations management (OM) and operations research (OR) perspective, is very limited. This conclusion is confirmed by the overview paper of Grieco et al. [8]. According to Grieco et al., the vast majority of the OR-related HHC studies focus on staff-to-patient allocation, visit scheduling, and the routing of visits, leading to more technical reviews concerning HHC routing and scheduling [9–11]. In contrast, only a few studies consider strategic and/or tactical decisions concerning team size and composition.

Below, we provide an overview of and discuss relevant studies that focus on resource dimensioning and team composition within a long-term care setting (i.e., residential and HHC). We opted for this scope because HHC is a prominent part of the Dutch long-term care (LTC) system. In addition, as resource dimensioning and team composition in an LTC setting is generally carried out at strategic and tactical levels, studies that focus on the operational level were not taken into account. In addition to resource dimensioning and team composition, the concept of 'economies of scale' will also be elaborated on as it plays an important role in the remainder of the paper.

From a healthcare-capacity-planning perspective, determining team sizes can be considered a resource dimensioning issue. Many studies have been devoted to resource dimensioning, most frequently for hospital capacity, of which a large share are quantitative in nature and stem from the domains of OR and OM.

Resource dimensioning at a strategic level involves structural decision-making on a relatively long time horizon (typically 1 year or more). Two examples of OR/OM studies involving residential care services at a strategic level are those of Christensen et al. and Moeke et al. [12,13]. Multiple quantitative studies have been conducted regarding economies of scale and scope from the perspective of the total organization (i.e., applying an aggregate perspective). Most of these studies make use of methods like regression analysis (e.g., [12]) or data envelopment analysis (e.g., [14]). Using a less aggregate approach, the study of red Moeke et al. aims to provide more insight into the effects of scale for small-scale living facilities in terms of waiting time and occupancy [13]. They present a comprehensive what-if analysis based on a discrete-event simulation model. When it comes to OR/OM literature regarding resource dimensioning on a strategic level in a home healthcare context, the districting problem is the most common area of focus (see, e.g., [15,16]). According to Benzarti et al., *districting a territory is a strategic decision that aims at grouping basic units (a set of patients) into larger clusters, i.e., districts, so that these districts are "good" according to relevant criteria. These criteria can be related to the activity, demography, or geographic characteristics of the basic units* [15]. In this paper, we essentially also try to determine the 'optimal size of a district', but our goal is to provide generic guidelines that abstract from the specific region. As such, the study presented in the current paper has a fundamentally different focus than the districting papers mentioned above.

The time horizon of decisions related to resource dimensioning at a tactical level is typically 3–12 months. OR/OM studies with a focus on resource dimensioning at a tactical level in a residential care context are scarce. The studies of Moeke et al. and Van Eeden et al. were the only ones we could find [17,18]. The study of Moeke et al. provides insights into how and why 'scale of scheduling' and the enlargement of care workers' jobs (blending tasks of different qualification levels) affect the number and type of staff required to meet the preferences (in terms of day and time) of nursing home residents [17]. The focus is on activities of daily living (i.e., activities like bathing or showering, dressing, getting in and out of bed or a chair, walking, using the toilet, and eating). The study of Van Eeden et al., on the other hand, focuses on determining the required amount of capacity regarding random care activities [18]. Based on the analysis of real-life 'call button' data, they present a queueing model that can be used by nursing home managers to determine the number of care workers required to meet a specific service level. As mentioned in the recent overview of Grieco et al., OR/OM studies with a focus on resource dimensioning at a tactical level are also scarce in a home healthcare context [8]. To the best of our knowledge, only the following three studies fall into this category: [19–21]. Each of the three studies propose a two-stage capacity planning approach based on (integer linear) stochastic programming. The model of Nikzad et al. considers decisions on districting, staff dimensioning, resource assignment, scheduling, and routing simultaneously [19]. Their results show that the algorithm is able to solve large instances. As such, it also considers the more strategic issue of districting. In the work of Restrepo et al., a two-stage stochastic programming model is presented for employee staffing and scheduling in a HHC context [20]. In this model, the issue of staff dimensioning is part of the first-stage decision process. Finally, Rodriguez et al. aim to determine the number of care workers required to balance the coverage of patients in a region and the workforce cost over several months [21]. We observe that these papers tend to focus on optimization rather than on providing generic capacity guidelines, which is our aim.

Team composition also plays an important role in creating effective and efficient LTC delivery systems (see e.g., [22]). In line with the objective of this study, our literature search focused on OR/OM studies that deal with determining the optimal skill-mix in an LTC context, where skill-mix refers to *the mix of staff in the workforce or the demarcation of roles and activities among different categories of staff* [23]. More specifically, regarding team composition, the focus in this study is on 'the mix of staff' in terms of qualification levels (see also Section 3). Despite determining the right staff mix being considered important, to the best of our knowledge, the work of Moeke et al. is the only OR/OM study that focuses on this issue in an LTC context [17].

Finally, we note that questions concerning resource dimensioning and 'team size' are intimately linked to the concept of economies of scale. For instance, for bed capacity decisions in hospitals (phrased as 'how many hospital beds' by Green [24]) it has long been recognized that smaller hospital units should have lower target occupancy rates to achieve the same levels of delay. More generally, economies of scale in resource planning describes the positive relationship between the performance of the planning outcome (in terms of efficiency or effectiveness) and the pooling of customer demands, along with the pooling of the required resources to serve those demands. Therefore, within the realm of resource planning, it also known as the 'pooling principle' [25–27]. From a mathematical perspective, the benefits of increasing scale are the consequence of a reduction in relative variability as the standard deviation of the sum of two random variables is smaller than the sum of the two standard deviations (if the coefficient of correlation is smaller than 1) [28]. We refer to the studies of Van Leeuwaarden and Whitt for a more elaborate exposition of the impact of scale in a queueing context [29,30].

1.2. Background: Practice

In the Netherlands, HHC services are provided to persons in need of care or support due to (chronic) illness, disability, or impairment. Determining eligibility for HHC services is carried out by the Centre for Healthcare Indication (CIZ). To receive paid home care, the CIZ must issue a so-called 'indication of need'. The services provided by HHC organizations must fit within the limitations of this indication of need (the type of care, amount of care, time period, etc.). In 2021, the Netherlands counted over 2500 HHC providers who collectively served about 585,000 people in the same year [31]. Especially, elderly people make use of HHC services. By 2021, roughly about 80% of the Dutch HHC clients were aged 66 and over, with an average age of 75. Most recipients are women (59%), which can be explained by the fact that life expectancy is higher for women [32].

Our partner HHC provider provides home, residential, custodial, personal, and informal care support to roughly 12,000 clients, with about 4000 employees (1600 FTE) and 1000 volunteers (2021 data). Regular home care is provided by a group of 55 teams. During the period 2020–2021, each team served 210 clients on average. The variation in client numbers across teams largely hinges on the intensity of care required by the clients and the population density of the relevant area. The total coverage area of the HHC teams is around 300 square kilometers. Table 1 provides an overview of the main characteristics per type of area (i.e., urban, suburban, and rural).

Table 1. General information per area type for the years 2020, 2021; all numerical values (except team count) represent the mean, with standard deviation in brackets.

Area Type	Teams	Planned Care (h/wk)	Clients	Clients/km^2
Urban	26	238 (51)	221 (51.4)	71 (31.4)
Suburban	18	224 (54)	238 (61.3)	11 (5.4)
Rural	11	213 (46)	176 (53.6)	3 (1.1)

Within each team, not every care worker is allowed to perform all tasks. Based on their education and expertise, care workers are hierarchically divided into three distinct qualification levels (QLs). Depending on the type of care, healthcare tasks are assigned to a healthcare worker with the required level of qualification. The hierarchical division of care workers' tasks is also referred to as differentiated practice (e.g., [17]). Table 2 shows the QLs relevant in the context of this study. Here, the three QLs are denoted as PV niveau 2+, PV niveau 3, and VP niveau 3, as described by our partner HHC organization. Note that 'PV' and 'VP' are Dutch abbreviations for 'persoonlijke verzorging' (personal care) and 'verpleegkundigde zorg' (nursing), respectively, whereas the number after 'niveau' (level) denotes the required skill level.

Table 2. Overview of qualification levels.

Qualification Level	Description	Type of Tasks	Proportion of Total Planned Care
1	PV niveau 2+	Personal Care	67%
2	PV niveau 3	Personal Care	9%
3	VP niveau 3	Nursing	24%

In the context of capacity planning, non-direct care activities should be taken into account for the working time of the care workers (e.g., [28]). Regarding the division of working time, we use the classification as presented in Figure 1. The percentages that correspond to the categories 'non-client related administration time', 'holiday and leave time', and 'sick leave' are according to the studies [5,33,34], respectively.

The sum of the first two categories is the time during which care workers are available; we will refer to this as the *effective capacity* (as opposed to categories three and four in which care workers are not available). In the remainder of this paper, we mainly consider the effective capacity, with a particular focus on direct care time (e.g., Section 3.1 below also only involves direct care). The holiday and (sick) leave time are assumed to be given.

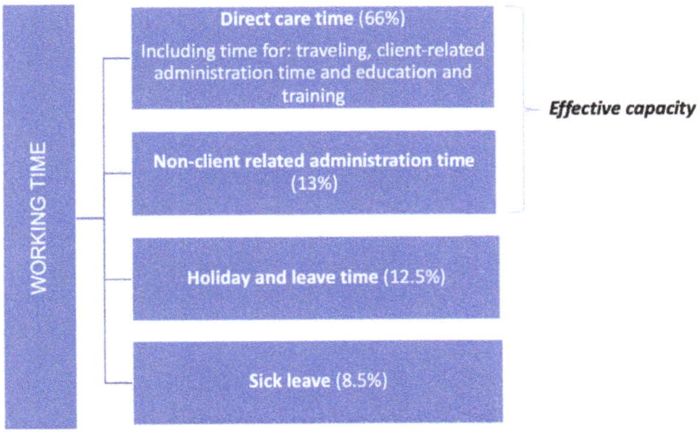

Figure 1. Distribution of working time across four categories.

1.3. Contribution

The blind spot in the existing literature, enhanced by the demand of our partner organization and the current challenges faced by Dutch HHC organizations, has been the primary motivation for a constructive research study whose results are presented and discussed in this paper. The aim of this paper is to provide guidance to managers and policy makers by formulating a set of six practically applicable principles that address issues on capacity planning regarding team size and composition in a HHC context. The team size concerns the required number of care workers per team, whereas the team composition refers to the mix of care workers (in terms of qualification levels) in each team and the demarcation of roles and activities among the different categories of care workers. To address the issue of 'the ideal team size', we do not necessarily restrict ourselves to the current division of teams; the goal is to provide insight into the impact of changing the amount of demand that should be served by a single team. This can be practically achieved by either (re-)designing the cooperation between teams or, more drastically, by splitting or merging teams or redesigning the current division (which relates to the districting problem; see, e.g., [8]).

The six principles originate from discussions with our partner HHC organization and are formalized in terms of elementary mathematical models that capture the fundamental elements. Furthermore, the principles are supported by real-life data and demonstrated using practice-based scenarios. The paper is of value to both the management of HHC organizations as well as the scientific research community. For management, the principles provide both guidance and quantitative support regarding decisions about the employment of capacity, including strategic questions concerning the 'ideal team size'. A particularly appealing property of the presented principles is that they support decision-making without the need for detailed data. For the scientific community, the data analysis offers insight into some key characteristics of HHC. Moreover, the models considered in this paper are of a fundamental nature; they may serve as inspiration and a starting point for more detailed modeling of the HHC demand and supply processes.

2. Methods

In accordance with the approach for constructive research presented by Kasanen et al., the following steps were followed [35]. With help of our partner HHC organization, we first identified a practical problem with research potential. Next, to gain a more comprehensive understanding of the topic, we conducted an extensive and systematic data analysis (see Section 3.1). To this end, we obtained data from our partner organization regarding all planned care activities of the years 2020 and 2021. For each single activity, we have, among others, an anonymized client ID, the date and day part, the duration, the qualification level, and the location (estimate). We note that we were unable to obtain historical data about the deployment and contracts of care workers (the capacity of the service system). As such, the number of care workers is based on generic estimations. As part of the data-validation process and the corresponding analysis, regular monthly validation sessions were conducted throughout the project. These sessions involved collaboration with professionals from our partner HHC organization. Guided by the data analysis outlined in Section 3.1 and in close interaction with our partner organization, we then developed six model-based principles (i.e., rules of thumb) (see Section 3.2). For these six principles, we formulated elementary mathematical models that capture the essential properties of each principle. Subsequently, using various forms of algebraic manipulations, we obtained the performance measures of interest for each model. Next, by using practice-based scenarios, we demonstrated the added value from a practical perspective (see Section 4). Finally, we discuss the applicability and scientific value of the presented principles (see Section 5).

3. Results

In Section 3.1, we present the results of our data analysis . Furthermore, the model-based principles are presented and elaborated on in Section 3.2.

3.1. Data Analysis

The aim of this subsection is to provide insight into the demand for home care, where the demand is defined as the planned HHC activities over time. Although the delivery of care is influenced by how capacity is deployed, we use the planned care activities as an approximation of the actual demand. For interpretation, it is useful to consider a period during which a client regularly receives the same type of care, which we refer to as a *case*. More specifically, a case is defined as care for one client at one given qualification level, for which the time difference between two subsequent visits does not exceed 30 days. In practice, one client may have multiple active cases simultaneously. We first consider the total demand for care (volume of care) revealing substantial variability in demand. Subsequently, we decompose the volume of care into its three primary ingredients: demand per case, the number of new cases per week, and the length of stay (LoS) per case.

3.1.1. Volume of Care

For the considered qualification levels, with a total of about 76%, the vast majority of the delivered care consists of personal care, i.e., PV niveau 2+ and PV niveau 3 (see Table 2 for further details). Personal care encompasses all actions and practices that individuals typically undertake to maintain their well-being. This includes not only basic personal hygiene routines, such as bathing, but also specialized personal care required to address health conditions, such as managing a stoma.

The distribution of care provided among teams, QLs, and area types is depicted in Figure A1, showing the aggregate demand over the years 2020 and 2021. In line with earlier observations, the distribution of care types over the three QLs remains predominantly occupied by personal care. Furthermore, no significant differences can be observed between the various area types. The average aggregate planned care per team is 228 h per week. For most teams, the demand is reasonably close to this average, albeit there are some smaller (teams 5, 27, and 28 have a total of less than 15k care hours), and larger (teams 4, 21, 23, 31, 32, 37, and 41 have more than 30k care hours) teams. In Figure 2, boxplots of the total weekly demand per team are depicted. As indicated by both the interquartile range and the differences between the upper and lower whiskers, there is considerable variability in the aggregate demand per team. In the figure, large volumes of weekly demand are typically associated with more variability, but this does clearly not apply to all teams. The weekly demand per team is more or less symmetric, with only a few teams exhibiting stronger degrees of skewness (left and right). Observe that the variability in weekly demand makes the efficient use of capacity challenging, as we will demonstrate in Sections 3.2.1 and 3.2.4.

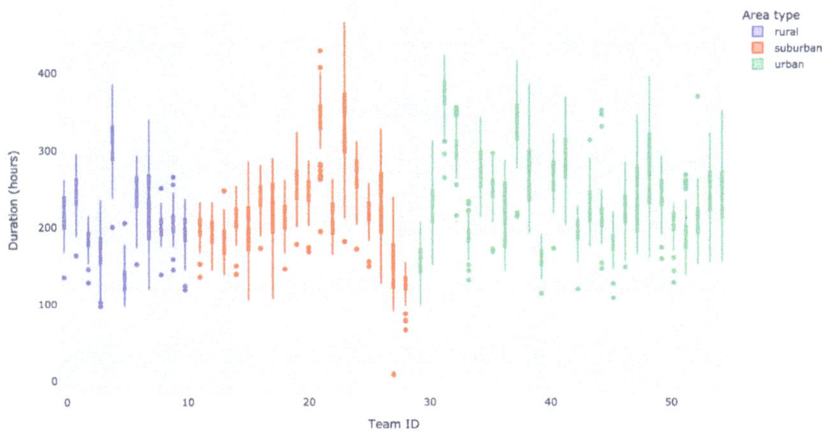

Figure 2. Boxplots of weekly demand for care services per team by area type; years = 2020 and 2021.

The total demand for care per weekday and for each part of the day is visualized in Figure 3. The demand over the course of the week is rather stable, with a decrease in demand during the weekend of about 19.3% compared to the weekdays. The differences in demand across the day are more noticeable. The vast majority of care is taking place in the morning (68.6%), followed by the evening (24.2%). Only 7.3% of the demand is provided during the afternoon. This uneven distribution of demand across the day may complicate the deployment of care workers, as we will demonstrate in Section 3.2.5.

3.1.2. Case Demand

The boxplot in Figure A2a describes the distribution of mean weekly care per case over all 55 teams. The median is about 3.3 h, with the lower and upper fences at 2.4 and 4.0 h, respectively. To put this into perspective, in the year of 2021, HHC clients in the Netherlands received an average of 6 h of care per week. However, the variation in the received amount of care was large. For example, terminally ill clients received 25 h of care per week, while frail elderly and chronically ill people who were in need of somatic and/or psycho-geriatric care for more than 3 months received 4 h of support per week [32]. Note that a client may have multiple cases simultaneously, making a comparison between care per case and care per client more difficult.

To visualize the variability in weekly planned care per case, Figure A2b depicts a boxplot of the variance-to-mean ratios (VMRs) of the weekly care per case of the 55 teams. The figure indicates that the variance in demand per case is roughly about four times the mean (50% of the values are between 3.1 and 4.5).

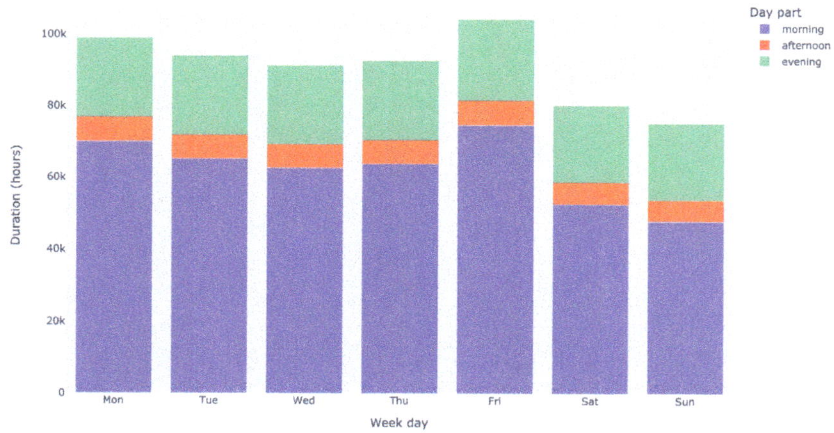

Figure 3. Total demand for care per week day by part of day; years = 2020 and 2021.

3.1.3. Arrival Rate

The boxplot in Figure A2c illustrates the distribution of mean weekly new case arrivals across the 55 HHC teams. The median number of mean weekly new case arrivals by team equals 3.6, with lower and upper fences at 1.0 and 6.5, respectively. The median of the 55 VMRs of the number of new cases is 1.4, and the VMRs are somewhat right skewed with a lower fence at 0.9 and an upper fence at 2.4 (Figure A2d). Note that there is thus some slight overdispersion compared to a Poisson arrival process.

3.1.4. Length of Stay

The LoS is here defined as the number of weeks between the start and conclusion of a given case. To estimate the distribution of the LoS and corresponding statistical measures, a Kaplan–Meier (KM) survival curve $\hat{S}(t)$ is constructed. This is the solid line in Figure A3. The curve of the tail distribution stops around the 100 week mark, which is the actual time range of the data set. This highlights a key challenge when estimating the mean and variance of the LoS as the data are both left- and right-censored.

A common approach to handling censored data is to fit a parametric distribution, such as the Weibull, to the non-parametric KM curve. Figure A3 depicts the Weibull fit to the KM curve for one care team. Although the quality of the fit seems to be (visually) acceptable for this particular case, an accurate estimation of the tail seems difficult, which in turn may severely impact the estimation of the mean and variance. For the analysis in Section 3.2, we therefore use an implied mean LoS.

3.2. Model-Based Principles

In this section, we formulate six key principles that can be used as a guideline for tactical and strategic decisions regarding the team size and composition. The principles are based on stylized models that capture the essential dynamics of the HHC process. For each principle, a more complex model can be constructed. However, our focus here is on simplicity, and we aim to facilitate a shift in the mindset of the HHC managers.

Below, we first state the principles in popular terms. More precise statements are presented in the subsequent Sections 3.2.1–3.2.6. In each subsection, we first present the model on which the principle is based, followed by a numerical illustration.

Principle 1 (Care demand). *The absolute variability in healthcare demand increases with scale, whereas the relative variability decreases with scale. As a consequence, the buffer capacity required to handle demand variability decreases with scale, but the possible reduction becomes smaller as the scale increases.*

Principle 2 (Travel time). *The travel time for an efficient routing strategy is roughly proportional to the square root of the service area and number of clients. Moreover, the travel time is not subject to economies of scale.*

Principle 3 (Effective capacity). *Small teams are more prone to lower levels of effective capacity than large teams as a result of variability in leave of absence and sick leave, whereas the differences between larger teams become smaller.*

Principle 4 (Team composition). *Small teams must deploy above-average numbers of high-level care workers to sufficiently cope with the variability in demand. As the scale increases, the amount of capacity required will move closer to the average workload for each qualification level.*

Principle 5 (Contract type). *There is a restriction on how many contracts can be full-time, if split shifts need to be prevented. The fraction of full time contracts can be increased by augmenting the number of client-related care activities during the afternoon.*

Principle 6 (Communication and management). *The complexity of managing a team increases rapidly with team size due to the number of possible interactions between team members. The complexity can be mitigated by splitting the team into smaller flexible sub-teams coordinated by a central managing post.*

3.2.1. Modeling Care Demand and Required Capacity

For Principle 1, we consider the amount of capacity that is required to keep home care accessible, i.e., avoid excessively long waiting lists. In particular, we determine the expectation and variability in the amount of care work that is offered. We use this to provide a rule of thumb for the required capacity that is provided by a rich literature on square-root staffing principles. Note that this principle relates to the direct care time in Figure 1 and the volume of care in Figure 2.

Model

First, we determine the demand for home care in terms of the required number of care hours per week if all demand can be met. Essentially, we interpret the demand for care as a discrete-time infinite-server queue, in which each server represents a single care hour per week. In particular, in line with Section 3.1, the three ingredients generating demand for care are (i) A_s, the number of new cases in week s; (ii) S_i, the length of stay (LoS) of case i (in weeks); and (iii) B_i, the demand for care per week of case i (in hours per week). We assume that the number of new clients, the LoS, and the case demand for care per week are all i.i.d. and mutually independent (see Remark 2 in case S_i and B_i are dependent). Moreover, we denote by m_a, m_s, and m_g their respective means, and by σ_a^2, σ_s^2, and σ_g^2 their respective variances.

Next, we determine the mean and variance of the demand. Interestingly, the variance of the demand in stationarity can be expressed in terms of the so-called Gini coefficient (see also [36]). This coefficient is related to the Lorenz curve, which is used in economics to represent the inequality in the distribution of wealth or income among the citizens of a country. Here, we use it for the inequality in the LoS S among cases. The Gini coefficient is defined as the area under the Lorenz curve. In particular, the Gini coefficient [37] is, in this case for a discrete random variable S,

$$G_s = 1 - \frac{1}{\mathbb{E}S} \sum_{k=0}^{\infty} \mathbb{P}(S > k)^2.$$

For short- to medium-term planning of capacity of several weeks ahead, it is of interest to consider the time-dependent demand N_t. Let $\hat{A}_0$ be the number of patients currently present, i.e., at time 0, and let S_i^r be their remaining LoS and $\hat{B}_i$ their case demand.

Lemma 1. *The mean and variance of the number of care hours t weeks from now is given by*

$$\mathbb{E}[N_t] = N_0\mathbb{P}(S^r \geq t) + m_a m_g \sum_{s=0}^{t-1} S(t-s) \tag{1}$$

$$\begin{aligned}\mathbb{V}\mathrm{ar}(N_t) &= S^r(t)(1-S^r(t))\sum_{i=1}^{\hat{A}_0}\hat{B}_i^2 + m_a(\sigma_g^2+m_g^2)\sum_{s=0}^{t-1}S(t-s) \\ &\quad + m_g^2(\sigma_a^2 - m_a)\sum_{s=0}^{t-1}S(t-s)^2\end{aligned} \tag{2}$$

with $S(t) = \mathbb{P}(S \geq t)$ *and* $S^r(t) = \mathbb{P}(S^r \geq t)$. *In stationarity, the mean and variance of the number of care hours reduce to*

$$\mathbb{E}[N] = m_a m_s m_g \tag{3}$$

$$\mathbb{V}\mathrm{ar}(N) = m_a m_s m_g\left[\frac{\sigma_g^2}{m_g} + m_g + m_g(1-G_s)\left(\frac{\sigma_a^2}{m_a} - 1\right)\right] \tag{4}$$

Proof. Consider the required demand in week t. We then have the following relation:

$$N_t = \sum_{i=1}^{\hat{A}_0}\mathbb{1}\{S_i^r \geq t\}\hat{B}_i + \sum_{s=0}^{t-1}\sum_{i=1}^{A_s}\mathbb{1}\{S_i \geq t-s\}B_i, \tag{5}$$

where S_i and B_i represent the LoS and weekly demand of the ith case arriving in that specific week. Observe that the first term represents demand from cases currently present, whereas the second term is due to cases that are yet to arrive. Using this relation, we may determine the first and second moment of the demand. More specifically, combining this relation with Wald's equation, we obtain

$$\begin{aligned}\mathbb{E}[N_t] &= \sum_{i=1}^{\hat{A}_0}\hat{B}_i\mathbb{P}(S^r \geq t) + \sum_{s=0}^{t-1}\mathbb{E}[A_s]\mathbb{P}(S \geq t-s)\mathbb{E}[B] \\ &= N_0\mathbb{P}(S^r \geq t) + m_a m_g\sum_{s=0}^{t-1}S(t-s).\end{aligned} \tag{6}$$

with N_0 the current demand for care and $S(t) = \mathbb{P}(S \geq t)$ the survival probability or tail distribution of the LoS.

Now, for the variance we distinguish again between cases currently present and newly arriving cases. Note that $\mathbb{1}\{S_i^r \geq t-s\}$ corresponds to a Bernoulli random variable with probability $S^r(t) = \mathbb{P}(S^r \geq t-s)$, from which we directly retrieve the variance.

For the cases that are yet to arrive, we use that if the random variable N is independent of the random variables $X_1, X_2, \ldots$, then $\mathbb{V}\mathrm{ar}(\sum_{k=1}^N X_k) = \mathbb{E}N\mathbb{V}\mathrm{ar}(X_1) + \mathbb{V}\mathrm{ar}N(\mathbb{E}X_1)^2$; see, e.g., ([38], Equation (A.10)). We will apply the above with $X_i = \mathbb{1}\{S_i \geq t-s\}B_i$. Note that $\mathbb{1}\{S_i \geq t-s\}$ corresponds to a Bernoulli random variable with probability $S(t-s) = \mathbb{P}(S \geq t-s)$. Moreover, observe that

$$\begin{aligned}\mathbb{V}\mathrm{ar}(\mathbb{1}\{S \geq t-s\}B) &= \mathbb{V}\mathrm{ar}(\mathbb{1}\{S \geq t-s\})\left(\mathbb{V}\mathrm{ar}B + (\mathbb{E}B)^2\right) + (\mathbb{E}\mathbb{1}\{S \geq t-s\})^2\mathbb{V}\mathrm{ar}B \\ &= S(t-s)(1-S(t-s))\left(\sigma_g^2 + m_g^2\right) + S(t-s)^2\sigma_g^2.\end{aligned}$$

Combining the above, we obtain

$$\begin{aligned}\mathbb{V}\mathrm{ar}(N_t) &= \sum_{i=1}^{\hat{A}_0} \hat{B}_i^2 \mathbb{P}(S^r \geq t)(1 - \mathbb{P}(S^r \geq t)) \\ &\quad + \sum_{s=0}^{t-1} \mathbb{E}A_s \Big[S(t-s)(1 - S(t-s)) \Big(\sigma_g^2 + m_g^2 \Big) + S(t-s)^2 \sigma_g^2 \Big] \\ &\quad + \mathbb{V}\mathrm{ar}(A_s) S(t-s)^2 m_g^2 \\ &= \sum_{i=1}^{\hat{A}_0} \hat{B}_i^2 S^r(t)(1 - S^r(t)) + m_a(\sigma_g^2 + m_g^2) \sum_{s=0}^{t-1} S(t-s) \\ &\quad + m_g^2(\sigma_a^2 - m_a) \sum_{s=0}^{t-1} S(t-s)^2, \end{aligned} \tag{7}$$

where the second equality follows from some rewriting.

For the stationary demand N, we let $t \to \infty$ in (6) and (7), yielding the result. □

Remark 1. *We note that the demand for home care is related to the number of customers in a discrete-time infinite-server queue with batch arrivals ($G^X/G/\infty$). The difference of such a queue with our setting is that we assume that every customer that arrives in the same batch has the same service time. In addition, we do not assume that a customer requires a server, that is, we allow for fractional values.*

Remark 2. *We note that it may be argued that S_i and B_i are dependent due to the type of care activity of case i. In that case, the demand per activity type can be analyzed first, yielding (3) and (4) for its mean and variance. Then, the total demand simply follows by aggregating over the activity types.*

The infinite-server queues provide some fundamental insight into how to choose the capacity in systems with a large but finite number of servers, through a rich literature on heavy-traffic approximations. These heavy-traffic approximations are typically in the Quality-and-Efficiency-driven (QED) regime. More specifically, the suggested heavy-traffic approximation for similar models (see, e.g., [39]) is

$$N_t \approx \mathcal{N}(\mathbb{E}[N_t], \mathbb{V}\mathrm{ar}(N_t)), \tag{8}$$

where $\mathcal{N}(\mu, \sigma^2)$ is a random variable of a normal distribution with mean μ and variance σ^2.

In [30], the author focuses on a rough characterization of the required service capacity to achieve a desired grade of service γ, where the grade of service is related to the probability of delay. Using (8), it can be seen that the approximate required capacity $t = 0, 1, \ldots$ weeks from now is $s_t = \rho_t + \gamma\sqrt{\rho_t z_t}$, which is also often referred to as the square-root staffing formula (which is intimately related to the QED regime). Here, $\rho_t = \mathbb{E}[N_t]$ is the expected demand in week t, and $z_t = \mathbb{V}\mathrm{ar}(N_t)/\mathbb{E}[N_t]$ is called the peakedness, or VMR, reflecting the variability in the aggregated demand process. Observe that with this choice of s_t, it holds that the probability that the demand exceeds capacity s equals $\mathbb{P}(N_t \geq s_t) = 1 - \Phi(\gamma)$. We note that there is now a substantial body of literature on such heavy-traffic approximations with many servers; see, e.g., the recent survey [29] and references therein. Moreover, similar types of asymptotic results have been derived for infinite-server queues with batch arrivals, see [39,40].

For the first principle, that is, the required capacity that HHC organizations need, we rely on the heavy-traffic approximations of many server queues. In particular, assuming that HHC organizations operate in a QED regime combined with Lemma 1, we can specify Principle 1 as follows.

Principle 1 (Care demand). *For some grade of service γ (typically $\gamma \in [0.5, 2]$), the required weekly capacity C is*

$$C = \rho + \gamma\sqrt{z\rho}, \tag{9}$$

where $\rho = m_a m_s m_g$ is the average demand, and z is the peakedness given by

$$z = \frac{\sigma_g^2}{m_g} + m_g + m_g(1 - G_s)\left(\frac{\sigma_a^2}{m_a} - 1\right). \tag{10}$$

Hence, the utilization of the capacity C is

$$\frac{\mathbb{E}[N]}{C} = \frac{1}{1 + \frac{\gamma\sqrt{z}}{\sqrt{\rho}}},$$

revealing economies of scale and diminishing returns.

Here, the peakedness z represents the variability in demand that results from variability in the arrival process, LoS, and case demand per week. To be precise, $\mathbb{V}\mathrm{ar}(N) = z\rho$. Observe that the first term in (9) ensures that the capacity is sufficient to handle the load on average, whereas the second term represents the safety capacity required to cover the variability in demand (in particular, the standard deviation of N is $\sqrt{z\rho}$). Hence, the safety capacity only grows with the square root of the offered load, providing opportunities for economies of scale.

The principle as stated above is formulated for a stationary system, i.e., for the long term in case of the absence of structural changes. For the short-term, in the order of weeks, the care demand depends on the current situation. The principle can easily be adapted by using $\mathbb{E}[N_t]$ and $z_t = \mathbb{V}\mathrm{ar}(N_t)/\mathbb{E}[N_t]$ instead of ρ and z, respectively.

Remark 3. *We note that our peakedness z is consistent with the $G/G/\infty$ results. Assuming $B_i \equiv 1$, (10) reduces to $z = 1 + (1 - G_s)(\frac{\sigma_a^2}{m_a} - 1)$. Moreover, due to the relation between interarrival times and number counts, it holds that $c_{IA}^2 = \sigma_a^2/m_a$, with c_{IA}^2 the squared coefficient of variation of the interarrival times. This corresponds to the classical result due to* [41]. *We refer to* [30,42] *for additional background and to* [36] *for the relation between the peakedness and the Gini coefficient.*

Application

In Figure 4, the utilization of capacity $\mathbb{E}[N]/C$ is illustrated as a function of the average weekly demand ρ in hours. This illustration is based on teams 5, 29, and 32, which were chosen based on their features depicted in Figure 2. In particular, team 5 is characterized by a relatively low volume of weekly demand ($\mathbb{E}[N] = 132.30$) and low variability ($z = 6.99$). Team 29 exhibits a moderate volume of weekly demand ($\mathbb{E}[N] = 231.59$) but experiences substantial variability ($z = 18.49$). Finally, team 32 has a high volume of weekly demand ($\mathbb{E}[N] = 370.87$) and a moderate level of variability ($z = 9.01$). For the three lines in Figure 4, the peakedness is held constant whereas average weekly demand varies. For each team, the utilization of capacity is marked for their current weekly demand and peakedness on the respective graph. As can be observed, the utilization of capacity increases with the average weekly demand, albeit at a decreasing rate, demonstrating economies of scale and the law of diminishing returns. This effect appears when comparing teams 5 and 32 since the utilization of capacity of team 32 is significantly higher than for team 5 due to a larger volume of weekly demand (whereas the peakedness is somewhat comparable). Although team 29 also has a larger volume of weekly demand than team 5, its utilization of capacity is lower due to the relatively high peakedness. This demonstrates that reducing the variability in weekly demand can also increase the utilization of capacity. Overall, we see that an average demand of at least a couple of hundred care hours per week seems desirable for an efficient HHC operation. This exceeds the current size of most teams.

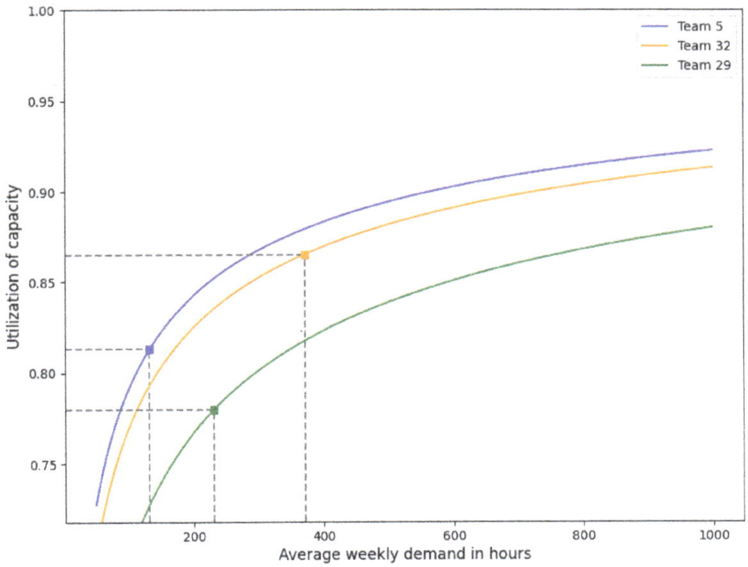

Figure 4. Utilization of capacity $\mathbb{E}[N]/C$ as a function of the average weekly demand ρ in hours, with $\gamma = 1$ based on the peakedness of teams 5, 29, and 32.

3.2.2. Modeling Travel Time

Regarding Principle 2, the travel time of care workers is considered to be part of the direct care time in Figure 1. In this subsection, we describe a rule of thumb for the amount of travel time during a day part.

Model

The approximation for the travel time depends on the number of clients with care activities n, the size of the service area A, and the number of care workers M. Essentially, the travel time is the result of determining a set of M routes that visit all n clients from a central location (office of the HHC organization). Without any further constraints, this corresponds to a Vehicle Routing Problem (VRP), with vehicles corresponding to care workers. Due to many practical constraints, such as qualification levels and time windows, there is now a large body of literature on the Home Healthcare Routing and Scheduling Problem (HHCRSP); see, e.g., [9,10]. As there are currently no approximations for the route length of the HHCRSP, we consider the length of the optimal route for the VRP. However, note that similar approximations remain valid for the Capacitated VRP [43] and some specific time window instances [44], such that the approximation seems reasonably robust.

For the case $M = 1$, already in 1959, [45] showed that the optimal tour in the classical TSP asymptotically converges to $k_l\sqrt{An}$ for $n \to \infty$ and the constant k_l. By now, there are various approximations [46], where many of them are of the following type:

$$\text{VRP} \approx k_l\sqrt{An} + k_c\bar{r}M, \tag{11}$$

where k_l and k_c are constants, and $\bar{r}$ is the average distance from clients to the central location. The coefficients reported in [46] vary from 0.44 to 0.59 for k_l and values close to 2 for k_c. Here, the first term corresponds to the length of the route required for visiting every client, whereas the second term relates to traveling from and to the central location.

The approximation (11) provides some interesting insights. First, the type of region (urban, suburban, and rural) influences the route length through the size of the area A, as may be expected. Second, as the number of visited clients n increases, the route length only increases with the square root of the number of clients. Hence, the travel time per client decreases and the relative amount of traveling becomes smaller. Finally, we give two illustrative examples to support the organizational decisions related to the team size.

Example: merging regions. Suppose that there are R identical neighboring regions, each with n clients, service area A, and M care workers. If the R regions are merged, there are nR clients, the service area is of size AR, and there are MR care workers. If the distance to the central location is the same, then the new total route length is

$$\text{VRP - merged} \approx k_l\sqrt{AR \times nR} + k_c\bar{r}MR = R\left(k_l\sqrt{An} + k_c\bar{r}M\right) = R \times \text{VRP}.$$

Hence, there is no efficiency gain in traveling when merging different regions. In fact, the distance to the central location may become larger, making it even worse.

Example: individual routes. Suppose that the n clients are randomly assigned to the M care workers. This may happen when clients are pre-assigned to care workers to provide continuity of care. As the clients of each care worker may be spread over the area, the traveling time of each care worker is now $k_l\sqrt{A \times n/M} + k_c\bar{r}$. Hence, the total route length is

$$\text{VRP - ind} \approx M \times \left(k_l\sqrt{A \times \frac{n}{M}} + k_c\bar{r}\right) = \sqrt{M} \times \text{VRP} + (1 - \sqrt{M})k_c\bar{r}M.$$

Apart from traveling from and to the central location, the route length becomes $\sqrt{M}$ times as large. Thus, pre-assigning clients to care workers may come at the cost of a considerable increase in traveling.

In practice, there can be various complicating factors, such as time windows and different qualification levels of tasks. However, the above examples and approximation provides some fundamental insight into routing to customers in a spatial area.

Principle 2 (Travel time). *The travel time for an efficient routing strategy is roughly* $VRP \approx k_l\sqrt{An} + k_c\bar{r}M$ *for constants* k_l *between 0.44 and 0.59, and* k_c *close to 2. Moreover, merging regions does not lead to a more efficient route.*

Application

The total distance travelled by the team of care workers per day is estimated for each team using approximation (11). The area A corresponds to Table 1; we used the source data to determine the number of client visits n per day as this does not follow (directly) from Table 1. The client count includes instances where the same client was visited multiple times during a single day. As the teams did not operate from a central location, the average distance from clients to the central location is set to 0 ($\bar{r} = 0$). Moreover, we took $k_l = 0.5$.

The average of the approximated travel distances per area type can be found in Table 3. The relative differences between area types seem consistent with what would be expected; the travel distances in rural areas are notably longer than in urban and suburban areas, although there are variations between teams. Overall, given the reasonably small numbers, the contribution of traveling on the direct care time seems to be modest.

Table 3. Travel distance approximation per area type; all numerical values represent the mean, with standard deviation in brackets.

Area Type	Active Clients per Day	Total Distance (km) per Day	Travel per Client
Urban	83 (18.6)	10.0 (9.1)	0.12
Suburban	76 (24.7)	14.0 (7.2)	0.18
Rural	69 (16.4)	26.5 (6.0)	0.39

3.2.3. Modeling Effective Capacity

Principle 3 concerns the availability of care workers. As visualized in Figure 1, care workers can be unavailable due to holiday and leave time (12.5%) and sick leave (currently 8.5%). The effective capacity P is defined as the fraction of time care workers are available, either for administration work or providing care to clients. Typically, management aims for a target effective capacity, where the mean effective capacity is currently 79% (see Figure 1). However, even if the target is met over the course of a year, a temporal shortage of care workers may occur due to randomness.

Model

To obtain insight into the impact of the team size on effective capacity, we consider the following stylized model. Let M be the total number of scheduled care workers during a period T, and let p be the probability that the care worker is present. The period T may either represent a single day, where M care workers are scheduled and $1-p$ is the probability of unexpected illness, or M may be the number of care workers over a longer period (e.g., summer holidays), and $1-p$ represents the probability a care worker is on leave. The number of care workers present $\tilde{M}$ then follows a Binomial(M,p) distribution. Consequently, the properties of the effective capacity $P=\tilde{M}/M$ follow directly from this observation.

Principle 3 (Effective capacity). *With p the probability that a care worker is present, the mean and variance of the effective capacity P are*

$$\mathbb{E}P = p, \qquad \text{and} \qquad \mathbb{V}\text{ar}(P) = \frac{p(1-p)}{M},$$

whereas $\mathbb{P}(P \le l)$, for $l \in [0,1]$, follows from (12). Hence, for larger team sizes M, there is less variability in the effective capacity.

In fact, from the above it follows that the standard deviation of P is linear in $1/\sqrt{M}$, showing economies of scale and the law of diminishing returns. Let us consider the impact of the team size M in more detail. We use the following representation for the binomial distribution, which also holds for non-integer M. For $l \in [0,1]$, the probability that the effective capacity is at most l equals

$$\mathbb{P}(P \le l) = \mathbb{P}(\tilde{M} \le lM) = \frac{B(lM+1,(1-l)M,p)}{B(lM+1,(1-l)M)}, \tag{12}$$

with

$$B(x,y,p) = \int_p^1 t^{x-1}(1-t)^{y-1}\mathrm{d}t$$

the incomplete Beta function and $B(x,y) = B(x,y,0)$.

Remark 4. *In practice, there may be variability in the number of working hours in period T of a care worker. Denote by w_i the number of working hours of care worker i. Then, $P = \sum_{i=1}^{M} w_i\tilde{M}_i/C$ with $C = \sum_{i=1}^{M} w_i$, where $\tilde{M}_i$ is a Bernoulli random variable with probability p. Thus, we have*

$$\mathbb{E}P = p, \qquad \text{and} \qquad \mathbb{V}\text{ar}(P) = p(1-p)\frac{\sum_{i=1}^{M} w_i^2}{C^2}.$$

If $w_i = O(1)$ as $C \to \infty$, then we still have that $\sigma_P = O(1)/\sqrt{C}$ for $C \to \infty$, with σ_P representing the standard deviation of P.

Application

Figure 5 visually represents the probability $\mathbb{P}(P \leq l)$ of having an effective capacity of at most l. In this case, we consider three thresholds: 50%, 60%, and 70%. The target effective capacity p is set at 79%. As an example, the two points in Figure 5 display the probability $\mathbb{P}(P \leq 0.6)$ for teams of size $M = 7$ and size $M = 19$. Those team sizes are based on a relative small team (team 5) and a larger team (team 32); the number of care workers per week is estimated by the ratio of the average weekly demand (Figure A1) and the average direct care time per week of a single care worker (estimated by our partner organization at 20 h per week). The figure shows that the probability of an effective capacity below 60% is around 0.21 for the small team, whereas this probability is only 0.05 for the larger team.

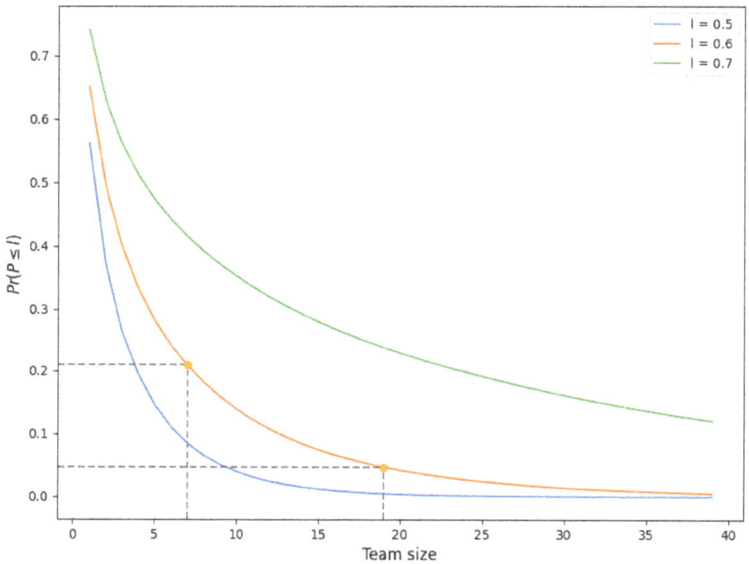

Figure 5. $\mathbb{P}(P \leq l)$ as a function of the team size M for effective capacity levels l of 50%, 60%, and 70% (with $p = 0.79$).

3.2.4. Modeling Required Capacity per Qualification Level

Principle 4 concerns the team composition and relates to the direct care time of Figure 1 again. In Section 3.2.1, we established that the distribution of the weekly demand N can be approximated by a normal distribution. Under this normality assumption, we determine the capacity per qualification level (QL) required to cover demand, taking the hierarchy in qualification levels into account.

Model

Let $Q = \{1, 2, \ldots, K\}$, $K \in \mathbb{N}$ be the set of qualification levels. We assume that there an ordering in QLs exists such that capacity of QL k can be deployed to cover the demand of all QLs $j \leq k$ as well. Denote N_k as the required demand for QL $k \in Q$ in a given week and assume that N_k is normally distributed with mean μ_k and variance σ_k^2. Next, let $C_k \geq 0$ be the capacity of QL k deployed over the given week. The quantities C_k can be viewed as (continuous) decision variables and should be chosen such that the capacities at least cover the average weekly demand per QL, whereas they also act as a buffer in case of demand fluctuations. Each unit of capacity of QL k comes at a cost $w_k \geq 0$, where we assume that $w_j \leq w_k$, if $j \leq k$. Due to the minimum size of contracts, if capacity of QL k is used (i.e., $C_k > 0$), then the corresponding capacity should at least be ℓ units.

Now, the (optimization) problem to determine the capacity per QL can be formally written as

$$\min \sum_{k \in Q} w_k C_k \tag{13}$$

$$\text{s.t. } C_k + e_k \geq \mu_k + \eta_\alpha \sigma_k, \qquad \forall k \in Q, \tag{14}$$

$$C_k \in \{0\} \cup [\ell, \infty), \qquad \forall k \in Q, \tag{15}$$

where $e_K = 0$ and $e_k := \mathbb{E}(\sum_{j>k} C_j - N_j - e_j)^+$, for $k < K$, is the excess capacity of QLs $k, \ldots, K$. Furthermore, $\eta_\alpha \geq 0$ in (14) is chosen such that $\Phi(\eta_\alpha) = 1 - \alpha$, with $\alpha \in (0, 1/2)$ to bound the probability of insufficient capacity. In particular, if (14) holds, then

$$\mathbb{P}(N_k > C_k + e_k) = 1 - \Phi\left(\frac{C_k + e_k - \mu_k}{\sigma_k}\right) \leq \alpha.$$

For the expected excess over C of a normally distributed random variable Y with mean μ and variance σ^2, we have

$$\mathbb{E}(C - Y)^+ = (C - \mu)\Phi\left(\frac{C - \mu}{\sigma}\right) + \frac{\sigma}{\sqrt{2}} e^{-\frac{1}{2}(\frac{C-\mu}{\sigma})^2}. \tag{16}$$

Observe that the optimization problem (13)–(15) has a simple closed-form solution in case $\ell = 0$. In that case, it is always beneficial to set the capacity of each QL at the lower bound implied by (14) since $w_j \leq w_k$, for $j \leq k$. In particular, the optimal solution to the optimization problem is then

$$C_k = \min\{0, \mu_k + \eta_\alpha \sigma_k - e_k\}, \tag{17}$$

which can be easily obtained by (backwards) induction using (16), starting at the highest QL K. The solution in (17) yields insight into the distribution in capacity over the QLs. Specifically, it follows directly that $C_K = \mu_K + \eta_\alpha \sigma_K$, implying that the highest QL has sufficient safety capacity. This may not hold for each individual QL, as capacity of higher QLs may be utilized.

Now, consider the capacity for QL k as a fraction of the total capacity, i.e., $C_k / \sum_{j \in Q} C_j$. To obtain insight into the impact of team size, we scale the demand by increasing the number of new cases m_a per week while keeping the case demand and LoS the same. In view of (3) and (4), the demand N_k is thus normally distributed with mean $m_a \mu_k$ and variance $m_a \sigma_k^2$. When m_a grows large, the optimal capacities are given by (17) as C_k will be larger than ℓ (we exclude the trivial case in which $\mu_k = 0$). Then, it clearly holds that $C_K = m_a \mu_K + \eta_\alpha \sigma_K \sqrt{m_a}$. Also, it may be verified by induction that the expected excess capacity $\mathbb{E}(C_k - N_k)^+ = \tilde{e}_k \sqrt{m_a}$ for the constant $\tilde{e}_k \geq 0$ that can be iteratively determined. Hence, $C_k = m_a \mu_k + \sqrt{m_a}(\sigma_k - \tilde{c}_k)$ for the constant $\tilde{c}_k \geq 0$. This implies that $C_k \leq m_a \mu_k + \eta_\alpha \sigma_k \sqrt{m_a}$ for $k = 1, \ldots, K-1$, meaning that any QL $k < K$ has relatively less overcapacity than the highest QL K. Moreover, $C_k / \sum_{j \in Q} C_j \to \mu_k / \sum_{j \in Q} \mu_j$ as $m_a \to \infty$, implying that the capacity ratios of the different QLs are equal to the demand ratios as the team size grows large.

Principle 4 (Team composition). *The optimal team composition to cover the demand of different qualification levels* $1, \ldots, K$ *can be obtained by the optimization problem (13)–(15). The highest qualification level has relatively high overcapacity* $C_K \geq \mu_K + \eta_\alpha \sigma_K$*, whereas for larger teams the optimal capacity ratios converge to the corresponding demand ratios* $C_k / \sum_{j \in Q} C_j \to \mu_k / \sum_{j \in Q} \mu_j$.

We like to emphasize that the principle above only relates to the delivery of care. Activities such as supervision are more often invested at higher QLs, but this is not yet incorporated as it depends on agreements within the HHC organization.

Application

In Figure 6, an example of the behavior of $C_k / \sum_{j \in Q} C_j$ is illustrated as m_a increases with $\eta_\alpha = 2$. The example is based on team 5 since it has a relatively low volume of average weekly demand and a relatively well-balanced ratio of QLs, as depicted in Figure A1. The optimal capacity ratio for the current demand per QL of team 5 (i.e., $m_a = 1$) is illustrated with a dashed vertical line. Moreover, the ratios in mean demand per QL, $\mu_k / \sum_{j \in Q} \mu_j$ are illustrated with corresponding dashed horizontal lines. To ensure that care workers can work at their own QL, we require that $C_k / \sum_{j \in Q} C_j$ is close to $\mu_k / \sum_{j \in Q} \mu_j$ for each QL. This implies that, for each QL, the solid lines should be close to the horizontal dashed lines in Figure 6. It can be observed that for smaller teams (lower values of m_a), there is a relatively large overcapacity for the highest QL due to a large relative variability in demand; see the capacity ratio (green solid line) for VP niveau 3 in Figure 6. Consequently, a large amount of the demand for the mid-tier QL (PV niveau 3, indicated in red in Figure 6) is covered by the excessive capacity of the highest QL. In this case, we see that the capacity ratio of the lowest QL (PV niveau 2+) is closest to the ratio in demand since the blue solid and dashed lines are relatively close to each other. For all QLs, the capacity ratios converge to the ratios in demand.

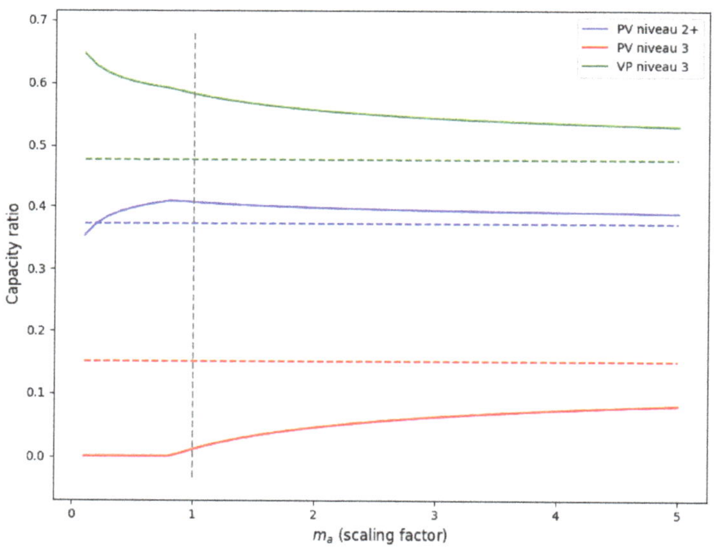

Figure 6. Ratio in capacity $C_k / \sum_{j \in Q} C_j$ as mean number of new clients m_a increases; dashed horizontal lines represent ratios in demand $\mu_k / \sum_{j \in Q} \mu_j$. Dashed vertical line corresponds to current demand of team 5.

3.2.5. Modeling Required Contract Type

Contract type affects all elements of Figure 1, but as far as Principle 5 is concerned, we focus on the demand pattern across the day of the direct care time, combined with the non-client related administration time. In particular, the relatively small fraction of work in the afternoon (see Figure 3) poses a challenge for offering large contracts.

Model

To quantify the impact of the demand pattern across the day on the mix of full-time and part-time contracts, we consider the following stylized example. We assume that *short* shifts take place during one day part (morning, afternoon, or evening) and are of equal length. A *long* shift covers a short shift and part of the afternoon work. In particular, we scale time such that the length of a short shift is the basic time unit. The length of a long shift equals $a > 1$ times the length of a short shift. Let $b_{FT} \geq 5$ and $b_{PT} \in (0, 5]$ denote the number of short shifts required for a full-time and part-time contract, respectively. We assume here that any care worker can at most structurally work 5 days per week. Moreover, denote by f_2 and f_0 the fraction of work that needs to be carried out during the afternoon (care activities during day part 2) or that can be scheduled at any moment (e.g., administration), respectively.

Principle 5 (Contract type). *All contracts can be full time if*

$$f_0 + f_2 \geq \min\left\{ \frac{b_{FT} - 5}{b_{FT} - b_{PT}}, 1 - \frac{1}{a} \right\}. \tag{18}$$

If (18) does not hold, then the maximum fraction of full-time contracts (p_{FT}) to avoid split shifts, due to the large fraction of client-related care activities in the morning and evening, satisfies

$$p_{FT} \leq \frac{(f_0 + f_2) b_{PT}}{b_{FT} - 5 + (b_{PT} - b_{FT})(f_0 + f_2)}. \tag{19}$$

'Proof' of Principle 5. Equation (19) follows by considering the amount of work that needs to be done during short shifts. Due to the structure of long shifts and the amount of work during the afternoon, the fraction of work during long shifts can be at most $(f_2 + f_0) \times a/(a-1)$. We assume that $f_2 + f_0 < 1 - 1/a$, as (18) holds otherwise and the result is trivial. Equivalently, the fraction of work during short shifts is at least $1 - (f_2 + f_0)a/(a-1)$. The total capacity is $M[b_{FT} p_{FT} + (1 - p_{FT}) b_{PT}]$, expressed in terms of number of short shifts, where M is the total number of care workers. Thus, the total amount of work that needs to be carried out during shorts shifts is $M[b_{FT} p_{FT} + (1 - p_{FT}) b_{PT}] \times (1 - (f_2 + f_0)a/(a-1))$.

Now, consider the maximum number of short shifts available as a result of p_{FT}. Consider a care worker with a full-time contract. To respect the contract hours, the number of short shifts x for a full-time contract should satisfy $x + (5 - x)a = b_{FT}$; hence, for a care worker with a full-time contract, there are $(5a - b_{FT})/(a-1)$ short shifts. Hence, the number of short shifts available is at most $M[p_{FT}(5a - b_{FT})/(a-1) + (1 - p_{FT}) b_{PT}]$. There should be a sufficient number of short shifts available to cover the amount of work. That is,

$$M\left[p_{FT} \frac{5a - b_{FT}}{a - 1} + (1 - p_{FT}) b_{PT}\right] \geq M[b_{FT} p_{FT} + (1 - p_{FT}) b_{PT}] \times \left(1 - (f_2 + f_0)\frac{a}{a-1}\right).$$

The inequality above can be rewritten as

$$p_{FT}(b_{FT} - 5 + (b_{PT} - b_{FT})(f_0 + f_2)) \leq (f_0 + f_2) b_{PT}.$$

In case $f_0 + f_2 \geq (b_{FT} - 5)/(b_{FT} - b_{PT})$, this equation holds for any $p_{FT} \in [0, 1]$ yielding (18). Otherwise, solving for p_{FT} yields (19). □

Application

In Figure 7, the right-hand side of the inequality in (19) is illustrated as a function of f_0 and f_2 for set values of $a = 1.5$, $b_{FT} = 8$, and $b_{PT} = 5$. These values correspond to short shifts of 4 h, long shifts of 6 h, full time contracts of 32 h per week, and part time contracts of 20 h per week. In the current situation, the fraction of work during the afternoon is $f_2 = 7.3\%$ (as shown in Figure 3). The left blue dot in Figure 7 indicates that only about 15% of the contracts can be full time if other work cannot be carried out during the afternoon. If all administrative work can be carried out during the afternoon ($f_0 = 13\%$), then the second blue dot shows that the maximum fraction of full-time contracts a HHC provider can offer is approximately 50%. As an example, if the desired maximum fraction of full-time contracts is 80%, then this can be achieved by increasing the fraction of work during the afternoon or any moment ($f_0 + f_2$) to approximately 32% (as indicated by the red star in

Figure 7). This can potentially be achieved by shifting work from the (late) morning or (early) evening to the afternoon.

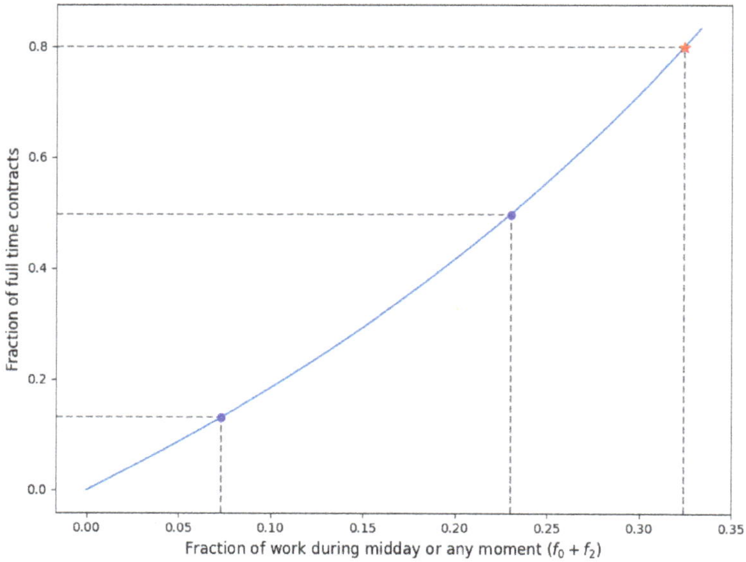

Figure 7. Maximum fraction of full-time contracts (upper bound of p_{FT} in (19)) as a function of available work during the afternoon or any moment ($f_0 + f_2$).

3.2.6. Modeling Complexity of Team Size

The principles of the previous subsections indicate that the efficiency of a team (almost) invariably increases as the team size grows. However, it is also intuitively clear that larger teams are harder to manage. With this in mind, Principle 6 focuses on the number of interactions that occur within a team. For example, in [47] the author concludes that smaller teams make for better team work, mainly because information sharing between team members and coordinating activities among team members becomes more difficult as the team size grows. Although the discussion in [47] concerns project teams in a broader sense, the idea of considering interactions also applies to a home care context as care workers discuss the health status of their clients and coordinate their schedules.

Model

To illustrate the number of interactions in a team, we may represent a team of size M as a graph, where each node represents a team member and each edge corresponds to a line of communication between team members (i.e., interaction). Under the assumption that such a graph is complete (i.e., each team member is able to communicate with all other members within the team), there are

$$\frac{M(M-1)}{2} \tag{20}$$

edges in total. We refer to Figure A4 for an illustration of a complete graph for $M = 5$ and $M = 10$. In terms of complexity, the number of interactions between a team of size M thus equals $\mathcal{O}(M^2)$. The blue line (for the complete team) in Figure 8 visualizes how the number of interactions increases as the team size M grows.

Both figures indicate that the difficulty of managing a team increases rapidly as the team size grows. However, it is difficult to determine an appropriate threshold that remains manageable based on the number of interactions as this will depend on the type of work and the realized and/or required number of interactions.

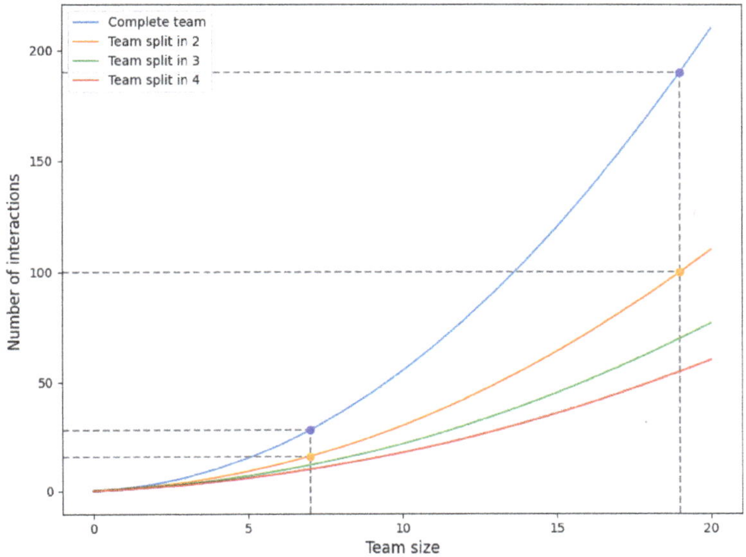

Figure 8. Number of interactions as a function of the team size (i.e., number of members) for a team where all members interact (complete team) and for teams that are split up and connected by a mediator.

The number of interactions within a large team can be reduced by splitting up the team into smaller (flexible) sub-teams and centrally connecting the sub-teams via a mediator. In practice, the individual sub-teams can still function as one team. The sub-teams should be sufficiently flexible such that they can also assist other teams when necessary where the information flow is via the mediator.

To determine the implications of this strategy in terms of complexity, consider k individual sub-teams of sizes $M_1, M_2, \ldots, M_k$, and let $M = M_1 + \cdots + M_k$. As mentioned, all team members within an individual team interact with each other but do not interact with members of another team. Moreover, we assume that there is one mediator that is able to interact with all members in each team.

Again, the number of interactions within sub-team $j \in \{1, 2, \ldots, k\}$ equals $M_j(M_j - 1)/2$, whereas the number of interactions with the mediator is equal to M. Hence, in total there are

$$M + \sum_{j=1}^{k} \frac{M_j(M_j - 1)}{2} \tag{21}$$

interactions taking place. In case the sub-teams are of equal size, that is, $M_j = \frac{1}{k}M$, then Equation (21) simplifies to

$$M + \frac{1}{2}M\left(\frac{1}{k}M - 1\right) = \frac{1}{2}M + \frac{1}{2k}M^2 = \frac{1}{2}M\left(1 + \frac{1}{k}M\right). \tag{22}$$

Clearly, the complexity is still equal to $\mathcal{O}(M^2)$; however, the number of interactions is reduced compared to a single large team, cf. (20). Specifically, as M grows the number of interactions reduces by a factor $\frac{1}{k}$ in the limit when k sub-teams connected via a mediator are created instead of a single large team:

$$\frac{\frac{1}{2}M(1+\frac{1}{k}M)}{\frac{1}{2}M(M-1)} \to \frac{1}{k} \text{ as } M \to \infty.$$

Principle 6 (Communication and management)**.** *The complexity of the number of interactions for a team of size M is $\mathcal{O}(M^2)$. However, by splitting the team into k flexible sub-teams of equal size, managed by one mediator, the number of interactions can be reduced by a factor k as M grows large.*

Application

The number of interactions is illustrated in Figure 8 in case of a single team (complete team) and for split ups in 2, 3 and 4 sub-teams of equal sizes. In the figure, we highlighted the cases of teams consisting of $M = 7$ and $M = 19$ members in total, which are based on teams 5 and 32, respectively (see Section 3.2.3). The blue dots represent the case of a single team (representing the current situation), whereas the orange dots demonstrate the number of interactions in the (hypothetical) scenario where the teams are split up into two equally sized sub-teams. The benefit of splitting up teams into (two) sub-teams is obviously greater for large teams than for small teams.

4. Practice Based Scenarios

It is clear from Principles 1, 3, and 4 that the efficiency of a team increases with team size. Conversely, Principle 6 illustrates the difficulty in managing larger teams; note that team size has no direct implications for Principles 2 and 5. Moreover, Principles 1, 3, and 4 are subject to the law of diminishing returns; most efficiency improvements can be achieved by merging relatively small teams into larger ones.

In practice, the capacity of a team can typically be increased by merging one team with another (i.e., pooling all team members of both teams to cover their shared demand). Naturally, this only makes sense when the geographical territories of the teams are closely situated. To illustrate how the principles in Section 3.2 can be used in practice, we consider a selection of 9 out of the 55 teams of the HHC organization. The 9 teams are merged one by one into larger teams, whereupon we consider the effects under Principles 1, 3, 4, and 6 at each step of the merging process. The merging process is illustrated in Figure 9, showcasing the centroid of the geographical locations of the nine selected teams (each labeled with its team ID). The marker size represents the mean weekly demand relative to the other teams. Each arrow indicates the next step in the merging process: starting with team 5, we first merge teams 5 and 15; subsequently, we merge team 39 with the cluster of $\{5, 15\}$, and so on. The characteristics of each team (including the mean weekly demand) can be found in Table 4.

The effects of Principles 1, 3, 4, and 6 are illustrated at each step in the merging process in Figure 10; starting from the left, each point indicates that another team is added to the cluster. Here, Figure 10a shows the utilization of capacity $\mathbb{E}[N]/C$, Figure 10b the probability that effective capacity falls below 60%, and Figure 10d the number of interactions within the team. Moreover, Figure 10c shows the difference between the capacity and demand ratio for each QL k, $(C_k/\sum_{j\in Q} C_j) - (\mu_k/\sum_{j\in Q}\mu_j)$, which is ideally just above zero for every QL. From the figures, we observe that there is a considerable improvement in capacity utilization, the risk reduction in shortage in effective capacity, and the capacity deviations in the first few steps of the merging process. However, the improvements diminish significantly following subsequent merging steps. Roughly, most of the improvements have been achieved after four teams have been merged, i.e., teams 5, 15, 39, and 41, corresponding to a total aggregate of almost 800 care hours per week. Moreover, the number of interactions is already significant for the combination of the four teams. This can be partly mitigated by splitting the combined team $\{5, 15, 39, 41\}$ into two flexible sub-teams managed by a central post (yellow line in Figure 10d).

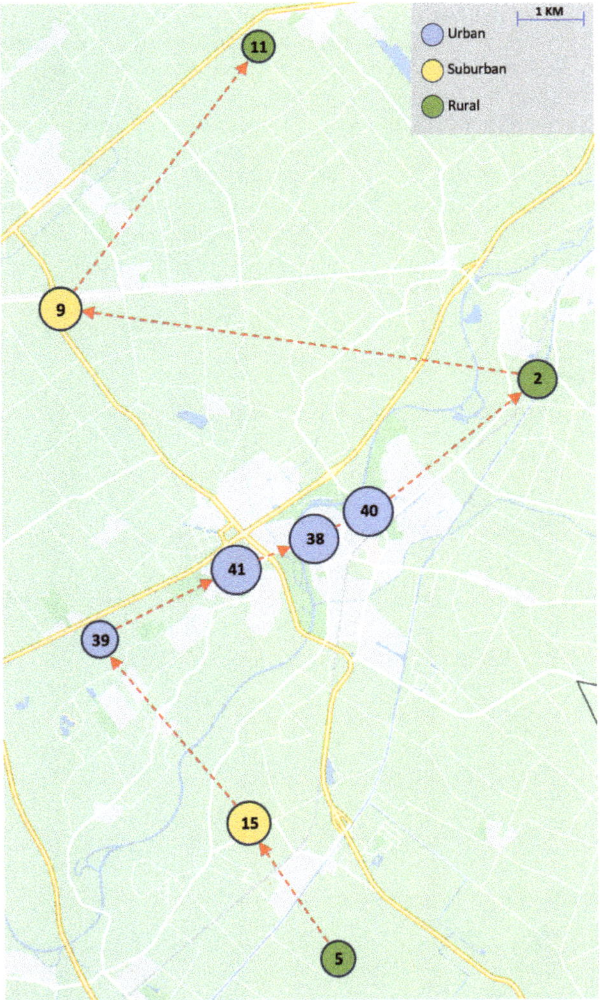

Figure 9. Geographical locations of the teams selected for the merging process.

Table 4. Characteristics of the teams selected for merging; see Section 3.2.1 for notation.

Team ID	Mean Demand	m_a	σ_a^2/m_a	m_g	σ_g^2/m_g	G_s	m_s (Implied)
2	183.46	1.99	1.10	3.61	3.18	0.79	25.50
5	132.30	1.58	1.30	3.00	3.72	0.74	27.93
9	206.06	3.69	1.12	3.24	3.13	0.78	17.25
11	125.41	2.43	1.64	3.06	1.97	0.79	16.85
15	211.13	3.06	1.28	2.78	2.15	0.77	24.81
38	268.71	3.64	1.78	3.82	3.23	0.81	19.32
39	159.07	3.49	1.68	2.68	2.51	0.78	17.03
40	265.53	3.04	1.19	3.60	3.50	0.75	24.29
41	290.75	5.33	0.90	3.31	3.44	0.82	16.49

To be more specific, when comparing team 5 to the combined team $\{5, 15, 39, 41\}$, we see in Figure 10 that there is a relative increase of 13% in capacity utilization; a relative decrease of 82% of overcapacity for PV niveau 2+ and 45% for VP niveau 3; and a relative decrease of 97% in probability that the effective capacity falls below a level of 60%. On the other hand, by merging all nine teams, the relative increase in capacity utilization only improves marginally by 3% (hence, ultimately giving a relative increase of 16%) compared to the situation with 4 teams merged. The improvements of merging 9 teams over the first 4 teams are 3% and 18% in terms of overcapacity of PV niveau 2+ and VP niveau 3, respectively, and a 2% reduction in risk of a low effective capacity. In line with earlier observations, we conclude that the majority of the benefits occur in the first few steps of the merging process. Finally, the combined team $\{5, 15, 39, 41\}$ has 441 possible interactions. Excluding team 41 would give a drop to 182 interactions (i.e., 68% reduction). Conversely, merging an additional team (team 38) results in 784 interactions (i.e., 78% increase). This shows that the impact on the number of interactions is severe.

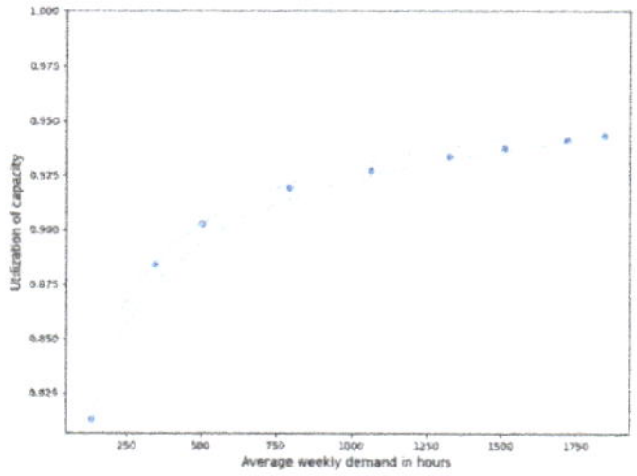

(**a**) Principle 1: utilization of capacity.

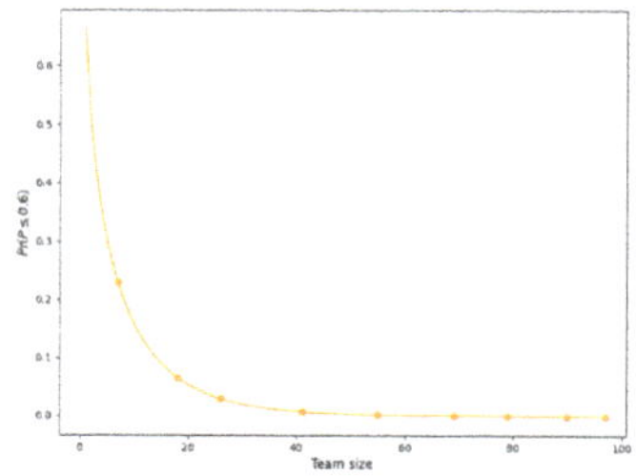

(**b**) Principle 3: risk of lack of effective

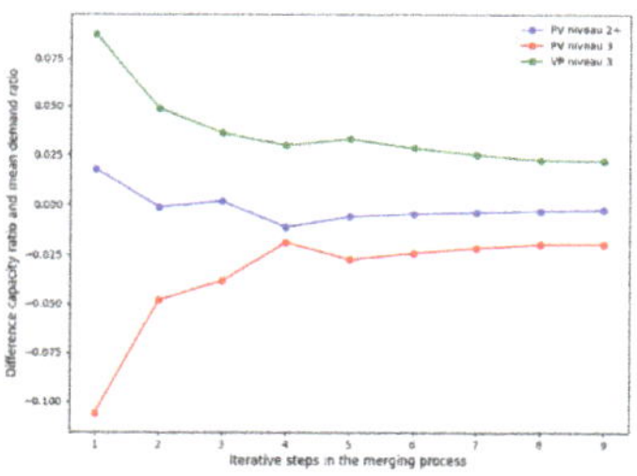

(**c**) Principle 4: capacity vs. demand per QL.

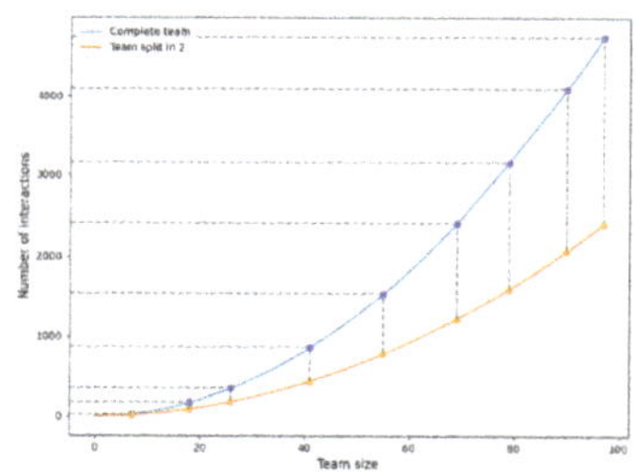

(**d**) Principle 6: number of interactions.

Figure 10. Illustration of Principles 1, 3, 4, and 6 at each step of the merging process; (**a**,**b**,**d**) correspond to Figures 4, 5, and 8, respectively, whereas (**c**) shows the difference between the ratios of optimal capacity $C_k / \sum_{j \in Q} C_j$ and mean demand $\mu_k / \sum_{j \in Q} \mu_j$ per QL.

The observation above intuitively indicates that merging teams 5, 15, 39, and 41 may produce an appropriate balance between efficiency and manageability. However, such decisions depend on the relative importance of the individual components. To formalize this idea, we consider the following weighted objective function that needs to be maximized:

$$\lambda_1 \frac{\mathbb{E}[N]}{C} + \lambda_3 \mathbb{P}(P > l) - \lambda_4 \sum_{k \in Q} \left(\frac{C_k}{\sum_{j \in Q} C_j} - \frac{\mu_k}{\sum_{j \in Q} \mu_j} \right)^+ - \lambda_6 \frac{M(M-1)}{2}. \quad (23)$$

Here, the first term is the utilization of capacity based on Principle 1, the second term is the probability that the effective capacity exceeds level $l \in [0, 1]$ based on Principle 3, the third term is the overcapacity of each qualification level relative to the mean demand based on Principle 4, and the fourth term is the number of (potential) interactions based on Principle 6. The weights $\lambda_i \geq 0$ represent the relative importance of component i. For the number of interactions, the weight λ_6 also serves as a scaling factor (as the units of the first three terms are in %). Note that each component completely depends on either team size or mean demand, which are both a direct consequence of the merging process. Hence, it is possible to find the optimal level at which teams need to be merged by evaluating the objective function at each step of the merging process. This idea is illustrated in Figure 11, where we set $\lambda_1 = \lambda_3 = \lambda_4 = 1$ and use different values of λ_6 to signify the impact of prioritizing team manageability. Clearly, the decision depends on the weights λ_i, reflecting the trade-off of the decision maker's policy. Nonetheless, Figure 11 indicates that the combination of only two or three teams might be ideal, corresponding to a total aggregate weekly demand of 350–500 care hours.

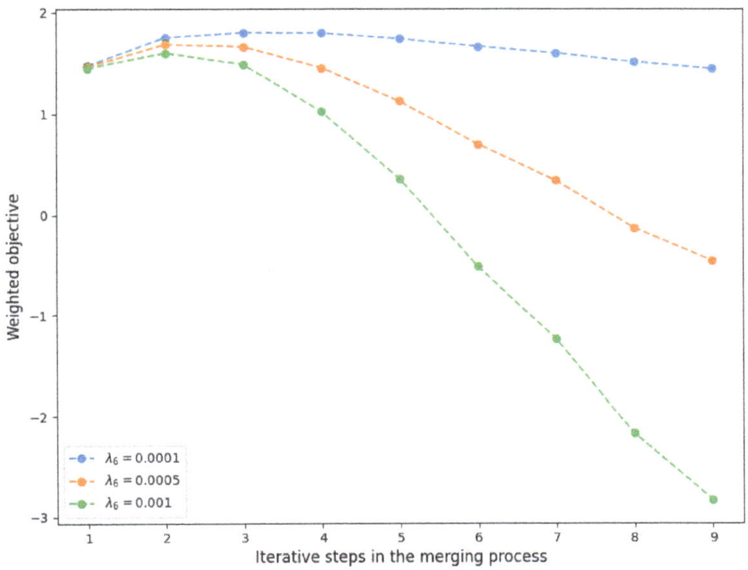

Figure 11. Objective function (23) at each step in the merging process for various weights of λ_6.

5. Discussion

The principles presented in Section 3.2 provide guidance to managers and policy makers when making decisions about team size and composition in the context of home healthcare. The principles reveal that efficiency improves with team size, albeit more prominently for smaller teams due to diminishing returns. Moreover, it is demonstrated that the complexity of managing and coordinating a team becomes increasingly more difficult as team size grows. An estimate for travel time is provided given the size and territory of a team, as well as an upper bound for the fraction of full time contracts, if split shifts are to be avoided.

In addition to the team size and composition, we provide some other interesting observations. First, we were able to quantify the variability in home-care demand and the corresponding capacity requirements per qualification level. Second, we provide a rough estimate of the total travel time as a function of client count, area size, and the number of available care workers. Somewhat surprisingly, travel times are hardly affected by the scale at which teams are organized, e.g., merging regions does in essence not lead to more efficient routes. Third, we touched upon a typical problem recognized by Dutch HHC organizations; due to the lack of care demand during the afternoon, part-time contracts are inevitable. We provide an upper bound for the number of full-time contracts based on the afternoon care demand and administration time.

Whereas the six principles provide valuable practical insights into team size and composition, it is crucial to place them in the right perspective. First of all, the principles are of a generic nature (which we consider as their strength), but their application depends on the specific context. Their implementation and corresponding effects will invariably be influenced by the context in which they are applied. Most notably, the impact of scale on manageability, cooperation, and the quality and efficiency of team work is difficult to quantify in general. Moreover, it is typically impossible to capture all of the details of the application within a model; after all, a model is a simplified representation of a real-life situation. See [48] for a plea of the application of deductive modeling. Hence, managers and policymakers should regard any results obtained from these models as estimations rather than absolute certainties.

As indicated above, we believe that there is great potential by increasing the scale at which HHC teams operate. At this point, we like to emphasize that multiple ways exist to organize healthcare on a larger scale, next to the 'straightforward' merging of teams. During the last decade, various strategies have been investigated to achieve economies of scale for hospital wards while mitigating their drawbacks; see, e.g., [49–52]. A common aspect is that each team does not necessarily need to operate at a large scale as long as some flexibility is organized such that teams cooperate when peaks in demand occur. We think that such a design might be a practical first step to improve efficiency in the context of HHC.

Besides creating practical value, our goal is to trigger the OR community to address tactical and strategic challenges that HHC organizations are facing. The presented data and principles provide a solid basis for further research in which the principles can be further explored and/or extended. For instance, one possible direction is to model the interplay between care demand and the available capacity in terms of a queueing model. Developing such a model is intricate as in practice the capacity will not be constant over time and the admission policy also plays a vital role (see e.g., [53]). Moreover, the team composition is fundamental to all scheduling and routing problems that differentiate between skill sets of care workers. Therefore, the process of determining the necessary capacity per qualification level as outlined in Principle 4 can potentially be improved by specifically customizing it to a direct application. Finally, team manageability is essential for establishing an 'ideal' team size as it acts as a natural counterbalance to the economies of scale implied by most other principles. Clearly, the increasing complexity of coordinating large teams should eventually lead to a decline in effectiveness. As a consequence, a thorough and comprehensive modeling and evaluation of team manageability from an OR perspective is necessary. It is worth highlighting that those subjects have received (almost) no attention within the existing OR literature, despite their significance.

6. Conclusions

In this contribution, six model-based principles (i.e., rules of thumb) are presented and illustrated using real-life demand data. These principles provide guidance to managers and policy makers when making decisions about team size and composition in the context of home healthcare. In particular, the principles involve insights in capacity planning (Principles 1 and 4), travel time (Principle 2), available effective capacity (Principle 3), contract types (Principle 5), and team manageability (Principle 6). The principles concerning capacity planning and effective capacity generally state that the efficiency of a team improves as team sizes increase (due to economies of scale). However, smaller teams benefit more from this effect than larger teams due to the law of diminishing returns. In contrast, larger teams also imply an increase in the complexity of team coordination. The principle on team manageability shows that the complexity increases in a quadratic fashion with team size. Overall, it seems that an ideally sized team should serve (at least) approximately a few hundreds care hours per week.

Author Contributions: Conceptualization, Y.C., W.t.H., R.B. and D.M.; methodology, Y.C., W.t.H., R.B. and D.M.; investigation, Y.C., W.t.H., R.B. and D.M.; formal analysis, Y.C., W.t.H. and R.B.; writing—original draft preparation, Y.C. and W.t.H.; writing—review and editing, Y.C., W.t.H., R.B. and D.M.; and funding acquisition, D.M. All authors have read and agreed to the published version of the manuscript.

Funding: This research was funded by the Netherlands Organization for Scientific Research (NWO) under the Living Lab Sustainable Supply Chain Management in Healthcare project (project number: 439.18.457).

Institutional Review Board Statement: Not applicable.

Informed Consent Statement: The data used for this study are anonymized and cannot be traced back to a person.

Data Availability Statement: Data are not publicly available.

Acknowledgments: The authors would like to thank the anonymous home care organization for their valuable contribution to this research.

Conflicts of Interest: The authors declare no conflict of interest.

Appendix A

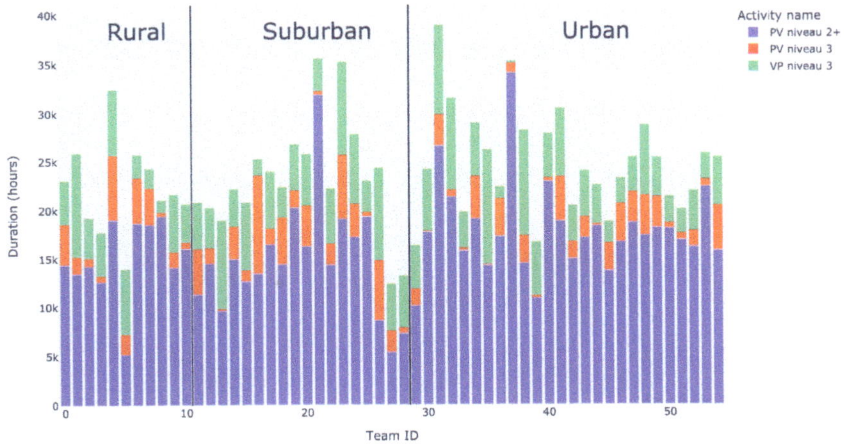

Figure A1. Total care duration per team by qualification level; years = 2020 and 2021.

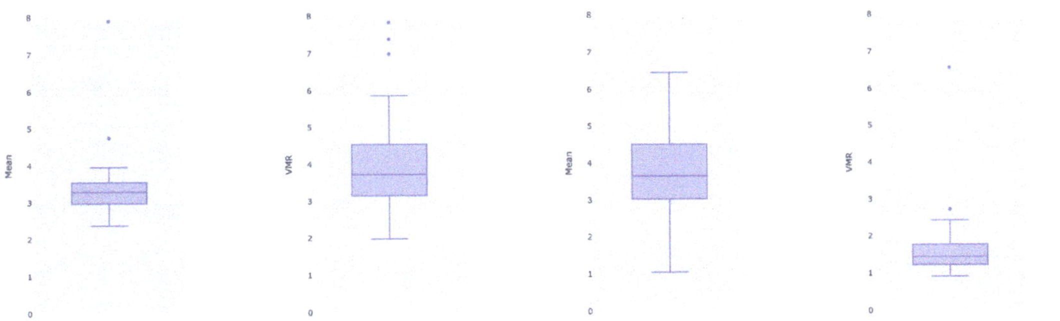

(**a**) Mean case demand. (**b**) VMR of case demand. (**c**) Mean arrival rate. (**d**) VMR of new cases.

Figure A2. Boxplots of selected summary statistics per team; years = 2020 and 2021.

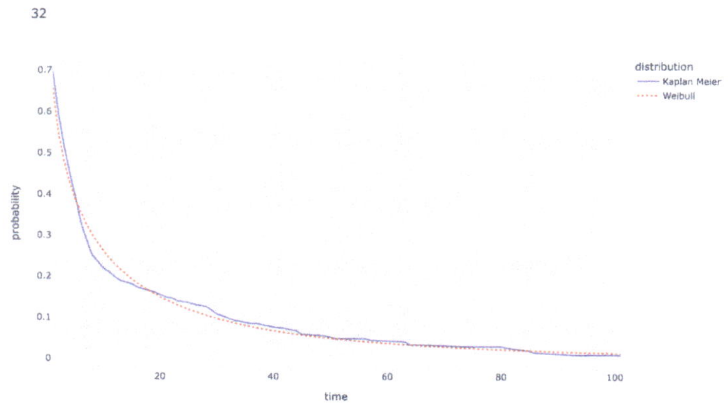

Figure A3. Example of LoS tail distribution for a specific team, time in weeks; years = 2020 and 2021.

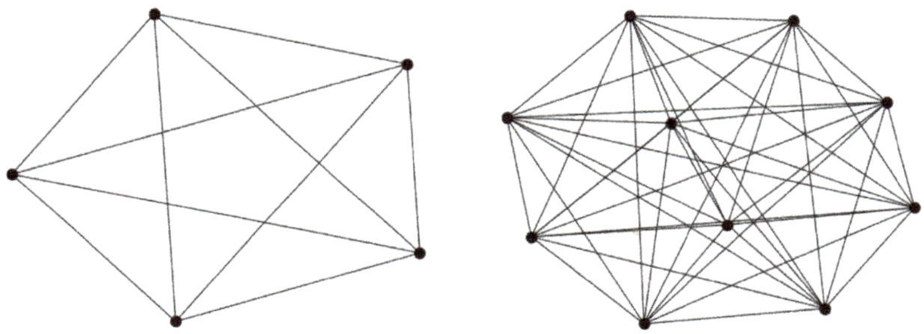

Figure A4. Complete graphs of size $M = 5$ (**left**) and $M = 10$ (**right**), illustrating the number of interactions.

References

1. Knight, S.; Tjassing, H. Health care moves to the home. *World Health* **1994**, *4*, 413–444.
2. CBS. 2021. Available online: https://www.cbs.nl/nl-nl/nieuws/2021/50/prognose-bevolkingsgroei-trekt-weer-aan (accessed on 3 September 2023).
3. Meerding, W.J.; Bonneux, L.; Polder, J.J.; Koopmanschap, M.A.; van der Maas, P.J. Demographic and epidemiological determinants of healthcare costs in Netherlands: Cost of illness study. *BMJ* **1998**, *317*, 111–115. . [CrossRef] [PubMed]
4. VWS. 2023. Available online: https://www.prognosemodelzw.nl/binaries/prognosemodelzw/documenten/brieven/2023/03/21/nieuwe-arbeidsmarktprognose-zorg-en-welzijn/Nieuwe+arbeidsmarktprognose+zorg+en+welzijn.pdf (accessed on 2 September 2023).
5. Vernet. 2023. Available online: https://zorgkrant.nl/arbeid-cao/16737-ziekte-verzuim-zorgsector-gestegen-naar-recordhoogte (accessed on 10 September 2023).
6. Hulshof, P.J.; Kortbeek, N.; Boucherie, R.J.; Hans, E.W.; Bakker, P.J. Taxonomic classification of planning decisions in health care: A structured review of the state of the art in OR/MS. *Health Syst.* **2012**, *1*, 129–175. [CrossRef]
7. Matta, A.; Chahed, S.; Sahin, E.; Dallery, Y. Modelling home care organisations from an operations management perspective. *Flex. Serv. Manuf. J.* **2014**, *26*, 295–319. [CrossRef]
8. Grieco, L.; Utley, M.; Crowe, S. Operational research applied to decisions in home health care: A systematic literature review. *J. Oper. Res. Soc.* **2021**, *72*, 1960–1991. [CrossRef]
9. Cissé, M.; Yalçındağ, S.; Kergosien, Y.; Şahin, E.; Lenté, C.; Matta, A. OR problems related to Home Health Care: A review of relevant routing and scheduling problems. *Oper. Res. Health Care* **2017**, *13*, 1–22. [CrossRef]
10. Di Mascolo, M.; Martinez, C.; Espinouse, M.L. Routing and scheduling in home health care: A literature survey and bibliometric analysis. *Comput. Ind. Eng.* **2021**, *158*, 107255. [CrossRef]
11. Fikar, C.; Hirsch, P. Home health care routing and scheduling: A review. *Comput. Oper. Res.* **2017**, *77*, 86–95. [CrossRef]
12. Christensen, E.W. Scale and scope economies in nursing homes: A quantile regression approach. *Health Econ.* **2004**, *13*, 363–377. [CrossRef]

13. Moeke, D.; van de Geer, R.; Koole, G.; Bekker, R. On the performance of small-scale living facilities in nursing homes: A simulation approach. *Oper. Res. Health Care* **2016**, *11*, 20–34. [CrossRef]
14. Ni Luasa, S.; Dineen, D.; Zieba, M. Technical and scale efficiency in public and private Irish nursing homes—A bootstrap DEA approach. *Health Care Manag. Sci.* **2018**, *21*, 326–347. [CrossRef] [PubMed]
15. Benzarti, E.; Sahin, E.; Dallery, Y. Operations management applied to home care services: Analysis of the districting problem. *Decis. Support Syst.* **2013**, *55*, 587–598. [CrossRef]
16. Ozturk, O.; Begen, M.A.; Zaric, G.S. Home Health Care Services Management: Districting Problem Revisited. In Proceedings of the Industrial Engineering in the Internet-of-Things World: Selected Papers from the Virtual Global Joint Conference on Industrial Engineering and Its Application Areas, GJCIE 2020, Online, 14–15 August 2020; Springer: Berlin/Heidelberg, Germany, 2022; pp. 407–421. [CrossRef]
17. Moeke, D.; Koole, G.; Verkooijen, L. Scale and skill-mix efficiencies in nursing home staffing: Inside the black box. *Health Syst.* **2014**, *3*, 18–28. [CrossRef]
18. van Eeden, K.; Moeke, D.; Bekker, R. Care on demand in nursing homes: A queueing theoretic approach. *Health Care Manag. Sci.* **2016**, *19*, 227–240. [CrossRef]
19. Nikzad, E.; Bashiri, M.; Abbasi, B. A matheuristic algorithm for stochastic home health care planning. *Eur. J. Oper. Res.* **2021**, *288*, 753–774. [CrossRef]
20. Restrepo, M.I.; Rousseau, L.M.; Vallée, J. Home healthcare integrated staffing and scheduling. *Omega* **2020**, *95*, 102057. [CrossRef]
21. Rodriguez, C.; Garaix, T.; Xie, X.; Augusto, V. Staff dimensioning in homecare services with uncertain demands. *Int. J. Prod. Res.* **2015**, *53*, 7396–7410. [CrossRef]
22. Koopmans, L.; Damen, N.; Wagner, C. Does diverse staff and skill mix of teams impact quality of care in long-term elderly health care? An exploratory case study. *BMC Health Serv. Res.* **2018**, *18*, 1–12. [CrossRef]
23. Buchan, J.; Calman, L. *Skill-Mix and Policy Change in the Health Workforce: Nurses in Advanced Roles*; OECD Publishing: Paris, France, 2005. [CrossRef]
24. Green, L.V. How many hospital beds? *Inq. J. Health Care Organ. Provis. Financ.* **2002**, *39*, 400–412. [CrossRef] [PubMed]
25. Cattani, K.; Schmidt, G.M. The pooling principle. *Informs Trans. Educ.* **2005**, *5*, 17–24. [CrossRef]
26. Joustra, P.; Van der Sluis, E.; Van Dijk, N.M. To pool or not to pool in hospitals: A theoretical and practical comparison for a radiotherapy outpatient department. *Ann. Oper. Res.* **2010**, *178*, 77–89. [CrossRef]
27. van Dijk, N.M.; van der Sluis, E. To pool or not to pool in call centers. *Prod. Oper. Manag.* **2008**, *17*, 296–305. [CrossRef]
28. Moeke, D.; Bekker, R. Capacity planning in healthcare: Finding solutions for healthy planning in nursing home care. In *Integrating the Organization of Health Services, Worker Wellbeing and Quality of Care*; Springer: Berlin/Heidelberg, Germany, 2020; pp. 171–195. [CrossRef]
29. van Leeuwaarden, J.; Mathijsen, B.; Zwart, A. Economies-of-Scale in many-server queueing systems: Tutorial and partial review of the QED halfin–whitt heavy-traffic regime. *SIAM Rev.* **2019**, *61*, 403–440. [CrossRef]
30. Whitt, W. Understanding the efficiency of multi-server service systems. *Manag. Sci.* **1992**, *38*, 708–723. [CrossRef]
31. NZA. Available online: https://www.nza.nl/zorgsectoren/wijkverpleging/kerncijfers-wijkverpleging (accessed on 10 January 2023).
32. Vektis. Available online: https://www.vektis.nl/intelligence/publicaties/factsheet-wijkverpleging-2022 (accessed on 10 January 2023).
33. De Veer, A.; Groot, K.d.; Brinkman, M.; Francke, A. *Administratieve Druk: Méér dan Kwestie van Tijd*; NIVEL: The Netherlands, 2017. Available online: https://www.nivel.nl/sites/default/files/bestanden/factsheet_administratie_druk.pdf (accessed on 1 August 2023).
34. FBZ. Available online: https://www.fbz.nl/caos/verpleeg-verzorgingshuizen-en-thuiszorg/ (accessed on 10 May 2023).
35. Kasanen, E.; Lukka, K.; Siitonen, A. The constructive approach in management accounting research. *J. Manag. Account. Res.* **1993**, *5*.
36. Bekker, R.; Koeleman, P. Scheduling admissions and reducing variability in bed demand. *Health Care Manag. Sci.* **2011**, *14*, 237–249. [CrossRef] [PubMed]
37. Dorfman, R. A formula for the Gini coefficient. *Rev. Econ. Stat.* **1979**, 146–149. [CrossRef]
38. Tijms, H. *A First Course in Stochastic Models*; John Wiley and Sons: Hoboken, NJ, USA, 2003. [CrossRef]
39. Pang, G.; Whitt, W. Infinite-server queues with batch arrivals and dependent service times. *Probab. Eng. Informational Sci.* **2012**, *26*, 197–220. [CrossRef]
40. Daw, A.; Pender, J. On the distributions of infinite server queues with batch arrivals. *Queueing Syst.* **2019**, *91*, 367–401. [CrossRef]
41. Borovkov, A. On limit laws for service processes in multi-channel systems. *Sib. Math. J.* **1967**, *8*, 746–763. [CrossRef]
42. Whitt, W. Heavy-Traffic Approximations for Service Systems With Blocking. *AT&T Bell Lab. Tech. J.* **1984**, *63*, 689–708. [CrossRef]
43. Akkerman, F.; Mes, M. Distance approximation to support customer selection in vehicle routing problems. *Ann. Oper. Res.* **2022**, 1–29. [CrossRef]
44. Figliozzi, M. Planning approximations to the average length of vehicle routing problems with time window constraints. *Transp. Res. Part Methodol.* **2009**, *43*, 438–447. [CrossRef]
45. Beardwood, J.; Halton, J.; Hammersley, J. The shortest path through many points. In *Mathematical Proceedings of the Cambridge Philosophical Society*; Cambridge University Press: Cambridge, UK, 1959; Volume 55, pp. 299–327. [CrossRef]

46. Mei, X.; Curtin, K.; Turner, D.; Waters, N.; Rice, M. Approximating the Length of Vehicle Routing Problem Solutions Using Complementary Spatial Information. *Geogr. Anal.* **2022**, *55*, 125–154. [CrossRef]
47. Hoegl, M. Smaller teams–better teamwork: How to keep project teams small. *Bus. Horizons* **2005**, *48*, 209–214. [CrossRef]
48. Gallivan, S. Challenging the role of calibration, validation and sensitivity analysis in relation to models of health care processes. *Health Care Manag. Sci.* **2008**, *11*, 208–213. [CrossRef]
49. Arabzadeh, B. Reconfiguration of Inpatient Services to Reduce Bed Pressure in Hospitals. Ph.D. Thesis, University of London, London, UK, 2022.
50. Bekker, R.; Koole, G.; Roubos, D. Flexible bed allocations for hospital wards. *Health Care Manag. Sci.* **2017**, *20*, 453–466. [CrossRef]
51. Best, T.J.; Sandıkçı, B.; Eisenstein, D.D.; Meltzer, D.O. Managing hospital inpatient bed capacity through partitioning care into focused wings. *Manuf. Serv. Oper. Manag.* **2015**, *17*, 157–176. [CrossRef]
52. Izady, N.; Mohamed, I. A clustered overflow configuration of inpatient beds in hospitals. *Manuf. Serv. Oper. Manag.* **2021**, *23*, 139–154. [CrossRef]
53. Koeleman, P.M.; Bhulai, S.; van Meersbergen, M. Optimal patient and personnel scheduling policies for care-at-home service facilities. *Eur. J. Oper. Res.* **2012**, *219*, 557–563. [CrossRef]

healthcare

MDPI

Article

The Role of Technology in Online Health Communities: A Study of Information-Seeking Behavior

LeAnn Boyce [1,*], Ahasan Harun [2], Gayle Prybutok [3] and Victor R. Prybutok [4]

1 Department of Advanced Data Analytics, Toulouse Graduate School, University of North Texas, Denton, TX 76201, USA
2 Department of Information Systems, Robert C. Vackar College of Business, University of Texas Rio Grande Valley, Edinburg, TX 78539, USA; ahasan.harun@utrgv.edu
3 Department of Rehabilitation and Health Services, College of Health and Public Service, University of North Texas, Denton, TX 76203, USA; gayle.prybutok@unt.edu
4 Department of Information Technology and Decision Sciences, G. Brint Ryan College of Business, University of North Texas, Denton, TX 76203, USA; victor.prybutok@unt.edu
* Correspondence: leann.boyce@unt.edu

Abstract: This study significantly contributes to both theory and practice by providing valuable insights into the role and value of healthcare in the context of online health communities. This study highlights the increasing dependence of patients and their families on online sources for health information and the potential of technology to support individuals with health information needs. This study develops a theoretical framework by analyzing data from a cross-sectional survey using partial least squares structural equation modeling and multi-group and importance–performance map analysis. The findings of this study identify the most beneficial technology-related issues, like ease of site navigation and interaction with other online members, which have important implications for the development and management of online health communities. Healthcare professionals can also use this information to disseminate relevant information to those with chronic illnesses effectively. This study recommends proactive engagement between forum admins and participants to improve technology use and interaction, highlighting the benefits of guidelines for effective technology use to enhance users' information-seeking processes. Overall, this study's significant contribution lies in its identification of factors that aid online health community participants in the information-seeking process, providing valuable information to professionals on using technology to disseminate information relevant to chronic illnesses like COPD.

Keywords: online forum; information-seeking behavior; online information seeking; online information-seeking behavior; online health information; online health communities

1. Introduction

The role of technology in healthcare continues to evolve, with online health communities (OHCs) emerging as a powerful platform for sharing knowledge and promoting collective action [1]. In particular, Facebook groups have become a significant source of health-related information, providing a sense of community and belonging for individuals facing medical challenges. However, several issues persist with OHCs, and there is a need for greater understanding and management of these communities. This study offers valuable insights into the factors that trigger contributors' online information-seeking behaviors within OHCs, specifically in the context of COPD, a chronic and incurable respiratory condition with significant economic and societal impact. The findings of this study bridge a critical gap in the understanding of OHCs and underscore the crucial role of technology in facilitating access to information and support for those in need, ultimately improving outcomes and reducing costs. This study's contribution is particularly significant in the context of Information Technology and People, focusing on technology, as it highlights the potential of technology to support those with significant medical challenges through innovative approaches to disseminating relevant information.

This study presents two primary objectives that significantly deviate from those of previous studies. First, this research assists healthcare professionals in enhancing their approach to COPD OHCs by considering age and gender factors. The proposed modifications are expected to optimize available resources and improve patient outcomes. Second, this study employs an importance–performance map analysis (IPMA) at the construct and indicator levels to obtain valuable insights into critical concerns related to online health information-seeking behavior. By comparing participants' comprehensive experiences with the average scores derived from latent variables that detail performance, the IPMA evaluates the importance of participants' involvement in the endogenous construct [2,3].

The following research questions (RQ) address these objectives and the research gap:

RQ1: Do age and gender influence online health information-seeking behavior?

RQ2: Do age and gender relate to external factors such as self-worth, perceived experience, perceived usefulness, and perceived ease of use?

This research sheds light on the utilization of current technologies by the public to fulfill their health information needs. It fills a significant research gap by enhancing the understanding of how medical professionals can serve their patients better by gaining insight into how their patients utilize technology. The findings of this study are expected to have significant implications for health practitioners, policymakers, and researchers alike, emphasizing the importance of incorporating age and gender factors in the design and deployment of online health information resources.

2. Literature Review

The Internet has become an essential resource for individuals seeking health information, with millions of people globally relying on online sources for guidance. The Digital 2022 Global Overview Report [4] indicates that around thirty-six percent of Internet users are actively searching for health information, and Foster's report [5] confirms this high engagement with health content on social media. On Facebook, with 2.91 billion users, over 1.8 billion engage in health-related groups monthly, forming over 10 million communities [6]. Jia, Pang, and Liu [7] found that over a quarter of health information consumers search for information online multiple times daily. Facebook groups, defined as communities offering belonging and connection, became critical support networks during the COVID pandemic, with most users participating in mutual support [8].

The relevance of online health communities is on the rise, but challenges remain. This study contributes to the literature on online health behavior triggers and the influence of disease-specific factors, with a focus on chronic illnesses like COPD. Our findings bridge a critical gap in the understanding of online health communities and offer actionable information for both medical and non-medical professionals. Moreover, this study highlights how technology aids in information dissemination and support network formation. The economic implications of COPD, costing USD 49.0 billion in 2020, are also addressed [9]. Despite OHCs' extensive use for various health issues (e.g., mental health [10,11], AIDS/HIV [12,13], and cancer [14,15]), their role in COPD management has been underexplored. These platforms offer not just disease-specific information but also emotional support and social interaction (refs. [16–19]), which are key to patient empowerment and improved quality of life. This study underscores technology's potential to reduce COPD's financial and societal impacts by connecting patients and facilitating information access.

2.1. Theoretical Background and Hypotheses

Our research team developed items based on a five-point Likert scale drawn from the extant literature to assess the survey constructs. In Table 1, the sources for the survey items are provided.

Table 1. Survey constructs, composite reliability, and AVE scores.

Constructs	Item Sources	Item Label	Loadings	Dillon–Goldstein's *p*	Average Variance Extracted (AVE)
Perceived ease of use	Ahadzadeh et al. [20]	PEOU1 PEOU2 PEOU3	0.775 0.881 0.897	0.889	0.728
Perceived usefulness	Ahadzadeh et al. [20]	PU1 PU2 PU3	0.864 0.900 0.895	0.917	0.786
Sense of self-worth	Yan et al. [21]	SSW1 SSW2	0.868 0.874	0.863	0.759
Perceived expertise	Durcikova et al. [22], Kollmann et al. [23]	PE1 PE2 PE3	0.801 0.828 0.895	0.880	0.709
Information-seeking behavior	Nambisan [16]	ISE1 ISE2 ISE3	0.881 0.880 0.836	0.900	0.750

For the relationships between the exogenous factors and the outcome variable (Figure 1), we propose the following hypotheses:

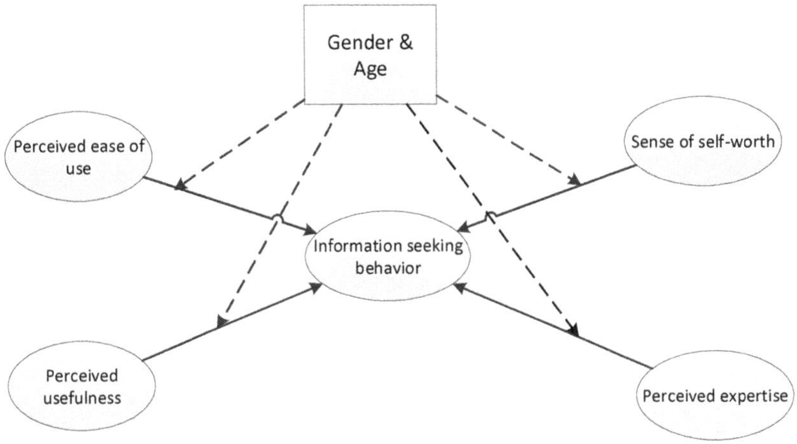

Figure 1. Theoretical framework.

H1. *Perceived ease of use (PEOU) plays a significant positive role in shaping the information-seeking behaviors of COPD forum users.*

H2. *Perceived usefulness has a significant positive effect on information-seeking behaviors.*

H3. *Perceived expertise (PE) plays a significant positive role in shaping the information-seeking behaviors of COPD forum users.*

H4. *Sense of self-worth (SSW) plays a significant positive role in shaping the information-seeking behaviors of COPD forum users.*

H5. *In the context of information-seeking behavior, the influence of determinants (PU, PEOU, SSW, and PE) is moderated by gender.*

H6. *In the context of information-seeking behavior, the influence of determinants (PU, PEOU, SSW, and PE) are moderated by age.*

2.2. Roles of Perceived Ease of Use and Perceived Usefulness (H1 and H2)

In this study, information-seeking effectiveness is defined as the comprehensive assistance provided to those with specific medical conditions, encompassing social and emotional support and critical health information based on the accuracy of information, details concerning rehabilitation, and access to other pertinent services [24]. Recent work has shown how online health information impacts patient decision-making and proactive engagement in health management within online health communities (OHC) [25]. The Technology Acceptance Model (TAM), developed by Davis [26], assesses how individuals perceive and adopt new technologies by examining perceived usefulness and ease of use [27]. OHCs facilitate patient and healthcare provider interaction via the Internet [28]. Research based on TAM suggests that perceived ease of use and usefulness positively influence technology use [29]. Perceived usefulness is defined as the extent to which an individual believes that utilizing a specific system or technology, such as an Online Health Community (OHC), will enhance the overall quality of their life. For a system, including an OHC, to be effective, it must either enhance or assist its users, consequently influencing the extent to which users actively contribute within the designated online platform, such as a Facebook group. On the other hand, perceived ease of use refers to the degree to which an individual perceives the online system as effortless to operate [30]. A good technological infrastructure, a favorable attitude toward technology, and a user-friendly, uncomplicated interface are anticipated to enhance the likelihood of adopting and using online resources. TAM's insights are instrumental in understanding interactions within OHCs, especially regarding technology's perceived benefits [30].

2.3. Role of Perceived Expertise (H3)

Perceived expertise in online health forums is the belief in one's capability to positively influence health outcomes. It is a key predictor of participation in online health communities, with a proven link between cancer management program involvement and perceived expertise [31]. Those with higher expertise are more likely to engage in their own disease management, utilizing various resources. The Internet's role as a primary health information source has been extensively researched. Lee, Niederdeppe, and Freres [32] note that the wealth of information online helps fill knowledge gaps, reducing feelings of uncertainty and despondency, particularly concerning COPD. The availability of such information has been linked to greater patient control, satisfaction, and empowerment and enhanced physician communication [33]. Consequently, this study examines the correlation between participants' perceived expertise in COPD Facebook groups and their online information-seeking behavior.

2.4. Role of Sense of Self-Worth (H4)

In this study, self-worth is operationalized as individuals' perception of their value addition to an online community by sharing knowledge [34]. This is based on Social Exchange Theory (SET), which explains social behavior as a series of transactions where participants engage in the reciprocal exchange of goods, which can manifest as either non-material or material entities [35], thus establishing equilibrium between the rewards gained and the costs incurred within these interactions. Yan et al. [21] view knowledge sharing as an exchange where the costs and benefits can be balanced. Here, an information need is any query requiring a response, with OHCs providing patients with the opportunity to obtain timely and effective answers to their questions, especially when access to their physicians is limited [36]. Social support is characterized by positive conversations that contribute to the well-being of participants, facilitating interactions among members who share similar illnesses. The multifaceted nature of social support includes attributes such as companionship, emotional support, and opportunities for socialization [37]. Sense of self-worth within SET is an individual's perceived impact on the group through their knowledge contributions [34,38]. Costs in OHCs, within the framework of SET, include the cognitive efforts of recalling past experiences, such as emotions like irritation, pain, and depression, and executional resources like time, money, and materials [39]. Additionally, participants' engagement in online communities is reinforced by their perceived elevated status within groups, which, in turn, boosts overall participation [38].

2.5. Role of Gender (H5)

Prior research on the moderating effect of gender on behavioral intention within diverse online environments has produced inconsistent results across different and, at times, similar applications. Researchers like Lian and Yen [40] and Tan and Ooi [41] report that gender does not moderate associations of perceived ease of use and perceived usefulness with users' behavioral intentions. Similarly, Kim [42] and Wong et al. [43] were not able to establish the moderating effect of gender on consumers' use of hotel email and tablet apps. Conversely, Mandari and Chong [44] and Acheampong et al. [45] report that the association between behavioral intention (BI) and PU was greater in male users, but the association between BI and ease of use was not as strong for males about mobile payments and mobile government service usage. Such findings, in the research of Tarhini et al. [46], were partly confirmed in the case of online learning. Their research discovered that associations between the adoption of eLearning technologies by students and perceived usefulness were unvarying between females and males. However, the association among eLearning adoption intention and perceived ease of use was greater for females [46]. The moderating effect of gender on online technologies and the use of information is therefore somewhat subjective and necessitates more examination in the context of COPD forum participants.

2.6. Role of Age (H6)

Age-related variances among humans within technology use are influenced by self-efficacy and life experience. Research indicates that older adults may feel too old to learn new technological skills, unlike younger adults, who are more eager to engage with and learn from new technologies [47,48]. However, the age-related effects on online behavior are not uniform. Tarhini et al. [46] found that in the context of eLearning, perceived usefulness correlates more with younger users' adoption intentions, while ease of use is more significant for older users. Similarly, Liebana-Cabanillas et al. [49] observed that while expertise, usefulness, and trust have less of an influence on older adults' purchase intentions online, ease of use affects both age groups equally. Lian and Yen [40] reported that age does not have any moderating impact on the usefulness of online shopping or on perceived ease of use (PEOU). In contrast, Kim [42] and Tan and Ooi [41] found no age moderation in the adoption of hotel tablet apps and online shopping or hotel tablet app adoption. Therefore, the moderating impact of age is relatively subjective and necessitates further attention in the context of COPD forum users.

3. Materials and Methods

3.1. Setting and Participants

To identify relevant online COPD communities, we conducted a systematic search for the keyword "COPD" in Facebook groups in August 2020. Our search yielded 95 groups that were specifically related to COPD. These groups varied in their objectives, ranging from providing emotional support to disseminating information about pulmonary rehabilitation, exercise, diet, and treatment options. Some groups also aimed to raise awareness of the disease and advocate for improved patient care. The membership of these groups ranged from 16 to 13,000 individuals, and the number of posts per day varied from 0 to 60.

3.2. Data Collection

Before collecting the data, the survey was reviewed by survey research experts and members of a PhD student research team with expertise in survey methods. This questionnaire was developed to collect data to measure the relationships in the proposed model to analyze the results between COPD Facebook groups. A 5-point Likert scale (5 = strongly agree, 4 = somewhat agree, 3 = neither agree nor disagree, 2 = somewhat disagree, and 1 = strongly disagree) was selected to measure the responses for all constructs.

The survey was revised based on the constructive feedback these individuals provided. IRB approval was obtained from the university, and a pilot test was conducted, resulting in slight re-framing and adjustments in the survey questions to improve the general clarity of the questionnaire. There were originally fifty questions, and after the review and pilot run, eleven of the questions were deleted. The survey was entered into Qualtrics. Please see the supplementary materials for the questions included in the survey.

To gather survey data, a licensed respiratory therapist on our research team accessed the identified Facebook COPD groups and posted the survey link with the group's approval. Out of the 66 groups contacted, 46 granted permission to post the survey link, and we successfully posted it in 32 groups. This approach allowed us to collect valuable data from online COPD OHCs and gain insights into the research questions that we aimed to address.

3.3. Analysis

Several analyses were conducted in this study on information-seeking behavior in COPD OHCs. These include:

Sample Size Determination: The determination of the sample size for the model was based on OLS regression properties.

Common Method Bias: Kock's conservative method was implemented to ensure that variance inflation factor values were below the threshold of five.

Non-Response Bias: A post hoc test comparing early and late respondents was carried out using an independent samples t-test.

Partial Least Squares Structural Equation Modeling (PLS-SEM): This was used for data analysis to develop a predictive model of information-seeking behavior, due to its appropriateness for predictive studies, stability with smaller sample sizes, and efficiency in analyzing models with convergence issues and complicated structural relationships.

Reflective Measurement Model: The reliability and validity of the constructs were evaluated using Dillon–Goldstein's rho for internal consistency and average variance extracted (AVE) for construct validity.

Structural Model Evaluation: The model's predictive value was assessed using a variance inflation factor (VIF), bootstrapping methods, and blindfolding for cross-validation.

Multi-Group Analysis: Measurement invariance across gender and age groups was tested using the Measurement Invariance of Composite Models (MICOM) process. The analysis allowed a comparison of path coefficients across groups since partial measurement invariance was achieved. Importance–performance map analysis (IPMA) was implemented to assess the diagnostic value of the model, focusing on 'information-seeking behavior' and its associations with other exogenous constructs. It also evaluated the importance and performance of these constructs within the structural model.

These analyses were integral to the study's aim of understanding and predicting information-seeking behavior within online COPD communities, and they provided a comprehensive evaluation of the model's reliability, validity, and predictive power.

4. Results

Determination of the sample for the model was based on the OLS regression properties [50]. Thus, this research required forty-one observations for identifying values of approximately 0.25, at the five percent significance level, with a statistical power of eighty percent [51]. After cleaning the data, there were two hundred and one usable responses for analysis. Thus, with a sample of two hundred and one, the minimum sample size to represent the population was far exceeded. The demographics of the participants were as follows: The proportion of females was seventy-eight percent and of males was twenty-two percent. Eleven percent of the study participants were between the ages of thirty-one to fifty-four years, forty-six percent were between the ages of fifty-five and sixty-four, thirty-five percent were between the ages of sixty-five and seventy-four, and eight percent were aged seventy-five years and above. The majority of the participants had less than fifty thousand dollars of yearly income.

Common method bias was addressed because participants' anonymity was assured, and all responses were de-identified before the data analysis. Common method bias was addressed by utilizing Kock's conservative method [52]. Kock proposed allowing a variance inflation factor under the threshold of five, which is also achieved in this study. A post hoc test was conducted to determine whether non-response bias could affect the generalizability of our findings. To accomplish this, early and late respondents were compared. As established in the research of Li and Calantone [53], the first seventy-five percent of the survey participants were designated early respondents, and the last twenty-five percent were designated late participants. No significant difference was found after comparing early and late respondents using an independent samples t-test. Thus, non-response bias was dismissed.

The data were analyzed using partial least squares structural equation modeling (PLS-SEM) for the following reasons. The primary objective of this study is to develop a predictive model of information-seeking behavior within COPD online communities. PLS-SEM is particularly appropriate for circumstances where prediction is the goal. Secondly, partial least squares structural equation modeling (PLS-SEM) employs a system of ordinary least squares regression that remains stable with smaller sample sizes, a finding confirmed through simulation analysis by Reinartz et al. [54]. Thirdly, relative to a covariance-based analysis, PLS-SEM is efficient in analyzing models where convergence may be a problem [50,55]. Wold's [56] research emphasized that PLS-SEM is optimal for a complicated structural relationship. Lastly, PLS path modeling integrates the values of latent variables, which are required for importance–performance map analysis.

4.1. *Reflective Measurement Model*

The reliability evaluation of each construct in the measurement model is also shown in Table 2. For assessing the reliability of internal consistency, the Dillon–Goldstein method was used, which additionally considers outer loadings as additional indicators. All constructs have composite reliability values over 0.7, and internal consistency reliability is also confirmed.

Table 2. Composite reliability and AVE scores.

Constructs	Dillon–Goldstein's ρ	Average Variance Extracted (AVE)
Information-seeking behavior	0.900	0.750
Perceived ease of use	0.889	0.728
Perceived expertise	0.880	0.709
Perceived usefulness	0.917	0.786
Sense of self-worth	0.863	0.759

An analysis of the average variance extracted (AVE) and the indicator reliability was also conducted to determine the validity of the reflective measurement model. Following the deletion of the items that failed to achieve the recommended value of 0.7, Table 2 presents the relevant themes of the retained survey items. While it is not recommended, an AVE value equal to or greater than 0.5 is considered acceptable because it suggests that the construct can explain over half of the variance associated with the indicator. Table 2 demonstrates that all constructs meet the 0.5 minimum value for AVE. Therefore, we assume that the convergent validity of our survey instrument is acceptable.

By analyzing indicator cross-loadings, we determined that discriminant validity was upheld. However, cross-loadings cannot indicate a lack of discriminant validity if two constructs are completely correlated. In addition, Table 3 also demonstrates that the indicators are accurate according to the Fornell–Larcker criterion [57]. The upper portion of Table 3 shows that the square root of the AVEs, shown on the diagonals for each construct, is greater than the correlations between the other latent variables. However, the Fornell–Larcker criterion performs poorly if construct indicator loadings differ slightly.

Table 3. Discriminant validity (Fornell–Larcker and HTMT criteria).

			Fornell–Larcker Criterion		
Constructs	Information-seeking behavior	Perceived ease of use	Perceived expertise	Perceived Usefulness	Sense of self-worth
Information-seeking behavior	0.866				
Perceived ease of use	0.719	0.853			
Perceived expertise	0.472	0.449	0.842		
Perceived Usefulness	0.635	0.622	0.460	0.886	
Sense of self-worth	0.561	0.549	0.423	0.505	0.871
			HTMT Criterion		
Information-seeking behavior	~				
Perceived ease of use	0.876				
Perceived expertise	0.580	0.561			
Perceived Usefulness	0.745	0.748	0.553		
Sense of self-worth	0.741	0.738	0.571	0.657	~

~ indicates it is not possible to have HTMT value with itself.

As a result, the heterotrait–monotrait correlation coefficients (HTMT) procedure [58] was applied and all the relationships were under the accepted value of 0.90, thus reinforcing discriminant validity (see the bottom portion of Table 3). Distribution was tested using bootstrapping to ensure that it was consistent with HTMT statistics. The confidence interval obtained from 5000 bootstrap samples substantiates that the HTMT values are significantly different, reinforcing discriminant validity. Therefore, the constructs are empirically distinct.

4.2. Structural Model Evaluation

The variance inflation factor (VIF) evaluated each construct for collinearity. Collinearity among the constructs is eliminated since the VIF values are below the threshold of five. Based on the bootstrap percentile confidence intervals, we determined whether the model's results were statistically significant (bias-corrected). Following Preacher and Hayes [59], 5000 bootstrap samples were run, with the original sample number of observations being included in each bootstrap sample. Table 4 illustrates the structural model relationships based on the 5000 bootstrap samples. Sixty-point two percent of the variation within the endogenous construct-information-seeking behavior is explained by the model.

Next, to assess the cross-validated redundancy, a blindfolding procedure with a distance of six as our predetermined distance was implemented. In other words, the combination of the in-sample and out-of-sample predictive powers should be higher than zero for an endogenous construct to define the predictive accuracy of a structural model [55]. In this research, the calculated statistic produced a value greater than zero. Thus, it was concluded that the model has predictive value. Additionally, when comparing the statistical values of information-seeking behavior with Hair's recommendations [55], it is apparent that the in-sample predictive power for information-seeking behavior was higher than the moderate level.

To assess the out-of-sample predictive power of the model, PLS predictive analysis was conducted with the default settings of ten folds and ten repetitions [60]. To analyze the results, the mean absolute prediction error (MAPE) values from both the PLS and LM analyses were examined, as well as the root mean square error (RMSE) and the predicted values from the PLS analysis. As can be seen in the lower portion of Table 3, all the values in the PLS analysis were greater than zero, indicating that the prediction errors created by the PLS-SEM results were less than the prediction errors created solely by relying on mean values. Additionally, the out-of-sample predictive power level was high regarding RMSE values at the indicator level since all three items of information-seeking behavior in the PLS-SEM model resulted in fewer prediction errors than the LM benchmark. At the indicator level, two of the three items exhibited similar behavior, indicating an acceptable degree of predictive power.

Table 4. Structural model results and out-of-sample predictive performance at indicator level.

Paths			Path Coefficient		Bias-Corrected 95% Confidence Interval	
Perceived ease of use → Information-seeking behavior			0.442 ***		[0.312, 0.578]	
Perceived expertise → Information-seeking behavior			0.099 **		[0.005, 0.192]	
Perceived usefulness → Information-seeking behavior			0.235 ***		[0.113, 0.363]	
Sense of self-worth → Information-seeking behavior			0.158 **		[0.031, 0.294]	
Items	PLS			LM			
	RMSE	MAPE	Q2_predict	RMSE	MAPE	$RMSE_{PLS}$—$RMSE_{LM}$	$MAPE_{PLS}$—$MAPE_{LM}$
ISE1	0.570	13.316	0.492	0.582	13.282	−0.012	0.034
ISE2	0.622	14.305	0.422	0.642	15.172	−0.020	−0.867
ISE3	0.623	14.512	0.388	0.644	14.614	−0.021	−0.102

*** $p < 0.01$; ** $p < 0.05$.

The above results confirm the influences of the constructs perceived ease of use, perceived usefulness, perceived expertise, and sense of self-worth on information-seeking behavior (H1, H2, H3, and H4).

4.3. Multi-Group Analysis

Invariance was evaluated using the Measurement Invariance of Composite Models (MICOM) process, which has three stages: 1. configural invariance evaluation, 2. compositional invariance evaluation, and 3. evaluation of the similarity of mean and variance values. In the event that stage 3 is not satisfied, a multi-group analysis can still be conducted [50]. In this case, partial measurement invariance is attained [50]. The PLS path models of this study, data treatments, and group-specific model approximations were the same about the algorithmic situations utilized for both gender and age groups (<65 years and 65 years+). Thus, configural invariance is confirmed. Compositional invariance was evaluated utilizing 1000 permutations [61] at the five percent significance level. The findings indicated that the p values were higher than 0.05, and the correlation was not substantially lower than 1, which validates compositional invariance. In the evaluation of the uniformity of variance and means throughout all age groups, we found that the permutation p values for the means in all constructs were higher than 0.05 and also higher for the variances for the information seeking, perceived expertise, and sense of self-worth constructs. For gender, the p-values for variances for all constructs were greater than 0.05, but all composite means were lower than 0.05.

Although full measurement invariance was not determined, the path coefficients for both gender and age groups can be compared since partial measurement invariance was determined at stages 1 and 2 [50]. To comply with the stringent guidelines for power analysis [50] and identify an R squared value of 0.25 at the one percent significance level and an eighty percent power level, forty-one observations per group were required. Adhering to these guidelines, the group sample sizes of one hundred and fifty-seven females and forty-four males are adequate. These guidelines are also met for age groups in that our study includes one hundred and fifteen participants who are sixty-four years old or younger and eighty-six participants who are sixty-five years old or older.

Table 5 shows the differences between male and female users in the following cases:

Table 5. Path coefficients for gender and age.

Paths for Gender	Path Coefficients (Male)	Bias-Corrected 95% Confidence Interval	Path Coefficients (Female)	Bias-Corrected 95% Confidence Interval
Perceived ease of use → Information-seeking behavior	0.332 ***	[0.093, 0.560]	0.487 ***	[0.345, 0.635]
Perceived expertise → Information-seeking behavior	0.080	[−0.104, 0.233]	0.117 *	[0.001, 0.229]
Perceived usefulness → Information-seeking behavior	0.353 ***	[0.093, 0.591]	0.192 ***	[0.060, 0.335]
Sense of self-worth → Information-seeking behavior	0.289 *	[0.012, 0.598]	0.089	[−0.059, 0.230]
Paths for Age	**Path Coefficients (64 Years or Less)**	**Bias-Corrected 95% C.I.**	**Path Coefficients (65+ Years)**	**Bias-Corrected 95% C.I.**
Perceived ease of use → Information-seeking behavior	0.468 ***	[0.304, 0.648]	0.420 ***	[0.225, 0.598]
Perceived expertise → Information-seeking behavior	0.162 **	[0.022, 0.284]	0.013	[−0.126, 0.145]
Perceived usefulness → Information-seeking behavior	0.085	[−0.060, 0.240]	0.408 ***	[0.218, 0.580]
Sense of self-worth → Information-seeking behavior	0.220 **	[0.032, 0.413]	0.091	[−0.051, 0.261]

*** $p < 0.01$; ** $p < 0.05$; * $p < 0.10$.

Perceived expertise has a stronger effect on information-seeking behavior for female participants than males. The impact of perceived expertise on the information-seeking behavior of male participants is insignificant.

Sense of self-worth has a stronger influence on information-seeking behavior for male participants than females, as there is no influence for female participants.

These results partly confirm that the influences of perceived expertise and sense of self-worth on information-seeking behavior are moderated by gender, partially supporting H5, since this is not the case with the effects of the constructs of perceived ease of use and perceived usefulness on information-seeking behavior.

In addition, Table 5 shows the following: Perceived expertise has a strong effect on information-seeking behavior for people who are sixty-four years old or younger. The impact of perceived expertise on information-seeking behavior in people who are sixty-five years old or older is statistically insignificant. The same was found for the relationship between a sense of self-worth and information-seeking behavior.

Perceived usefulness has a strong effect on information-seeking behavior for people who are sixty-five years old or older but not for those who are sixty-four years old or younger.

Thus, age moderates the influences of perceived expertise, perceived usefulness, and sense of self-worth on information-seeking behavior. Age does not moderate the relationship between information-seeking behavior and perceived ease of use. Therefore, H6 is partially supported.

4.4. *Importance–Performance Map Analysis (IPMA)*

To assess the diagnostic value of our models, a post hoc study employing the IPMA was conducted as proposed by Martilla and James [62]. The evaluation was based on the PLS estimates, emphasizing the importance of each construct in the existing relationships, and average values denoting performance. Specifically, the IPMA focused on the final main construct, 'information-seeking behavior,' examining its associations with other exogenous constructs and the performances of the currently hypothesized relationships within these exogenous experiences.

The total effects of predominant relationships within the structural model were evaluated and revealed the variance of the main construct, information-seeking behavior. Before calculating the averages of each indicator to represent performance, dissimilar scores of each of the latent variables and the indicators with scores between 0 to 100 were standardized [63]. Figure 2 demonstrates that, at the construct level, perceived expertise is located on the far left of the graph. This means that this construct is of lesser significance regarding information-seeking behavior relative to the other constructs. Figure 2 shows that perceived ease of use is situated on the far-right section of the graph. This indicates that information seekers in the Facebook COPD online community deem perceived ease of use as the most significant factor.

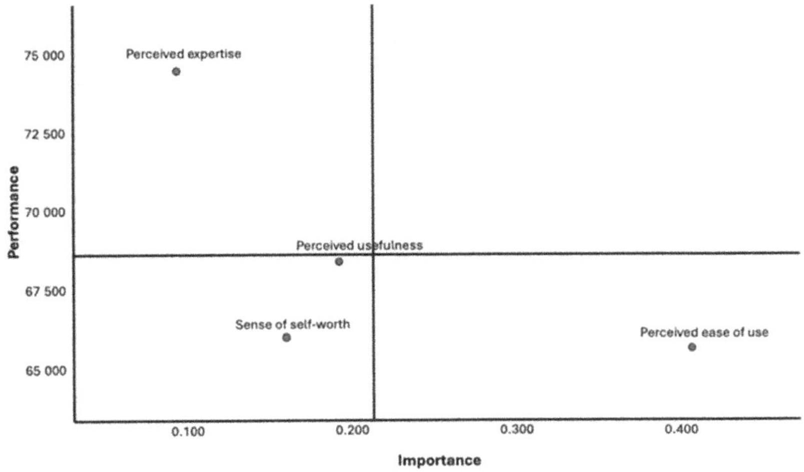

Figure 2. IPMA construct level.

5. Discussion

As we transition to discussing the implications of our findings, it is essential to highlight the pivotal role of interface design in user engagement within disease-specific online health communities (OHCs). Figure 3 emerges as a crucial element in our analysis, illustrating the areas within forum design that require enhancement to facilitate improved information-seeking behavior. This section will delve into the nuances of these findings, exploring the impact of perceived ease of use, usefulness, and self-worth on user participation. Moreover, we will examine how demographic variables such as age and gender differentially shape information-seeking activities, underscoring the importance of tailored approaches in the development and management of OHCs. Our discussion will draw upon these insights to propose practical strategies for medical professionals and forum administrators to foster a supportive and effective environment for patients and caregivers in these digital spaces.

Although many studies have been conducted on various online health communities, little research has focused on creating and managing disease-specific online health communities. As a result, more information is needed on the factors that trigger online information-seeking by participants within OHCs. This research investigated the extent and manner in which exogenous factors within a disease-specific OHC influence participants' online information-seeking behaviors.

Relevant constructs from the existing literature were utilized to develop and evaluate this theoretical framework. Consequently, this study sheds new light on the information-seeking behavior of a disease-specific community. Thus, this research provides a valuable perspective to medical professionals on implementing the proposed outline, which can increase the quality of life of patients, their caregivers, and their families.

According to this analysis, perceived ease of use is the strongest predictor of information-seeking behavior. Consequently, perceived ease of use should be given high priority. Additionally, perceived usefulness and sense of self-worth correlate positively and have significant predictive power. Further, our results confirm a positive relationship between perceived expertise and information-seeking behavior. These results provide insight into the thought processes of the forum participants and emphasize the need to focus on the participants' experiences to achieve a successful outcome. A systematic evaluation of the comparative effects of exogenous factors on information-seeking behavior within disease-specific Facebook groups is provided by this research.

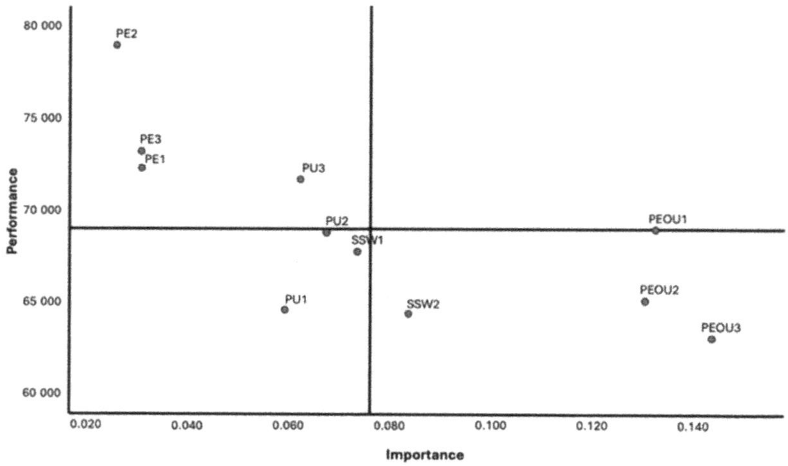

Figure 3. IPMA indicator level.

This research provides a theoretical framework emphasizing the importance of concentrating on these factors to design a successful approach to positively impacting disease-specific OHCs. To facilitate decision-making, the constructs should be considered within the context of an integrated model, such as the one developed in our study. Based on IPMA, this research provides insight into how to encourage disease-specific Facebook group participants' information-seeking behaviors. As shown in Figure 2, it is pertinent to emphasize that perceived expertise is less significant than other factors when considering information-seeking behaviors. In addition, the sense of self-worth construct performs significantly below average, as indicated on the IPMA's y-axis. For this reason, concentrated effort is necessary to improve its performance. In the future, additional research should be conducted to improve the construct's present performance for perceived ease of use in light of its placement on the y-axis.

Information seeking is influenced most by the indicator which corresponds to skillfully searching COPD-related information (PEOU3). As a result, it is imperative to continue focusing on improving its current performance. In addition, there is a need to enhance the opportunities for interaction between participants (PEOU1). This is crucial since this indicator is the second most significant factor. Currently, however, it is only performing at an average level, as illustrated by the y-axis in Figure 3. In the same way, Figure 3 shows how forums (PEOU2) can be improved significantly by improving navigation. As a result, it is critical to pay attention to those factors that contribute significantly to the information-seeking behavior of forum participants.

Further insights are provided by the secondary analysis from a gender-based perspective. Males and females have substantially different associations between perceived expertise and information-seeking behavior. In addition, the effect of sense of self-worth significantly differs between males and females. Information-seeking behaviors are influenced differently by perceptions such as perceived usefulness and perceived expertise between participants who are 64 years old or younger and participants who are 65 years old or older. Medical and non-medical professionals can use these insights to provide a pleasant experience for disease-specific Facebook participants while searching for information. While a specific feature may be prioritized to improve performance, the time and money needed to encourage such actions may not be worthwhile. Thus, it is possible to develop a comprehensive plan for practical approaches by using this blueprint:

- Implement the model as a benchmark in various online forums by distributing survey questions to provide a benchmarking environment.
- Develop a plan for forum administrators and moderators, which encourages frequent exchanges with participants and positively impacts the thought processes of disease-specific information seekers.

Additional textual data were collected that allowed the completion of a qualitative analysis for comparison with the findings. The qualitative analysis supported the main themes identified in the current research. For example, it was found that gender differences existed, and females tended to seek information more than males. In addition, revisiting the site using this mixed method approach allowed us to obtain longitudinal data and confirmed the stability of the findings over time. So, the finding that females reach out more than males was again confirmed.

6. Limitations and Future Work

This study presents a theoretical evaluation framework for information-seeking behavior in disease-specific online forums and evaluates the impact of age and gender on user behavior within the context of the model. Despite the limitations of self-reported data collected via online questionnaires [64], this study significantly contributes to the understanding of disease-specific support groups on Facebook. Future research should analyze other disease-specific online health communities both within and outside of Facebook using this model. Additionally, implementing other advanced statistical models, such as multilevel modeling (MLM) or latent growth modeling, would help us to gain a greater understanding of the complexities of information-seeking behaviors within OHCs. Lastly, consideration of the education level, socioeconomic status, or health literacy of those surveyed would provide a broader range of moderating variables.

7. Conclusions

The study employed cross-sectional survey data analyzed using partial least squares structural equation modeling, multi-group analysis, and importance–performance maps, resulting in the validation of the proposed model. The statistical methods used in this study ensured that the predictions made by the research are reliable. The research concluded with significant findings, notably that age and gender influence online health information-seeking behavior. It was discovered that perceived expertise and sense of self-worth differed based on the way each gender seeks information. Specifically, perceived expertise is more influential for women, while sense of self-worth is more influential for men. Lastly, this study highlights that while age moderates how perceived expertise, usefulness, and self-worth influence this behavior, it does not affect the impact of perceived ease of use.

The knowledge gained from this study is crucial for creating and managing online health communities (OHCs), with implications for both medical professionals and non-medical professionals. Medical professionals can recommend credible online health communities to patients and provide them with an "information prescription" for optimal patient outcomes. Technology professionals can use this study's findings to develop novel approaches for disseminating relevant information to individuals with chronic diseases, such as COPD.

Moreover, the study highlights the potential of technology in improving outcomes for caregivers, patients, and their families. Forum administrators and moderators can use our findings to enhance the interaction opportunities, navigation, and perceived expertise of community members, thereby positively impacting information-seeking behaviors.

In conclusion, this study provides significant insights into the information-seeking behavior of disease-specific forum users, with implications for the development and management of OHCs. Our findings have important implications for both medical and technology professionals, highlighting the potential of technology to improve outcomes for individuals with chronic diseases.

Supplementary Materials: The following supporting information can be downloaded at: https://www.mdpi.com/article/10.3390/healthcare12030336/s1.

Author Contributions: Conceptualization, L.B.; Methodology, L.B.; Software, L.B. and A.H.; Validation, A.H.; Formal Analysis, A.H.; Investigation, L.B.; Resources, L.B.; Data Curation, L.B.; Writing—Original Draft Preparation, L.B. and A.H.; Writing—Review and Editing, G.P. and V.R.P.; Visualization, A.H.; Supervision, G.P. and V.R.P.; Project Administration, L.B. All authors have read and agreed to the published version of the manuscript.

Funding: This research received no external funding.

Institutional Review Board Statement: This study was conducted according to the guidelines of the Declaration of Helsinki and approved by the Institutional Review Board of University of North Texas (IRB-19-176, dated 17 June 2020).

Informed Consent Statement: Informed consent was obtained from all subjects involved in this study.

Data Availability Statement: Dataset available on request from the authors.

Conflicts of Interest: The authors declare no conflicts of interest.

References

1. Gerzema, J. Harris Poll COVID-19 Tracker Wave 103. 2022. Available online: https://theharrispoll.com/briefs/COVID-19-tracker-wave-103/ (accessed on 19 December 2023).
2. Boyce, L.; Harun, A.; Prybutok, G.; Prybutok, V.R. Exploring the factors in information seeking behavior: A perspective from multinational COPD online forums. *Health Promot. Int.* **2022**, *37*, daab042. [CrossRef]
3. Harun, A.; Rokonuzzaman, M.; Prybutok, G.; Prybutok, V.R. Influencing perception of justice to leverage behavioral outcome: A perspective from restaurant service failure setting. *Qual. Manag. J.* **2018**, *25*, 112–128. [CrossRef]
4. We Are Social. *Digital-2022-Global-Overview-Report*; We Are Social: London, UK, 2022.
5. Foster, C. *Social Media And Healthcare: 10 Insightful Statistics*; MedicalGPS: Nashville, TN, USA, 2021.
6. Martin, M. *39 Facebook Stats That Matter to Marketers in 2022*; Facebook: Melon Park, CA, USA, 2022.
7. Jia, X.; Pang, Y.; Liu, L.S. Online health information seeking behavior: A systematic review. *Healthcare* **2021**, *9*, 1740. [CrossRef]
8. Facebook. *Findings from our Facebook Communities Insights Survey Facebook*; Facebook: Melon Park, CA, USA, 2020.
9. Centers for Disease Control and Prevention. *COPD Costs*; Centers for Disease Control and Prevention: Atlanta, GA, USA, 2019.
10. Yao, X.; Yu, G.; Tang, J.; Zhang, J. Extracting depressive symptoms and their associations from an online depression community. *Comput. Hum. Behav.* **2021**, *120*, 106734. [CrossRef]
11. Liu, J.; Kong, J. Why Do Users of Online Mental Health Communities Get Likes and Reposts: A Combination of Text Mining and Empirical Analysis. *Healthcare* **2021**, *9*, 1133. [CrossRef]
12. Gadgil, G.; Prybutok, G.; Prybutok, V. Qualitative investigation of the role of quality in online community support for people living with HIV and AIDS. *Qual. Manag. J.* **2018**, *25*, 171–185. [CrossRef]
13. Mo, P.K.H.; Coulson, N.S. Are online support groups always beneficial? A qualitative exploration of the empowering and disempowering processes of participation within HIV/AIDS-related online support groups. *Int. J. Nurs. Stud.* **2014**, *51*, 983–993. [CrossRef]
14. Chee, W.; Lee, Y.; Ji, X.; Chee, E.; Im, E.-O. The preliminary efficacy of a technology-based cancer pain management program among Asian American breast cancer survivors. *Comput. Inform. Nurs.* **2020**, *38*, 139–147. [CrossRef]
15. Lee, Y.; Kamen, C.; Margolies, L.; Boehmer, U. Online health community experiences of sexual minority women with cancer. *J. Am. Med. Assoc.* **2019**, *1*, 759–766. [CrossRef]
16. Nambisan, P. Information seeking and social support in online health communities: Impact on patients' perceived empathy. *J. Am. Med. Inform.* **2011**, *18*, 298–304. [CrossRef]
17. Sharma, S.; Khadka, A. Role of empowerment and sense of community on online social health support group. *Inf. Technol. People* **2019**, *32*, 1564–1590. [CrossRef]
18. Chen, Q.; Jin, J.; Yan, X. Understanding online review behaviors of patients in online health communities: An expectation-disconfirmation perspective. *Inf. Technol. People* **2021**, *35*, 2441–2469. [CrossRef]
19. Johnston, A.; Worrell, J.; Gangi, P.; Wasko, M. Online health communities: An assessment of the influence of participation on patient empowerment outcomes. *Inf. Technol. People* **2013**, *26*, 213–235. [CrossRef]
20. Ahadzadeh, A.; De, M.; Sharif, S.; Ong, F. Integrating Health Belief Model and Technology Acceptance Model: An investigation of health-related internet use. *J. Med. Internet Res.* **2015**, *17*, e45. [CrossRef]

21. Yan, Z.; Wang, T.; Chen, Y.; Zhang, H. Knowledge sharing in online health communities: A social exchange theory perspective. *Inf. Manag.* **2016**, *53*, 643–653. [CrossRef]
22. Durcikova, A.; Gray, P. How Knowledge validation processes affect knowledge contribution. *J. Manag. Inf. Syst.* **2014**, *25*, 81–108. [CrossRef]
23. Kollman, T.; Hasel, M.; Breugst, N. Competence of IT professionals in e-business venture teams: The effect of experience and expertise on preference structure. *J. Manag. Inf. Syst.* **2014**, *25*, 51–80. [CrossRef]
24. Nath, C.; Huh, J.; Adupa, A.K.; Jonnalagadda, S.R. Website sharing in online health communities: A descriptive analysis. *J. Med. Internet Res.* **2016**, *18*, e5237. [CrossRef]
25. Sinha, A.; Porter, T.; Wilson, A. The use of online health forums by patients with chronic cough: Qualitative study. *J. Med. Internet Res.* **2018**, *20*, e19. [CrossRef]
26. Davis, F.D. Perceived usefulness, perceived ease of use, and user acceptance of information technology. *MIS Q.* **1989**, *13*, 319–340. [CrossRef]
27. Lazard, A.J.; Watkins, I.; Mackert, M.S.; Xie, B.; Stephens, K.K.; Shalev, H. Design simplicity influences patient portal use: The role of aesthetic evaluations for technology acceptance. *J. Am. Med. Inform. Assoc.* **2016**, *23*, 157. [CrossRef]
28. Hodgkin, P.; Horsley, L.; Metz, B. *The Emerging World of Online Health Communities*; SSIR: Stanford, CA, USA, 2018.
29. Mailizar, M.; Burg, D.; Maulina, S. Examining university students' behavioural intention to use e-learning during the COVID-19 pandemic: An extended TAM model. *Educ. Inf. Technol.* **2021**, *26*, 7057–7077. [CrossRef]
30. Matthews, S.D.; Proctor, M.D. Public health informatics, human factors and the end-users. *Health Serv. Res. Manag. Epidemiol.* **2021**, *8*, 23333928211012226. [CrossRef]
31. Vydiswaran, V.G.; Reddy, M. Identifying peer experts in online health forums. *BMC Med. Inform. Decis. Mak.* **2019**, *19*, 68. [CrossRef]
32. Lee, C.; Niederdeppe, J.; Freres, D. Socioeconomic Disparities in Fatalistic Beliefs About Cancer Prevention and the Internet. *J. Commun.* **2012**, *62*, 972–990. [CrossRef]
33. Petric, G.; Atanasova, S.; Kamin, T. Impact of Social Processes in online health communities on patient empowerment in relationship with physician: Emergence of functional and dysfunctional empowerment. *J. Med. Internet Res.* **2017**, *19*, e74. [CrossRef]
34. Wu, P.; Zhang, R.; Luan, J. The effects of factors on the motivations for knowledge sharing in online health communities: A benefit-cost perspective. *PLoS ONE* **2023**, *18*, e0286675. [CrossRef]
35. Homans, G.C. Social behavior as exchange. *Am. J. Sociol.* **1958**, *63*, 597–606. [CrossRef]
36. Solberg, L.B. The benefits of online health communities. *Virtual Mentor* **2014**, *16*, 270–274.
37. Wang, X.; Zhao, K.; Street, N. Analyzing and predicting user participations in online health communities: A social support perspective. *J. Med. Internet Res.* **2017**, *19*, e130. [CrossRef]
38. Bock, G.; Zmud, R.W.; Kim, Y.; Lee, J. Behavioral intention formation in knowledge sharing: Examining the roles of extrinsic motivators, social-psychological forces, and organizational climate. *MIS Q.* **2005**, *29*, 87–111. [CrossRef]
39. Hatamleh, I.; Safori, A.; Habes, M.; Tahat, O.; Ahmad, A.; Abdallah, R.; Aissani, R. Trust in social media: Enhancing social relationships. *Soc. Sci.* **2023**, *12*, 416. [CrossRef]
40. Lian, J.; Yen, D.C. Online shopping drivers and barriers for older adults: Age and gender differences. *Comput. Hum. Behav.* **2014**, *37*, 133–143. [CrossRef]
41. Tan, G.W.; Ooi, K. Gender and age: Do they really moderate mobile tourism shopping behavior? *Telemat. Inform.* **2018**, *35*, 1617–1642. [CrossRef]
42. Kim, J. An extended technology acceptance model in behavioral intention toward hotel tablet apps with moderating effects of gender and age. *Int. J. Contemp. Hosp. Manag.* **2016**, *28*, 1535–1553. [CrossRef]
43. Wong, K.; Teo, T.; Russo, S. Influence of gender and computer teaching efficacy on computer acceptance among Malaysian student teachers: An extended technology acceptance model. *Australas. J. Educ. Technol.* **2012**, *28*, 1190–1207. [CrossRef]
44. Mandari, H.E.; Chong, Y. Gender and age differences in rural farmers' intention to use m-government services. *Electron. Gov.* **2018**, *14*, 217–239. [CrossRef]
45. Acheampong, P.; Li, Z.; Hiran, K.K.; Serwaa, O.E.; Boateng, F.; Bediako, I.A. Examining the intervening role of age and gender on mobile payment acceptance in Ghana: UTAUT Model. *Can. J. Appl. Sci. Technol.* **2018**, *6*, 141–151.
46. Tarhini, A.; Hone, K.; Liu, X. Measuring the moderating effect of gender and age on e-Learning acceptance in England: A structural equation modeling approach for an extended Technology Acceptance Model. *J. Educ. Comput. Res.* **2014**, *51*, 163–184. [CrossRef]
47. Phillips, L.W.; Sternthal, B. Age differences in information processing: A perspective on the aged consumer. *J. Mark. Res.* **1977**, *14*, 444–457. [CrossRef]
48. Fang, J.; Wen, C.; George, B.; Prybutok, V. Consumer heterogeneity, perceived value, and repurchase decision-making in online shopping. *J. Electron. Commer. Res.* **2016**, *17*, 116–131.
49. Liébana-Cabanillas, F.; Sánchez-Fernández, J.; Muñoz-Leiva, F. Antecedents of the adoption of the new mobile payment systems: The moderating effect of age. *Comput. Hum. Behav.* **2014**, *35*, 464–478. [CrossRef]
50. Hair, J.F.; Sarstedt, M.; Ringle, C.M.; Gudergan, S. *Advanced Issues in Partial Least Squares Structural Equation Modeling*; Sage: Los Angeles, CA, USA, 2018.

51. Cohen, J. A power primer. *Psychol. Bull.* **1992**, *112*, 155–159. [CrossRef]
52. Kock, N. Common method bias in PLS-SEM: A full collinearity assessment approach. *Int. J. e-Collab.* **2015**, *11*, 1–10. [CrossRef]
53. Li, T.; Calantone, R.J. The impact of market knowledge competence on new product advantage: Conceptualization and empirical examination. *J. Mark.* **1998**, *62*, 13. [CrossRef]
54. Reinartz, W.; Haenlein, M.; Henseler, J. An empirical comparison of the efficacy of covariance-based and variance-based SEM. *Int. J. Res. Mark.* **2009**, *26*, 332–344. [CrossRef]
55. Hair, J.F.; Risher, J.J.; Sarstedt, M.; Ringle, C.M. When to use and how to report the results of PLS-SEM. *Eur. Bus. Rev.* **2019**, *31*, 2–24. [CrossRef]
56. Wold, H. Partial Least Squares. In *Encyclopedia of Statistical Sciences*; Kotz, S., Johnson, N.L., Eds.; Wiley: Hoboken, NJ, USA, 1985; pp. 581–591.
57. Fornell, C.; Larcker, D.F. Evaluating structural equation models with unobservable variables and measurement error. *J. Mark. Res.* **1981**, *18*, 39. [CrossRef]
58. Henseler, J.; Ringle, C.M.; Sarstedt, M. A new criterion for assessing discriminant validity in variance-based structural equation modeling. *J. Acad. Mark. Sci.* **2015**, *43*, 115–135. [CrossRef]
59. Preacher, K.J.; Hayes, A.F. Asymptotic and resampling strategies for assessing and comparing indirect effects in multiple mediator models. *Behav. Res. Methods* **2008**, *40*, 879–891. [CrossRef]
60. Shmueli, G.; Sarstedt, M.; Hair, J.F.; Jun-Hwa Cheah Ting, H.; Vaithilingam, S.; Ringle, C.M. Predictive model assessment in PLS-SEM: Guidelines for using PLSpredict. *Eur. J. Mark.* **2019**, *53*, 2322–2347. [CrossRef]
61. Chin, W.W.; Dibbern, J. An introduction to a permutation based procedure for multi-group PLS analysis: Results of tests of differences on simulated data and a cross cultural analysis of the sourcing of information system services between Germany and the USA. In *Handbook of Partial Least Squares*; Springer: Berlin/Heidelberg, Germany, 2009; pp. 171–193.
62. Martilla, J.A.; James, J.C. Importance-Performance analysis. *J. Mark.* **1977**, *41*, 77–79. [CrossRef]
63. Anderson, E.W.; Fornell, C. Foundations of the American Customer Satisfaction Index. *Total Qual. Manag.* **2000**, *11*, 869–882. [CrossRef]
64. Podsakoff, P.M.; Organ, D.W. Self-reports in organizational research: Problems and prospects. *J. Manag.* **1986**, *12*, 531–544. [CrossRef]

healthcare

MDPI

Article

From Mandate to Choice: How Voluntary Mask Wearing Shapes Interpersonal Distance Among University Students After COVID-19

Yi-Lang Chen [1,*], Che-Wei Hsu [1,2] and Andi Rahman [1,3]

1 Department of Industrial Engineering and Management, Ming Chi University of Technology, New Taipei 243303, Taiwan; m10218009@mail2.mcut.edu.tw (C.-W.H.); m09218051@mail2.mcut.edu.tw (A.R.)
2 Quanta Computer Inc., Taoyuan 33377, Taiwan
3 Department of Industrial Engineering, Andalas University, Padang 25175, Indonesia
* Correspondence: ylchen@mail.mcut.edu.tw

Abstract

Background/Objectives: As COVID-19 policies shift from government mandates to individual responsibility, understanding how voluntary protective behaviors shape social interactions remains a public health priority. This study examines the association between voluntary mask wearing and interpersonal distance (IPD) preferences in a post-mandate context, focusing on Taiwan, where mask wearing continues to be culturally prevalent. **Methods:** One hundred university students (50 males, 50 females) in Taiwan completed an online IPD simulation task. Participants adjusted the distance of a virtual avatar in response to targets that varied by gender and mask status. Mask-wearing status upon arrival was recorded naturally, without manipulation. A four-way ANOVA tested the effects of participant gender, participant mask wearing, target gender, and target mask wearing on the preferred IPD. **Results:** Voluntary mask wearing was more common among female participants (72%) than males (44%). Mask-wearing individuals maintained significantly greater IPDs, suggesting heightened risk perception, whereas masked targets elicited smaller IPDs, possibly due to social signaling of safety. Gender differences emerged in both protective behavior and spatial preferences, with females showing stronger associations between mask use and distancing behavior. **Conclusions:** These findings offer actionable insights into how voluntary behavioral adaptations continue to shape spatial interaction norms after mandates are lifted. The integration of real-time simulation and statistical modeling highlights the potential of digital behavioral tools to support culturally adaptive, person-centered public health strategies.

Keywords: interpersonal distance (IPD); mask-wearing choice; public health behavior; participant gender; target gender

1. Introduction

The COVID-19 pandemic fundamentally reshaped human social behavior, with interpersonal distance (IPD) emerging as a central aspect of public health strategies [1,2]. IPD—defined as the physical space that individuals maintain between themselves and others during social interactions—has been widely used as an indicator of perceived risk and engagement in protective behaviors [3,4]. Examining how protective behaviors are associated with spatial preferences is essential for public health planning, as these associations may reflect underlying psychological processes that support adherence to health guidelines [5].

The relationship between mask wearing and IPD can be understood through several interconnected psychological frameworks. Risk compensation theory suggests that when individuals adopt one protective behavior, such as mask wearing, they may adjust other behaviors—like social distancing—accordingly [6]. Masks also function as visual cues that may signal health consciousness and perceived risk to others. Upon encountering a masked individual, people may interpret the behavior as indicating heightened caution, potentially prompting an increased distance, or as a sign of responsibility, possibly reducing the perceived threat and allowing closer proximity [7–9]. Protection motivation theory further proposes that protective behaviors are associated with both threat and coping appraisals, implying that voluntary mask wearers may perceive a greater threat and therefore prefer larger IPDs [10].

During the pandemic, numerous studies examined how mandated mask wearing was associated with changes in IPD, reporting mixed results across cultural and situational contexts [11–16]. However, these investigations primarily addressed behaviors influenced by governmental mandates rather than voluntary choices. As societies transition from mandate-driven to choice-driven protective practices, an important knowledge gap remains: how is voluntary mask wearing—reflecting personal risk assessment and health consciousness—related to IPD preferences in post-pandemic social interactions?

This question has important implications for public health policy. Gaining insights into how voluntary protective behaviors are associated with one another can help to inform future pandemic preparedness strategies. In addition, the continued presence of altered IPD preferences may be linked to long-term effects on social functioning and psychological well-being [17,18]. The transition from mandated to voluntary mask wearing offers a natural context to explore how individual differences in risk perception and cultural norms are related to spatial behavior.

Research on post-pandemic IPD has produced mixed findings, emphasizing the importance of distinguishing between mandated and voluntary protective behaviors. Welsch et al. [11] found that IPD preferences in Germany did not return to pre-pandemic levels even after restrictions were lifted, suggesting persistent behavioral adaptation. In contrast, Chen et al. [15] reported a rapid reduction in perceived IPD among young Taiwanese individuals following the removal of mask mandates, highlighting cultural and demographic variability in behavioral persistence. These contrasting results underscore the need to examine voluntary protective behaviors independently of compliance-driven responses, as voluntary behaviors may reflect more stable, intrinsic motivations that persist beyond external mandates. While existing studies offer useful insights into pandemic-era spatial behavior, few have explored how voluntary mask wearing—as a marker of intrinsic motivation rather than compliance—is associated with IPD in post-mandate contexts. The present study directly addresses this gap by examining the bidirectional relationship between voluntary protective choices and spatial preferences, offering insights into sustained behavioral adaptations that extend beyond policy enforcement.

Previous research has identified key demographic factors associated with protective behaviors and spatial preferences. Gender differences in health-related behaviors and COVID-19 risk perception have been consistently observed, with females generally exhibiting greater compliance and higher risk awareness [5,15,19,20]. Age-related variation in interpersonal space preferences has also been noted, with younger individuals displaying distinct spatial behavior patterns [21,22]. However, how voluntary mask wearing interacts with these demographic factors in post-mandate contexts remains insufficiently explored.

The distinction between mandated and voluntary protective behaviors is theoretically important, as voluntary behaviors are more likely to reflect intrinsic motivation, personal risk perception, and individual health beliefs rather than external compliance [23]. When individuals choose to wear masks voluntarily, this decision may signal a sustained perception of threat and a protective orientation that could also be associated with spatial behaviors, such as IPD preferences. However, existing research has not sufficiently examined this bidirectional relationship between voluntary mask adoption and spatial preferences—a relationship that may reflect the complex interplay between individual protective strategies and perceived social comfort.

This research addresses a critical need to understand how cultural norms and individual autonomy interact in shaping post-pandemic social adaptation. In post-mandate contexts, voluntary protective behaviors can serve as indicators of sustained risk awareness and social responsibility, making their examination essential in developing long-term public health strategies that uphold personal choice while supporting community well-being. This theoretical gap is particularly relevant in post-pandemic Taiwan, where voluntary mask wearing has become embedded in everyday social norms. Several factors appear to contribute to the continued use of masks in Taiwan and other East Asian societies. A long-standing tradition of mask wearing during respiratory illness seasons has been reinforced by experiences during the COVID-19 pandemic [24]. The cultural emphasis on collective well-being and social harmony has helped to normalize mask use as a symbol of mutual respect and health consciousness [25]. Additionally, positive experiences with mask wearing—particularly in crowded public spaces—have facilitated its incorporation into daily routines [26,27]. Taiwan's post-mandate environment thus offers a unique context in which to explore how voluntary mask wearing has shifted from policy-driven behavior to a culturally integrated practice.

This study addresses key knowledge gaps by examining how voluntary mask-wearing behavior is associated with IPD preferences in a post-mandate context, with the goal of providing evidence-based insights for public health policy and spatial management. We aimed to explore how individuals' voluntary mask-wearing choices relate to IPD preferences, assess the social signaling effects of encountering masked versus unmasked individuals, and identify gender-specific patterns that may inform actionable recommendations for public health practitioners and policymakers.

We recruited 100 university students (50 males, 50 females) and recorded their spontaneous mask-wearing behavior upon arrival at the experimental site, allowing for the naturalistic observation of personal protective decisions. By analyzing IPD preferences in response to virtual targets differing in gender and mask status, we examined how voluntary protective behaviors are related to spatial judgments in a post-mandate setting. This design enabled us to investigate both how individuals' own mask-wearing statuses corresponded with their preferred IPDs and how exposure to masked versus unmasked targets influenced their spatial behavior.

Grounded in risk compensation theory, social signaling theory, and protection motivation theory, we proposed four testable hypotheses. We hypothesized that individuals who voluntarily wore masks would maintain larger IPDs than non-mask wearers, reflecting heightened risk perception and a broader protective orientation. Encountering masked targets was expected to result in reduced IPDs, as mask wearing may signal safety and social responsibility. We further hypothesized that gender would be associated with both voluntary mask-wearing prevalence and the strength of the relationship between protective behaviors and spatial preferences, with females expected to show higher mask adoption rates and stronger associations. Finally, we anticipated that these behavioral patterns would produce measurable effect sizes sufficient to inform evidence-based recommendations for public space design and health communication strategies.

2. Materials and Methods

This study employed an observational experimental design to examine how voluntary mask-wearing behavior is associated with IPD preferences in post-pandemic contexts. To capture natural protective behavior, participants' mask-wearing statuses were recorded upon arrival without manipulation. They then completed an online IPD simulation task, adjusting the distance of a virtual avatar in response to targets that varied by gender and mask status. This approach allowed for the analysis of both how individuals' own mask-wearing behavior corresponded with their spatial preferences and how masked versus unmasked targets influenced IPD judgments. In doing so, the study directly addressed the relationship between voluntary protective behaviors and emerging social spatial norms. Ethical approval was obtained from the Ethics Committee of Chang Gung University, Taiwan, and all procedures were conducted in accordance with the 2013 World Medical Association Declaration of Helsinki and relevant institutional guidelines.

2.1. Participants

A total of 100 participants—equally divided between males and females—were enrolled in an online test. All were undergraduate or graduate students who reported no cognitive or psychological impairments. The average (standard deviation) ages were 21.4 (2.2) years for males and 20.9 (1.8) years for females. All participants were right-handed and unfamiliar with the target individuals used in the simulation. Data collection was conducted in September 2023, following Taiwan's phased lifting of mask mandates. This transition began on 17 April 2023, when the government removed most public mask-wearing requirements. Although certain settings, particularly healthcare facilities, retained mandates until 19 May 2024, mask wearing in most public spaces had largely shifted to a matter of personal choice during our data collection period. This timing enabled the study to examine voluntary mask-wearing behavior in a transitional social context—when external mandates had been lifted for most environments, but institutional requirements remained in select locations. Informed consent was obtained from all participants, including consent for the publication of identifying information and images in an open-access format.

While this sample offers valuable insights into young adult behavior within the Taiwanese context, the exclusive recruitment of university students from a single country may limit the generalizability of the findings to other populations, age groups, or cultural settings. The relatively homogeneous demographic profile—young, educated, and Taiwanese—should be taken into account when interpreting the results, as voluntary protective behaviors and spatial preferences may differ across socioeconomic, educational, and cultural backgrounds.

2.2. Experimental Setting

Although the pandemic had subsided, we employed an online test to collect IPD data, following the approach used by Chen and Rahman [5], to allow for comparison with prior studies. The online IPD measurement protocol gained widespread use during the pandemic and was adapted from the original paper-and-pencil methods developed by Hayduk [28] and Xiong et al. [29]. Our version of the test, widely accepted in both clinical and applied research settings [21], was implemented using Axure RP 11, a rapid prototyping tool (Version 11, Axure Software Solutions, San Diego, CA, USA).

During the test, participants used a computer cursor to move a virtual subject (avatar) toward a designated target. To avoid influencing distance judgments, the directional arrow between the avatars was hidden once movement began. No numerical cues were given regarding the distance between avatars; instead, participants relied solely on spatial perception as the avatar advanced. They were instructed to stop at a point that felt comfortable but had just begun to feel slightly uncomfortable—consistent with definitions used in prior studies [2,5,20,30–32]. The final avatar distance was converted to the psychological IPD using a 1:7.2 scale ratio. The starting point of 55.5 cm corresponded to an approximate real-world separation of 4 m between the participant and target [2,32]. Reliability was confirmed in a pilot study, which yielded a satisfactory intraclass correlation coefficient of 0.85 across repeated trials.

2.3. Targets

A male and a female, both 22 years old, were selected as target subjects, with respective heights of 176 cm and 160 cm. Both individuals were Taiwanese, ensuring demographic consistency with the participant population and cultural context of the study. Each subject was photographed wearing casual clothing with no accessories. Using a digital camera (Sony HDR-XR260; Sony, Tokyo, Japan), sagittal-view images were captured under four conditions—two based on gender and two on mask-wearing status—following the methodology used by Chen and Rahman [5], as illustrated in Figure 1. Throughout the image capture process, the subjects maintained neutral facial expressions. These photographs were then used as digital stimuli in the online test. To standardize the visual presentation, the images of the male and female targets were scaled to screen heights of 24.4 cm and 22.2 cm, respectively. The surgical masks worn in the masked conditions were plain blue and unembellished, representative of the typical face coverings used during the COVID-19 pandemic.

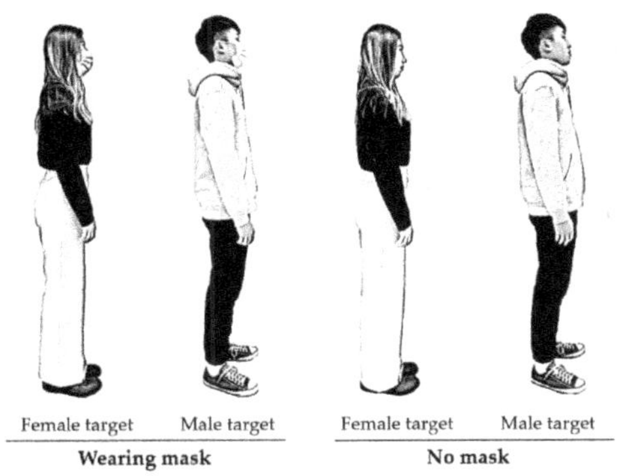

Figure 1. Images of the targets under different testing conditions (2 genders × 2 mask-wearing statuses), post-processed and manually redrawn to anonymize identities.

Several limitations related to the visual stimuli should be acknowledged. The use of only two target individuals with neutral expressions and standardized attire may not fully represent the diversity of social cues that influence IPD judgments in real-world settings. Moreover, the static nature of photographic stimuli—although beneficial for experimental control—differs from dynamic, face-to-face interactions, where movement, facial expressions, body language, and the situational context can influence spatial decision making. These limitations may have shaped participants' perceptions of the social signals conveyed by mask wearing and could impact the ecological validity of the findings.

2.4. Procedure

The primary aim of this study was to examine how participants' voluntary mask-wearing behavior was associated with their IPD preferences. Upon arrival at the experimental site, the experimenter visually recorded whether each participant was wearing a face mask. No instruction was given to wear or remove a mask, allowing for natural variations in protective behavior. Participants remained under observation throughout the session to ensure that those who arrived wearing a mask retained it during the entire experiment. No participant changed their mask status during testing.

Before the session began, all participants underwent a health screening to confirm that they were asymptomatic for respiratory illnesses, including cold, fever, COVID-19, and related conditions. This screening ensured that mask-wearing decisions reflected voluntary protective behavior and perceived risk, rather than immediate health-related needs. After screening, standardized instructions were provided. Participants were told that they would use a computer mouse to move a side-profile avatar toward a target person shown on the screen and should stop at the point where they would begin to feel uncomfortable if the interaction were occurring in real life (Figure 2). They were instructed to imagine that the approaching avatar represented themselves, and the static image represented another person. This procedure was adapted from previous studies on virtual IPD assessment [2,28].

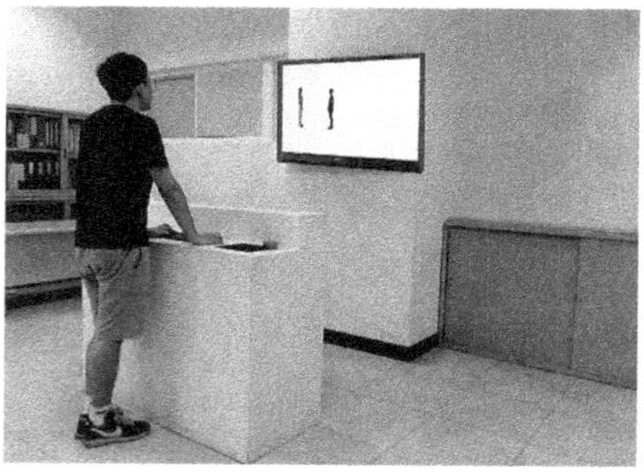

Figure 2. Schematic illustration of the experimental layout and testing procedure.

Each participant completed 12 trials, including three repeated measures for each of the four target conditions (2 genders × 2 mask statuses). Target presentations were randomized, and rest intervals of at least three minutes were included between trials to minimize fatigue or habituation effects. At the start of each trial, participants viewed frontal images of the target under all four conditions to facilitate the visualization of the scenario. They then performed the IPD task by adjusting the avatar's horizontal position to the point just before discomfort. Minor final adjustments were allowed, and the system automatically recorded the chin-to-chin distance between avatars. These values were subsequently converted to real-world measurements using a 1:7.2 scaling ratio to calculate the psychological IPD.

2.5. Statistical Analysis

The independent variables in the test included participant gender, participant mask status, target gender, and target mask status, while the dependent variable was the interpersonal distance (IPD), measured in centimeters. Data were analyzed using SPSS 23.0 (IBM, Armonk, NY, USA), with the significance level (α) set at 0.05. Because participant mask status was nested within gender, an unbalanced four-way nested ANOVA was conducted to evaluate the effects of the independent variables on IPD. In this model, participant gender and participant mask status were treated as between-subject factors, while target gender and target mask status served as within-subject factors. Additionally, two separate three-way ANOVAs were performed for male and female participants, respectively, followed by post hoc comparisons using independent t-tests. Effect sizes were reported using η^2 values. Prior to analysis, the Kolmogorov–Smirnov test confirmed that all numerical variables were normally distributed (all $p > 0.05$), and Levene's test indicated homogeneity of variances across groups (all $p > 0.05$), supporting the use of ANOVA procedures. No missing data were identified, as all participants completed the full experimental protocol, with valid IPD measurements recorded for all 12 trials (three repetitions × four target conditions).

3. Results

Figure 3 presents the proportions of male and female participants who wore masks upon arrival at the experimental site and throughout the experiment. A higher percentage of female participants (72%, $n = 36$) wore masks compared to male participants (44%, $n = 22$). Overall, 58% of the sample chose to wear masks despite the absence of a mandate, with the mask-wearing prevalence significantly higher among females than males.

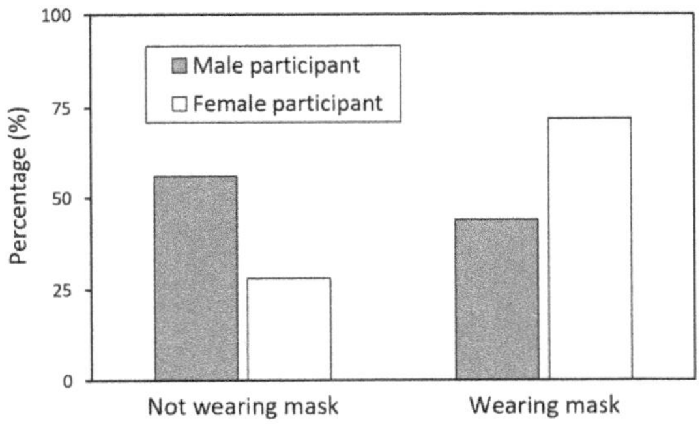

Figure 3. Proportions of mask wearing by gender. Female participants demonstrated significantly higher voluntary mask wearing (72%, $n = 36$) compared to males (44%, $n = 22$), $\chi^2 = 7.84$, $p < 0.01$. The overall prevalence of mask use among all participants was 58% (58 out of 100).

Table 1 summarizes the results of the four-way ANOVA conducted on IPD measurements. Participant gender ($p < 0.05$), participant mask status ($p < 0.001$), and target mask status ($p < 0.001$) were all significantly associated with differences in IPD, while target gender did not yield a significant main effect. Figure 4 illustrates these main effects, showing that male participants, masked individuals, and unmasked targets were associated with greater IPD values compared to their respective counterparts. In addition, Table 1 reveals a significant interaction between participant gender and target gender ($p < 0.05$), warranting further analysis to explore this relationship.

Table 1. Results of four-way ANOVA on interpersonal distance.

Source	F	*p*-Value	η^2
Participant gender (PG)	17.47	<0.05	0.022
Participant mask (PM)	35.29	<0.001	0.044
Target gender (TG)	1.09	0.298	0.001
Target mask (TM)	35.78	<0.001	0.045
PG × PM	1.86	0.173	0.014
PG × TG	4.52	<0.05	0.018
PG × TM	0.09	0.765	<0.001

Table 1. *Cont.*

Source	F	p-Value	η^2
PM × TG	0.34	0.559	<0.001
PM × TM	0.06	0.800	<0.001
TG × TM	0.01	0.909	<0.001
PG × PM × TG	0.01	0.906	<0.001
PG × PM × TM	0.40	0.527	0.001
PG × TG × TM	0.07	0.797	<0.001
PM × TG × TM	0.03	0.857	<0.001
PG × PM × TG × TM	0.01	0.924	<0.001

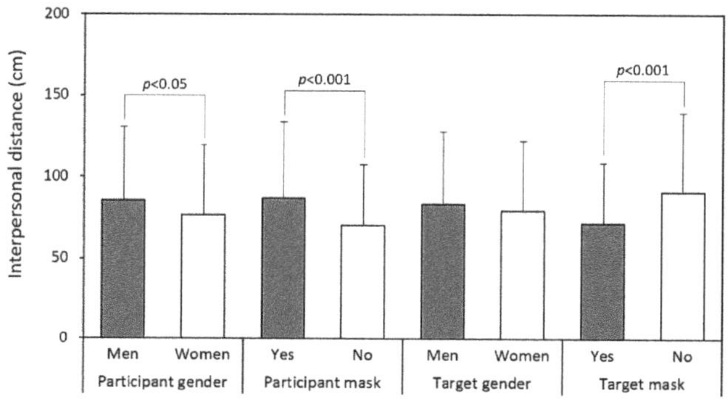

Figure 4. Main effects of the examined independent variables on interpersonal distance.

Table 2 presents the results of the three-way ANOVA conducted separately for each participant gender. The effect of the target gender on IPD differed by participant gender, reaching significance for female participants ($p < 0.05$) but not for males ($p = 0.430$). Among female participants, the smallest IPD was observed when interacting with female targets, while the remaining three target combinations yielded nearly identical IPD values (Figure 5). Figure 6 further illustrates the significant differences in IPDs between masked and unmasked participants across both genders, with all paired comparisons reaching significance among female participants.

Table 2. Results of three-way ANOVA on interpersonal distance within each participant gender group.

Source	F	p-Value	η^2
Male participants			
Participant mask (PM)	11.11	<0.001	0.028
Target gender (TG)	0.62	0.430	0.002
Target mask (TM)	20.93	<0.001	0.052
PM × TG	0.12	0.734	<0.001
PM × TM	0.08	0.782	<0.001
TG × TM	0.07	0.787	<0.001
PM × TG × TM	0.04	0.841	<0.001
Female participants			

Table 2. *Cont.*

Source	F	*p*-Value	η^2
Participant mask (PM)	25.41	<0.001	0.062
Target gender (TG)	4.78	<0.05	0.015
Target mask (TM)	15.38	<0.001	0.038
PM × TG	0.24	0.628	0.001
PM × TM	0.37	0.541	0.001
TG × TM	0.01	0.921	<0.001
PM × TG × TM	<0.01	0.954	<0.001

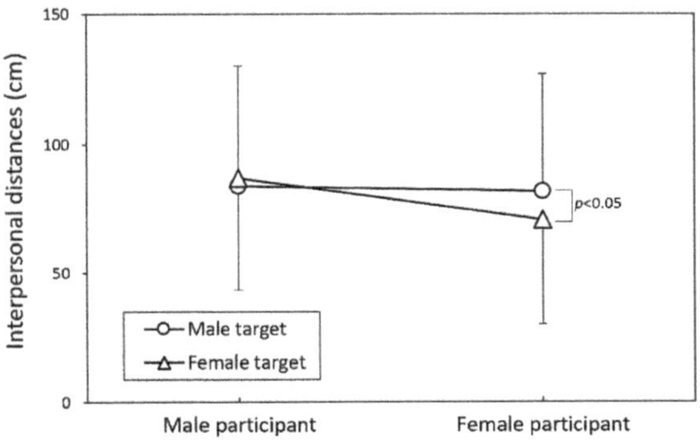

Figure 5. Comparison of interpersonal distance across participant genders in relation to target genders.

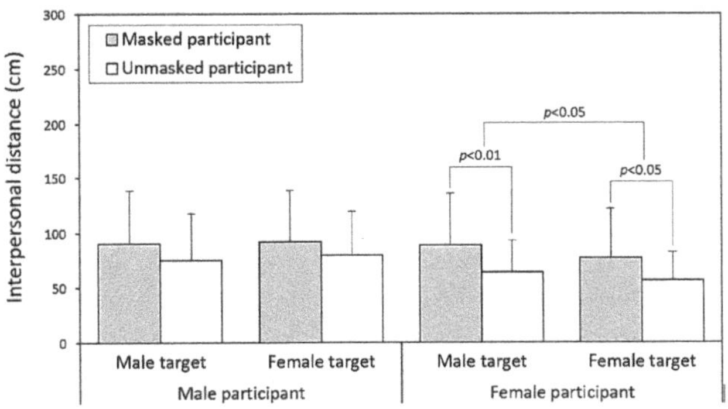

Figure 6. Pairwise comparisons of interpersonal distance values across participant mask-wearing statuses, based on independent t-tests conducted for each test condition.

4. Discussion

This study provides new insights into how voluntary mask wearing is associated with IPD in post-pandemic contexts. Although mask wearing is now a matter of personal choice rather than public mandate, our findings suggest that it remains meaningfully related to social spacing behaviors—potentially reflecting both risk perception and comfort in social interactions. The observed patterns align with our study's hypotheses, supporting possible associations between voluntary protective behaviors and IPD preferences, without implying direct causal relationships.

One key finding concerns the contrasting patterns associated with participant and target mask wearing. As shown in Table 1 and Figure 4, participants who wore masks tended to maintain larger IPDs than those who did not. This may reflect heightened risk perception or a general preference for increased personal space among individuals who choose to wear masks. Previous studies have noted that mask wearers often perceive themselves as more vulnerable to illness and consequently maintain greater distances from others [3,33]. In contrast, encountering a masked target was associated with a reduced IPD (71.6 cm vs. 90.6 cm), suggesting that masks may also function as prosocial signals that convey safety or trustworthiness [3,8]. This dual role—as both a protective barrier and a social signal—is consistent with earlier research indicating that masks can simultaneously communicate caution when worn and trustworthiness when observed [3,34,35].

Notably, before the COVID-19 pandemic, mask wearing was often interpreted as a sign of illness or heightened risk, contributing to social avoidance and psychological barriers [36,37]. Whether masks will eventually revert to their pre-pandemic connotations or continue to reflect new social meanings remains an open question worthy of continued investigation.

Gender differences further highlight the complexity of mask wearing's relationship with IPD. As shown in Figure 3, female participants were significantly more likely to voluntarily wear masks than male participants (72% vs. 44%), consistent with research suggesting that women tend to perceive greater health risks and adopt protective behaviors more frequently [20]. In addition, female participants exhibited smaller IPDs when interacting with other females, whereas the IPDs across other gender combinations were relatively uniform (Figure 5). This may reflect gender-based comfort and affiliation cues that continue to shape spatial preferences, even in a post-mandate environment. Prior studies on social bonding and gender norms indicate that women often maintain closer IPDs with same-gender individuals [2,38,39], which may help to explain the reduced IPD observed in female–female interactions in this study.

Our results contribute to the growing body of literature on the long-term effects of pandemic-induced behavioral adaptations. Kühne et al. [8] demonstrated that face masks can have both prosocial and antisocial effects depending on the context. Our findings reflect this complexity: voluntary mask wearing was associated with larger IPDs, suggesting a tendency toward increased social distancing among mask wearers—potentially indicating elevated risk perception or a protective orientation. Conversely, encountering a masked target was associated with smaller IPDs, suggesting that masks may function as prosocial signals that convey trust and safety. This dual pattern implies that the social meaning of voluntary mask wearing may depend on the perspective—whether one is the wearer or the observer.

These observed differences in IPD suggest that the pandemic may have contributed to lasting changes in how individuals regulate physical proximity, especially in cultures where mask wearing has become normalized [19]. Previous studies indicate that prolonged shifts in IPD may be influenced by prior experiences with public health crises, reinforcing more cautious spatial behavior over time [13,14]. Cultural norms also play an important role in shaping post-pandemic protective behaviors. In East Asian societies such as Taiwan, mask wearing has long been a social norm and may influence both the decision to wear a mask voluntarily and individuals' comfort in close interpersonal situations. These cultural factors should be considered when interpreting the generalizability of the present findings.

While this study offers valuable insights into how voluntary mask wearing relates to IPD, several limitations should be noted. First, although the use of an online simulation aligns with validated protocols in earlier research, it may not fully replicate the complexity of real-world social interactions. Dynamic factors such as facial expressions, movement, or environmental context are not captured in this format. The use of only two avatar targets—both with neutral expressions and standardized clothing—also limits the ecological validity, as characteristics like emotional displays, perceived attractiveness, or social status may influence IPD judgments. Additionally, although surgical masks were used consistently, research suggests that the mask color and type can elicit different psychological responses. Future studies could benefit from incorporating immersive virtual reality and a more diverse array of stimuli to enhance the realism and generalizability.

Second, the observational design of this study precludes causal inference. Participants were not randomly assigned to mask-wearing conditions; instead, their mask status was recorded upon arrival. While this naturalistic approach increases the ecological validity, it introduces potential self-selection bias, as mask-wearing decisions may be influenced by unmeasured factors such as risk perception, anxiety, past infection experiences, or regional background. These variables were not assessed. The study also lacked counterbalancing of mask conditions or matching between participant and avatar characteristics (e.g., gender or mask status), which limits interpretation regarding possible social mirroring effects. Additionally, although mask usage was monitored throughout the session, it was not strictly enforced or recorded during task execution. Finally, because the study was conducted in Taiwan—where mask wearing remains socially normative—the findings may not generalize to populations with different cultural or pandemic-related experiences. Future research should incorporate randomized designs, individual psychological measures, and cross-cultural comparisons to better understand how voluntary protective behaviors continue to shape interpersonal dynamics.

Understanding the long-term implications of voluntary protective behaviors is essential as societies adapt to the aftermath of the pandemic. While our results reveal meaningful associations between voluntary mask wearing and IPD preferences, these should be interpreted as correlational rather than causal. Future research should examine whether these behavioral patterns persist or diminish over time and explore how cultural, contextual, and individual-level factors—such as personality traits, perceived vulnerability, and previous health experiences—contribute to the adoption and maintenance of voluntary protective behaviors. Such investigations would offer deeper insights into the evolving relationships among public health practices, social norms, and risk perception in a post-pandemic society.

5. Conclusions

Our findings demonstrate that voluntary mask wearing remains significantly associated with IPD preferences in post-pandemic contexts. Female participants exhibited higher voluntary mask adoption rates (72% vs. 44%), and those who wore masks tended to maintain greater IPDs. In contrast, encounters with masked targets were associated with smaller IPDs, suggesting a nuanced dual role for masks in post-pandemic social interactions. These patterns offer evidence-based insights to inform public health strategies and the design of social spaces.

Public health authorities may benefit from recognizing the behavioral clustering observed among voluntary mask wearers, who tend to exhibit sustained protective behaviors. Given the substantial gender differences in mask adoption, gender-sensitive approaches should be considered in future public health messaging and intervention design. In spatial planning, social environments could be adapted to accommodate IPD differences—approximately 20 cm—between masked and unmasked interactions by incorporating flexible, modular layouts. Additionally, the observed social signaling effects—where masked individuals create a perceived zone of safety—can inform crowd flow and space allocation strategies in both public and private settings.

The shift from mandated to voluntary protective behaviors presents an opportunity to develop sustainable, choice-driven frameworks for future public health preparedness. Understanding how voluntary behaviors reshape social spatial norms is essential in creating culturally adaptive strategies that support community health resilience while respecting individual autonomy. For policymakers, these findings underscore the importance of integrating voluntary protective behavior patterns into pandemic response planning, implementing gender-sensitive public health measures, and designing adaptable environments that reflect the dual signaling effects of mask wearing in post-pandemic life. These quantifiable behavioral trends offer a practical foundation for evidence-informed social policy and spatial management in future public health contexts.

Author Contributions: Y.-L.C. provided the conceptualization. Y.-L.C. and C.-W.H. designed the investigation. C.-W.H. and A.R. performed the experiment, supervised data acquisition, and analyzed the data. C.-W.H. wrote the original draft. Y.-L.C. reviewed and edited the final manuscript. All authors have read and agreed to the published version of the manuscript.

Funding: This research was partially supported by the National Science and Technology Council (NSTC), Taiwan, grant number 110-2221-E-131-025-MY3, and the APC was also funded by the NSTC.

Institutional Review Board Statement: This research was approved by the Ethics Committee of Chang Gung Memorial Hospital, Taiwan (code: 20200114b0d001, 17 January 2022) and was conducted according to the guidelines of the Declaration of Helsinki.

Informed Consent Statement: Informed consent was obtained from all participants involved in the study.

Data Availability Statement: The data are available upon reasonable request to the corresponding author.

Acknowledgments: The authors would like to thank all participants for their contributions to the study.

Conflicts of Interest: Author Che-Wei Hsu was employed by Quanta Computer Inc. The remaining authors declare that the research was conducted in the absence of any commercial or financial relationships that could be construed as a potential conflict of interest.

References

1. Sajed, A.; Amgain, K. Coronavirus disease (COVID-19) outbreak and the strategy for prevention. *Eurasian J. Med. Sci.* **2020**, *2*, 1–3. [CrossRef]
2. Lee, Y.C.; Chen, Y.L. Influence of wearing surgical mask on interpersonal space perception between Mainland Chinese and Taiwanese people. *Front. Psychol.* **2021**, *12*, 692404. [CrossRef] [PubMed]
3. Cartaud, A.; Quesque, F.; Coello, Y. Wearing a face mask against COVID-19 results in a reduction of social distancing. *PLoS ONE* **2020**, *15*, e0243023. [CrossRef]
4. Kroczek, L.O.; Böhme, S.; Mühlberger, A. Face masks reduce interpersonal distance in virtual reality. *Sci. Rep.* **2022**, *12*, 2213. [CrossRef]
5. Chen, Y.L.; Rahman, A. Effects of target variables on interpersonal distance perception for young Taiwanese during the COVID-19 pandemic. *Healthcare* **2023**, *11*, 1711. [CrossRef]
6. Hagger, M.S.; Smith, S.R.; Keech, J.J.; Moyers, S.A.; Hamilton, K. Predicting social distancing intention and behavior during the COVID-19 pandemic: An integrated social cognition model. *Ann. Behav. Med.* **2020**, *54*, 713–727. [CrossRef]
7. Yin, W.; Lee, Y.C. How different face mask types affect interpersonal distance perception and threat feeling in social interaction. *Cogn. Process.* **2024**, *25*, 477–490. [CrossRef] [PubMed]
8. Kühne, K.; Fischer, M.H.; Jeglinski-Mende, M.A. During the COVID-19 pandemic participants prefer settings with a face mask, no interaction and at a closer distance. *Sci. Rep.* **2022**, *12*, 12777. [CrossRef]
9. Saint, S.A.; Moscovitch, D.A. Effects of mask-wearing on social anxiety: An exploratory review. *Anxiety Stress Coping* **2021**, *34*, 487–502. [CrossRef]
10. Carbon, C.C. Wearing face masks strongly confuses counterparts in reading emotions. *Front. Psychol.* **2020**, *11*, 566886. [CrossRef] [PubMed]

11. Welsch, R.; Wessels, M.; Bernhard, C.; Thönes, S.; Von Castell, C. Physical distancing and the perception of interpersonal distance in the COVID-19 crisis. *Sci. Rep.* **2021**, *11*, 11485. [CrossRef] [PubMed]
12. Yuan, J.; Zou, H.; Xie, K.; Dulebenets, M.A. An assessment of social distancing obedience behavior during the COVID-19 post-epidemic period in China: A cross-sectional survey. *Sustainability* **2021**, *13*, 8091. [CrossRef]
13. Sun, J.; Guo, Y. Influence of tourists' well-being in the post-COVID-19 era: Moderating effect of physical distancing. *Tour. Manag. Perspect.* **2022**, *44*, 101029. [CrossRef]
14. Savadori, L.; Lauriola, M. Risk perceptions and COVID-19 protective behaviors: A two-wave longitudinal study of epidemic and post-epidemic periods. *Soc. Sci. Med.* **2022**, *301*, 114949. [CrossRef] [PubMed]
15. Chen, Y.L.; Lee, Y.C.; Hsu, C.W.; Rahman, A. Perceived interpersonal distance changes in young Taiwanese pre and post SARS-CoV-2 pandemic. *Sci. Rep.* **2024**, *14*, 610. [CrossRef]
16. Georgescu, R.I.; Bodislav, D.A. The psychological and neurological legacy of the Covid-19 pandemic: How social distancing shaped long-term behavioral patterns. *Encyclopedia* **2025**, *5*, 60. [CrossRef]
17. Holt, D.J.; Zapetis, S.L.; Babadi, B.; Zimmerman, J.; Tootell, R.B. Personal space increases during the COVID-19 pandemic in response to real and virtual humans. *Front. Psychol.* **2022**, *13*, 952998. [CrossRef]
18. Layden, E.A.; Cacioppo, J.T.; Cacioppo, S. Loneliness predicts a preference for larger interpersonal distance within intimate space. *PLoS ONE* **2018**, *13*, e0203491. [CrossRef]
19. Tan, J.; Yoshida, Y.; Ma, K.S.K.; Mauvais-Jarvis, F.; Lee, C.C. Gender differences in health protective behaviours and its implications for COVID-19 pandemic in Taiwan: A population-based study. *BMC Public Health* **2022**, *22*, 1900. [CrossRef]
20. Lewis, A.; Duch, R. Gender differences in perceived risk of COVID-19. *Soc. Sci. Q.* **2021**, *102*, 2124–2133. [CrossRef]
21. Iachini, T.; Coello, Y.; Frassinetti, F.; Senese, V.P.; Galante, F.; Ruggiero, G. Peripersonal and interpersonal space in virtual and real environments: Effects of gender and age. *J. Environ. Psychol.* **2016**, *45*, 154–164. [CrossRef]
22. Mirlisenna, I.; Bonino, G.; Mazza, A.; Capiotto, F.; Cappi, G.R.; Cariola, M.; Valvo, A.; Francesco, L.D.; Monte, O.D. How interpersonal distance varies throughout the lifespan. *Sci. Rep.* **2024**, *14*, 25439. [CrossRef]
23. Lee, S.Y.; Ham, J.H.; Park, H.K.; Jang, D.H.; Jang, W.M. Association between risk perceptions of COVID-19, political ideology, and mask-wearing behavior after the outbreak: A cross-sectional survey in South Korea. *Risk Manag. Healthc. Policy* **2024**, *17*, 1659–1668. [CrossRef]
24. Zhang, N.; Liu, X.; Gao, S.; Su, B.; Dou, Z. Popularization of high-speed railway reduces the infection risk via close contact route during journey. *Sustain. Cities Soc.* **2023**, *99*, 104979. [CrossRef]
25. Biggio, M.; Bisio, A.; Bruno, V.; Garbarini, F.; Bove, M. Wearing a mask shapes interpersonal space during COVID-19 pandemic. *Brain Sci.* **2022**, *12*, 682. [CrossRef] [PubMed]
26. Yu, X.; Chen, C.H.; Xia, Z.; Wang, C.; Xiong, W. Interpersonal distance perception during the normalization of an pandemic situation: Effects of mask—wearing and vaccination. *PsyCh J.* **2023**, *13*, 190–200. [CrossRef] [PubMed]
27. Kühne, K.; Jeglinski-Mende, M.A. Refraining from interaction can decrease fear of physical closeness during COVID-19. *Sci. Rep.* **2023**, *13*, 7700. [CrossRef]
28. Hayduk, L.A. Personal space: Where we now stand. *Psychol. Bull.* **1983**, *94*, 293–335. [CrossRef]
29. Xiong, W.; Phillips, M.; Wang, Z.; Zhang, Y.; Cheng, H.; Link, B. Stigma and discrimination associated with mental illness and other stigmatizing conditions in China using two cultural-sensitive measures of stigma: Interpersonal distance and occupational restrictiveness. *Psychol. Med.* **2021**, *51*, 2804–2813. [CrossRef]
30. Adams, L.; Zuckerman, D. The effect of lighting conditions on personal space requirements. *J. Gen. Psychol.* **1991**, *118*, 335–340. [CrossRef]
31. Nandrino, J.L.; Ducro, C.; Iachini, T.; Coello, Y. Perception of peripersonal and interpersonal space in patients with restrictive-type anorexia. *Eur. Eat. Disord. Rev.* **2017**, *25*, 179–187. [CrossRef] [PubMed]
32. Yu, X.; Xiong, W.; Lee, Y.C. An investigation into interpersonal and peripersonal spaces of Chinese people for different directions and genders. *Front. Psychol.* **2020**, *11*, 981. [CrossRef] [PubMed]
33. Chu, D.K.; Akl, E.A.; Duda, S.; Solo, K.; Yaacoub, S.; Schünemann, H.J.; SARS-CoV-2 Systematic Urgent Review Group Effort (SURGE) Study Authors. Physical distancing, face masks, and eye protection to prevent person-to-person transmission of SARS-CoV-2 and SARS-CoV-2: A systematic review and meta-analysis. *Lancet* **2020**, *395*, 1973–1987. [CrossRef]
34. Chen, C.Y.C.; Lei, M. Psychosocial factors associated with mask-wearing behavior during the COVID-19 pandemic. *Psychol. Health Med.* **2022**, *27*, 1996–2006. [CrossRef]
35. Zhang, B.; Li, Z.; Jiang, L. The intentions to wear face masks and the differences in preventive behaviors between urban and rural areas during COVID-19: An analysis based on the technology acceptance model. *Int. J. Environ. Res. Public Health* **2021**, *18*, 9988. [CrossRef]
36. Abney, K. "Containing" tuberculosis, perpetuating stigma: The materiality of N95 respirator masks. *Anthropol. S. Afr.* **2018**, *41*, 270–283. [CrossRef]

37. Burgess, A.; Horii, M. Risk, ritual and health responsibilisation: Japan's 'safety blanket' of surgical face mask-wearing. *Sociol. Health Illn.* **2012**, *34*, 1184–1198. [CrossRef] [PubMed]
38. Hall, E.T. *The Hidden Dimension*; Doubleday: Garden City, NY, USA, 1966.
39. Aiello, J.R. Human Spatial Behavior. In *Handbook of Environmental Psychology*; Stokols, D., Altman, I., Eds.; Wiley: New York, NY, USA, 1987; Volume 1, pp. 389–504.

healthcare

MDPI

Perspective

Sharing Data and Transferring Samples Within Pediatric Clinical Studies: How to Overcome Challenges and Make Them a Science Opportunity

Annalisa Landi [1], Federica D'Ambrosio [2], Silvia Faggion [2], Francesca Rocchi [3], Carla Paganin [3], Maria Grazia Lain [4], Adriana Ceci [1] and Viviana Giannuzzi [1,*] on behalf of the EPIICAL Consortium

1 Fondazione per la Ricerca Farmacologica Gianni Benzi Onlus, 70124 Bari, Italy; al@benzifoundation.org (A.L.); adriceci.uni@gmail.com (A.C.)
2 Fondazione Penta ETS, 35127 Padova, Italy; federica.dambrosio@pentafoundation.org (F.D.); silvia.faggion@pentafoundation.org (S.F.)
3 Ospedale Pediatrico Bambino Gesù, 00152 Roma, Italy; francesca.rocchi@opbg.net (F.R.); carla.paganin@opbg.net (C.P.)
4 Fundação Ariel Contra o SIDA Pediátrico, Maputo P.O. Box 2822, Mozambique; mlain@arielglaser.org.mz
* Correspondence: vg@benzifoundation.org; Tel.: +39-080-902-6797

Abstract: EPIICAL (Early treated Perinatally HIV-Infected individuals: Improving Children's Actual Life) is a consortium of European and non-European research-driven organizations inter-connected with the aim of establishing a clinical and experimental platform for the early identification of novel therapeutic strategies for the pediatric Human Immunodeficiency Virus (HIV). Within the EPIICAL project, several pediatric clinical studies were conducted, requiring the collection and transfer of biological samples and associated data across boundaries within and outside Europe. To ensure compliance with the applicable rules on pediatric data and sample transfer and to support the efforts of academic partners, which may not always have the necessary expertise and resources in place for designing, managing and conducting multi-national studies, the consortium established a dedicated expert Working Group. This group has guided the consortium since the start of the project through the complexities of the ethical and regulatory aspects of international clinical studies. The group provided support in the design and preparation of the prospective and retrospective multi-center and multi-national pediatric studies with a focus on the clinical study protocols, informed consent and assent forms. In particular, well-structured informed consent and assent templates were developed, and data sharing and material transfer agreements were set up to regulate the transfer of samples among partners and sites. We considered that such support and the implementation of ad hoc agreements could provide effective practical solutions for addressing ethical and regulatory hurdles related to sharing data and transferring samples in international pediatric clinical research.

Keywords: pediatric clinical studies; transfer of samples; data sharing; regulatory; ethics

1. Introduction

Early treated Perinatally HIV-Infected individuals: Improving Children's Actual Life —EPIICAL [1]—is a consortium of European Union (EU) and non-European (non-EU) research-driven organizations and academic institutions aiming at implementing a predictive platform for the early identification of novel therapeutic strategies for children affected by the human immunodeficiency virus (HIV). It foresaw the design and conduct of studies in pediatric HIV populations in Europe, Africa and Asia. This involves developing and applying statistical and mathematical modeling to data derived from cohorts of early treated infants and children to identify virological, immunological and transcriptomic profiles associated with early control of HIV infection after antiretroviral therapy (ART) initiation as well as viral control following ART interruption.

EPIICAL consists of a large number of partners from all over the world and has been running for eight years.

The foresight of such a consortium was to anticipate potential ethical and regulatory issues related to the planned pediatric studies and to involve experts in the field from the outset of activities. Therefore, in the framework of the EPIICAL project, a Working Group (WG) with ethics and regulatory experts was set up to ensure that all relevant rules are complied with.

This paper aims to describe our experience coming from the EPIICAL project as an extensive work aimed to investigate and address the challenges related to the transfer of samples and associated data across boundaries within and outside Europe in the context of pediatric clinical studies. Possible solutions to overcome them will be emphasized as well. These would result in useful tools and strategies for other researchers working in different disease areas.

2. Setup of the Activities

Biological samples, like blood, tissue, urine and saliva are commonly used in biomedical research and their analyses provide key outputs in clinical studies. Regulatory, legal and ethical considerations, including but not limited to informed consent, assent from minors and data protection, particularly with respect to long-term storage of samples and related data, must be taken into account [2,3].

Several challenges can be identified when dealing with the transfer of samples and associated data across boundaries in the context of clinical studies. Among them, ethical challenges relate to the privacy of individuals and data control [4] and the respect for informed consent; furthermore, the regulatory challenges associated with the application of national provisions ruling the transfer of samples and associated data make the situation even more complex.

Such challenges are emphasized when vulnerable subjects, such as minors, are involved [3].

International clinical studies might represent a further complication since the ethics, regulatory and data protection framework regarding the sharing of samples and associated data for scientific purposes seems scattered among EU and non-EU countries [5]. In fact, countries have different laws regarding the use of clinical samples, especially when dealing with children. In addition, language barriers further complicate the conduct of multi-national studies.

The implementation of multi-national collaborative projects with a focus on data and sample sharing often faces regulatory roadblocks that slow progress. This has been exacerbated by the entry into force of the European General Data Protection Regulation Reg (EU) 2016/679 (GDPR) [6], which, by leaving a significant part of decision-making to the Member States, has led to confusion and bureaucratic complexity, particularly when non-EU partners are involved [7]. Although there is a lack of harmonized frameworks or guidelines across the world, there are many strategies that might be implemented to address the challenges outlined above. First of all, the transparency of the information to be provided to the study subjects and/or to their parents/legally designated representatives regarding the transfer and use/future use of samples and associated data to achieve the study purposes (e.g., analysis in specialized laboratories) is needed. This information shall always be included in the study protocol with a description of how data and samples are processed, as well as in the informed consent form of the study participants or their parents/legally designated representatives. When seeking consent, the use, storage, and possible future use of the material should also be explained [3]. Moreover, when dealing with minors, children should participate in the informed consent and assent process according to their age and understanding and receive age-appropriate information about what will happen in the study as well [3]. Finally, we considered that ad hoc agreements regulating the sharing of samples and associated data shall be set up to ensure the lawful sharing of data and samples among sites and countries. These agreements constitute mechanisms to ensure uniformity of data and sample access across projects and countries and may be regarded as consistent basic agreements for addressing data and material sharing globally [8].

The dedicated WG supported the investigators in the relevant ethical and regulatory applications during the whole duration of the clinical studies and deemed it necessary to involve the Sponsor's representatives in the group from the beginning. It started its activities by providing support in the design and preparation of the EPIICAL prospective and retrospective multi-center and multi-national pediatric studies. They involved both EU and non-EU countries: South Africa, Mozambique, Mali, Uganda, Thailand, Italy, the United Kingdom, Spain and the United States.

The group followed a centralized approach, ensuring uniform ethical standards across all countries and sites, as described below:

- The applicable regulatory and ethics provisions were identified through an analysis of the international framework: the Helsinki Declaration for Ethics in Human Subjects (2013) [9]; International Ethical Guidelines for Health-related Research Involving Humans CIOMS-WHO (2016) [10]; Additional Protocol to the Oviedo Convention on biomedical research (2005) [11]; European Commission Ethical considerations for clinical trials on medicinal products conducted with minors (2017) [12]; and European General Data Protection Regulation Reg (EU) 2016/679 (GDPR) [6]. They were considered to complement the national frameworks. In particular, the 2017 EC considerations for clinical trials in minors [12] were followed to verify the limit of blood amount to be taken from minors, while the CIOMS WHO guidelines [10] were followed for implementing separate consent for genetic testing.
- A core package of documents was prepared to submit the studies to the competent Ethics Committees in all clinical sites involved in compliance with the national rules and international standards.
- The clinical study protocol was reviewed and any necessary amendments were made to align it with local requirements and to develop and release a unique version for all sites.
- Data and sample flows were identified for all the EPIICAL studies to better illustrate the ethics and regulatory needs, including those specifically related to the transfer of health and genetic data with non-EU countries.
- Informed consent and assent templates were prepared to be adapted to local requirements, and support was given to implement data protection and confidentiality rules. Considering that the studies foresaw the transfer of samples and associated data, information on the transfer was provided to study participants in the parent information sheet and informed consent forms for minors.
- A Standard Operating Procedure was released on the management of personal data and samples and on consent requirements in 2018. Then, once GDPR [6] entered into force, a letter was prepared for the investigators to help them fully comply with the new EU privacy legislation and implement data protection and confidentiality rules.

3. Informed Consent and Assent

We deemed a well-structured informed consent template as the most suitable solution to address the national differences and then overcome the related challenges in samples and data sharing. For this reason, in the framework of the EPIICAL project, a parent information sheet and informed consent form template were prepared (available as Supplementary Materials). Given the pediatric specificities of the EPIICAL studies, the information sheet and informed consent form were addressed to the parents/legally designated representatives of the minor patients.

The information sheet included all the relevant information on the study and the use of samples and associated data, including information about the transfer; in particular, it included the following:

- The type of samples and data to be collected and shared.

- The purposes of the transfer (i.e., analysis in specialized laboratories).
- The rights of children, including the subject's confidentiality and all the rights under GDPR.
- The commitment of the Sponsor to ensure compliance with the applicable data protection rules.
- The explanation of the adoption of de-identification measures to protect patients' privacy.
- The storage location and duration of the data and samples and the countries/cities where the laboratories are located.
- The future use of remaining samples and the availability to be recontacted for possible further testing and then refreshing consent.

Study participants were also reassured that the Ethics Committee(s) approved the study and would approve any possible modification to the study, e.g., transfers to other locations not defined yet at the start of the study and new tests on the remaining samples.

In order to apply the minimization principle (as stated in the GDPR [6]), study participants were informed that only information essential for the purposes of the study would be collected.

Patients and their parents/legal guardians were informed of their right to withdraw at any time and without giving a reason for the decision, including the destruction of the remaining samples and associated data, unless already analyzed.

A granular consent section was foreseen to allow participants to make some choices related to the use of their samples and associated data. These choices included the transfer of samples to specific laboratories for analysis, the re-use of remaining samples and associated data and the performance of genetic testing. With reference to this latter point, participants shall be informed about any possible unexpected or incidental findings coming out from the research and if any treatment or preventive measures are available. This information was collected. Parents/legal guardians were also given the chance to refuse the inclusion of their children's data in an aggregated and anonymized form within reports/articles prepared for dissemination and communication purposes. The possibility to be re-contacted for further research studies was added as well.

Finally, in the event that the parent/legal guardian was unable to read and sign the parent information sheet and the informed consent form, the consent process implemented in EPIICAL foresaw (1) the involvement of a person in charge of reading and explaining the contents of the information sheet and (2) the thumbprint of the parent/legal guardian accompanied by the name and signature of a witness, defined as "a person independent from the research team or any team member and who was not involved in obtaining consent" to provide written consent. This provision was sourced from the EU Clinical Trials Regulation (CTR) [13], which rules interventional clinical trials in the EU.

Furthermore, considering the nature of EPIICAL studies, assent form templates were prepared for children and adolescents as well (available as Supplementary Materials). Plain and clear language was used to provide information to children according to their age and maturity. The study procedures and transfer of samples to other laboratories were explained.

Children were informed that they could choose not to take part in the study or to change their minds at any time without providing a reason. The basic concept of privacy was also included in the form to confirm that their identity shall be kept secret. Finally, they were informed that when they reach the age of maturity, they will have the possibility to re-evaluate their participation and to consent or object to any further use of their data.

4. Data Sharing Agreement

Clinical data from EPIICAL studies were entered by the study team at each participating center into a centralized database provided by the Sponsor (REDCap).

Each site was responsible for entering the data collected at their site, with access restricted to the dataset pertaining to their own patients. Access to REDCap was granted only to the clinical site's staff trained in the study protocol and the use of the database.

Access was provided via email with a username and a temporary password, to be replaced before their first login, adhering to the security criteria established by the Sponsor.

REDCap automatically prompted the user to update the password every ninety days.

Each patient enrolled in the study was assigned an alphanumeric code based on the principle of pseudonymization.

As part of the project activities (labs, center for statistical analysis, etc.), access to the database was also granted to other consortium partners following the same procedures outlined above. Depending on the delegated tasks, each partner was given access only to the dataset necessary to perform their specific activities as required by the study protocols.

A Data Sharing Agreement (DSA) was prepared for each EPIICAL study to regulate the data flow, as required by the GDPR [6]. The DSA focuses on EU privacy legislation since the Sponsor and some parties involved in the study were based in the EU, which means that the GDPR applies. Moreover, since the Sponsor is responsible for the conduct of the study and the activities delegated to the institutions involved in it, the Sponsor had to ensure compliance with the GDPR for all processing activities, regardless of whether they were carried out in the EU or outside the EU.

As a preliminary step, the study data flows were mapped, with parties being either senders/exporters or recipients/importers based on the role of each party in the study according to the protocol (clinical site, laboratory, chief investigator, etc.) and on the type of personal data being processed.

Following that, the DSA allocates the privacy roles of the parties according to each party's contribution to the study, defines the study processing activities' details (nature and purpose(s), categories of data subjects, categories of the data processed, frequency of transfer, data retention period) and sets out the obligations the parties are subject to when performing the personal data processing activities necessary to conduct the study. Such obligations include the responsibility of the parties to implement and maintain technical and organizational measures to ensure the security of personal data and the protection of data subjects' rights and freedoms.

Importantly, the DSA also regulates the transfer of personal data to third countries, ensuring that any transfer of personal data to a third country or an international organization within the study takes place in compliance with the GDPR.

Last but not least, on the assumption that by being based outside of the EU, many parties may not be familiar with the EU privacy legislation, some training materials were provided as an annex to the DSA, with the aim of helping parties get a better understanding of the basic concepts of the GDPR and thus of their obligations under the DSA.

5. Material Transfer Agreements

The setup of Material Transfer Agreements (MTAs) was considered relevant in the framework of the multi-national transfer of samples and associated data when conducting pediatric clinical studies, especially if it involves non-EU countries.

Therefore, for the EPIICAL studies, MTA templates were developed starting from the model provided by Mascalzoni et al. [8] to regulate the transfer of human samples among partners and concerned clinical sites (available as Supplementary Materials). They complemented the research project collaboration agreements, and the above-mentioned DSA set up by the Sponsor.

Two main figures were identified for each site transferring samples and associated data: the provider, the registered legal entity in charge of providing biospecimens and associated data to the recipient, and the recipient, the registered legal entity in charge of receiving biospecimens and associated data from the provider.

Information about the Sponsor of the study and the coordinating and principal investigators was included, as well as the definitions of specific terms (e.g., provider, recipient, informed consent, etc.).

The agreement included information and declarations from the provider and from the recipient.

The provider is required to do the following:

- Confirm the alignment of the regulatory and ethical framework of the country concerned with the international provisions concerning medical research.
- Guarantee research quality, security and privacy protection.
- Confirm that the international transfer of biospecimens and personal data is allowed.
- Ensure compliance with the international quality standards for human biological materials and the specific methods/measures applicable to the type of biospecimens.
- Describe the legal basis for the storage and distribution and for allowing biospecimens and data sharing by stating that informed consent was obtained from subjects or their parents/legal representatives in case of minors. It was accompanied by the informed assent, where required.
- Include information on the expected number of individuals providing data and samples as well as on the type of data (e.g., outcomes of clinical/laboratory/instrumental analyses, medical records, genetic testing results, Case Report Forms) and samples (e.g., blood samples, tissue type, cell preparation, DNA, RNA, protein)
- Describe the applied de-identification measures as well as information on the storage location and the modalities of transfer. Details about shipping and the applicable regulations (e.g., the International Air Transport Association, the European Agreement on International Carriage of Dangerous Goods) are requested.
- Define what happens at the end of the agreement with the shared data and samples. Two options are proposed: to destroy or return them to the provider. A written notification/certification with the confirmation of the destruction/anonymization is mandatory at the end of the agreement.

The recipient is required to do the following:

- Confirm compliance with applicable regulations, policies and guidelines, as well as with the study protocol.
- Declare that data and samples will be used only for the purposes established in the agreement and in the framework of the EPIICAL project and that they will not be transferred to other facilities or institutions without written consent from the provider.
- Undertake not to use data and samples in case of withdrawn consent and then destroy or return them.

Import and export licenses were also necessary, when requested by national laws, to make the transfer across boundaries of biospecimens lawful.

6. Discussion and Conclusions

The EPIICAL experience highlights well-known challenges related to the transfer of samples and associated data within pediatric clinical studies and reveals solutions proposed by the authors on how to overcome them and make them a scientific opportunity for researchers and healthcare professionals.

Firstly, we believe that the involvement of ethics and regulatory experts from the study design stage is relevant and valuable in supporting the design and conduct of studies and providing continuous advice to the study team. It allowed for the smoother execution of study activities to set up and conduct multi-national studies.

Such an involvement is intended to ensure that all study activities are performed according to the applicable rules and ethical standards, reduce differences and inequities across countries from different political and economic settings. This could be particularly challenging for academic partners, who may not always have the necessary expertise and resources in place for designing and managing multi-national studies [5,14]. Therefore, public–private collaborations or collaborations among different stakeholders, possibly in the framework of research funds, would be crucial for the future.

We emphasized that clear and easily accessible information related to the transfer of samples and associated data in the context of clinical studies must be provided in the informed consent and assent forms and that MTA and DSA represent useful means to regulate the transfer of samples among countries and institutions as well as to regulate the data flow, as required by the GDPR. Of course, setting up these agreements was not an easy task to do. This was mainly due to the lack of common internationally agreed rules and a consequent lack of harmonization of the regulatory framework across countries involved in multi-national clinical studies. In fact, such agreements were set up considering and incorporating all the applicable legislation.

A homogeneous support group aimed at guiding and monitoring the research can reduce differences and inequalities and ensure transparency in human research and ethical principles, including scientific partners from countries considered both rich and poor. Furthermore, a well-structured submission package streamlines the ethical submission process and reduces the time required for ethics committees to approve the study. Additionally, awareness of regulatory procedures might facilitate the sharing of samples and associated data.

Table 1 provides an overview of the ethics and regulatory issues that arose during our pediatric research project in the geographical areas involved and how they were addressed through the careful regulatory frameworks established by the consortium. For example, we consider the preparation of a letter for investigators, with practical information on how to comply with GDPR (e.g., how to modify the informed consent and assent processes and documents), as one of the "success stories" of this work. This is because we shared such a letter even before the full application of the 'new rule', i.e., GDPR. Another example is the agreement that was reached among clinicians and regulatory experts on the type of clinical studies foreseen in the project. Discussion and consultation of relevant applicable documents were adopted to solve the challenge.

Our experience has highlighted that real global harmonization of multi-national, multi-continental clinical studies not investigating any medicine is difficult to reach without a global regulatory framework like the ICH, and this becomes even more relevant in the light of the growing use of multi-sources data (e.g., studies involving primary and secondary data sources). Harmonization should also be pursued considering the international dimension of scientific research [7].

As a future direction, close collaboration and efficient communication between the study team and the regulatory/ethics experts should be pursued, achieved and maintained for the whole duration of the clinical studies. We consider this as a relevant action, considering that ethics and regulatory activities need timely planning (e.g., obtaining ethics approval, protocol amendments, etc.), especially in case of new ideas or changes to the original plans. Furthermore, a set of expected outcomes and key performance indicators could be identified and measured during a multi-national clinical study [15] to value and monitor the work done from an ethics/regulatory WG and to promptly identify issues and related solutions.

EXPECTED OUTCOMES:

- To accelerate the ethics approval and/or competent authority authorization;
- To reduce the number of requests for modifications/integrations from ethics committees and competent authorities;
- To speed up the start of data and sample sharing and, therefore, of their analysis.

KEY PERFORMANCE INDICATORS:

- Number of periodical group meetings, number of requests for support received from Sponsor or investigators and time to resolve a request for ethics/regulatory support;
- Number of requests for clarification/document modifications received by ethics committees and/or competent authorities out of the number of applications;
- Time for agreeing DSAs and MTAs.

Table 1. Ethics and regulatory issues arose during the pediatric research project in the geographical areas involved.

<table>
<tr><th>Continent</th><th>Ethics/Regulatory Issues</th><th>Solutions</th></tr>
<tr><td>America</td><td>Acceptance of EU standards for clinical research, data protection and confidentiality</td><td>In the agreements:<ul><li>To refer to the international standards, e.g., ICH, "as implemented in the national legislation".</li><li>To specify that provisions apply "to the extent the EU rule is compatible with the national laws".</li></ul></td></tr>
<tr><td>Africa</td><td>Storage of samples abroad for future studies not permitted.</td><td>Biospecimens for future studies only stored locally at the clinical sites.</td></tr>
<tr><td>America</td><td>Need to comply with local laws and requirements.</td><td>The researchers were asked to comply with both EU and local laws.</td></tr>
<tr><td>Africa, Europe</td><td>Divergent classification of the clinical study (observational, non-interventional, non-pharmacological, etc.).</td><td>Upfront agreed classification among clinicians and regulatory experts on the type of clinical studies foreseen in the project, i.e., non-pharmacological clinical study.</td></tr>
<tr><td>Africa, Europe</td><td>Need to limit blood withdrawals from children according to their age and weight.</td><td>Agreement among clinicians and regulatory experts to follow European ethical recommendations on pediatric studies regarding blood withdrawals from children.</td></tr>
<tr><td>Africa, Europe</td><td>Need to transfer samples outside the country in compliance with applicable laws.</td><td>To set up regulatory-sounded Material Transfer Agreements for sharing samples.</td></tr>
<tr><td>Europe</td><td>Results of the studies mandatorily shared with parents/legal representatives.</td><td>Procedure specified in the informed consent process: parents/legal representatives informed about their right to receive study results in the informed consent document.</td></tr>
<tr><td>Europe</td><td>Future uses of samples and related data not to be broad but related to the original study and approved by an ethics committee.</td><td>Future uses of samples and data specified in protocol and informed consent documents, as approved by an ethics committee.</td></tr>
<tr><td>Europe</td><td>Informed consent more user-friendly language, limiting medico-legal terminology wherever possible.</td><td rowspan="2">Informed consent and assent documents adapted to use user-friendly language, minimizing medico-legal terminology and revised by ELSI experts.</td></tr>
<tr><td>Europe</td><td>Need to use user-friendly language in informed assent documents.</td></tr>
<tr><td>Africa, America, Europe</td><td>Need to update EU laws because of modifications, e.g., Directive 95/46/EC repealed by GDPR.</td><td>Investigators provided with practical information on how to comply with GDPR requirements on informed consent and assent process and documents, in particular with those not already included in the studies.</td></tr>
</table>

These metrics, as well as others related to the execution phases of a pediatric clinical study (set up, enrolment, conduct, etc.), should be regularly measured and published.

The best possible guidance on how to deal with any ethical or regulatory issues that may arise during the study can only be provided if the regulatory team is promptly informed about them.

This work aimed to provide the scientific community with some learnings on how to build a strong consortium in the framework of pediatric studies and how to manage the ethics and regulatory issues related to pediatric samples and data sharing. This can also help to speed up study procedures and strategies.

Supplementary Materials: The following supporting information can be downloaded at: https://www.mdpi.com/article/10.3390/healthcare12232473/s1, Template S1: EPIICAL informed consent template; Template S2: EPIICAL assent template; Template S3: EPIICAL DSA MTA template.

Author Contributions: Conceptualization, A.L., A.C. and V.G.; methodology, V.G.; validation, A.L., F.D. and S.F.; writing—original draft preparation, A.L.; writing—review and editing, F.D., S.F., C.P., F.R., M.G.L., A.C. and V.G.; supervision, V.G. All authors have read and agreed to the published version of the manuscript.

Funding: The EPIICAL project is funded through an independent grant by ViiV Healthcare UK: "Research Collaboration Funding Agreement between Fondazione Penta and ViiV Healthcare UK Limited, made and entered into as of the 9th day of February, 2016, and subsequent amendments".

Institutional Review Board Statement: Not applicable.

Informed Consent Statement: Not applicable.

Data Availability Statement: No generated data.

Conflicts of Interest: The authors declare no conflicts of interest.

References

1. Epiical—The EPIICAL Project. Available online: https://www.epiical.org/ (accessed on 22 April 2024).
2. Giannuzzi, V.; Landi, A.; Bartoloni, F.; Ceci, A. A Review on Impact of General Data Protection Regulation on Clinical Studies and Informed Consent. *J. Clin. Res. Bioeth.* **2018**, *9*, 327.
3. Giannuzzi, V.; Stoyanova-Beninska, V.; Hivert, V. Editorial: The use of real world data for regulatory purposes in the rare diseases setting. *Front. Pharmacol.* **2022**, *13*, 1089033. [CrossRef] [PubMed]
4. Shahin, M.H.; Bhattacharya, S.; Silva, D.; Kim, S.; Burton, J.; Podichetty, J.; Romero, K.; Conrado, D.J. Open Data Revolution in Clinical Research: Opportunities and Challenges. *Clin. Transl. Sci.* **2020**, *13*, 665–674. [CrossRef] [PubMed]
5. Giannuzzi, V.; Felisi, M.; Bonifazi, D.; Devlieger, H.; Papanikolaou, G.; Ragab, L.; Fattoum, S.; Tempesta, B.; Reggiardo, G.; Ceci, A. Ethical and procedural issues for applying researcher-driven multi-national pediatric clinical trials in and outside the European Union: The challenging experience of the DEEP project. *BMC Med. Ethics* **2021**, *22*, 49. [CrossRef] [PubMed]
6. Regulation (EU) 2016/679 of the European Parliament and of the Council of 27 April 2016 on the Protection of Natural Persons with Regard to the Processing of Personal Data and on the Free Movement of Such Data, and Repealing Directive 95/46/EC (General Data Protection Regulation) (OJ L 119 04.05.2016), p. 1. Available online: http://data.europa.eu/eli/reg/2016/679/oj (accessed on 22 April 2024).
7. Vlahou, A.; Hallinan, D.; Apweiler, R.; Argiles, A.; Beige, J.; Benigni, A.; Bischoff, R.; Black, P.C.; Boehm, F.; Céraline, J.; et al. Data Sharing Under the General Data Protection Regulation: Time to Harmonize Law and Research Ethics? *Hypertension* **2021**, *77*, 1029–1035. [CrossRef] [PubMed]
8. Mascalzoni, D.; Dove, E.S.; Rubinstein, Y.; Dawkins, H.J.; Kole, A.; McCormack, P.; Woods, S.; Riess, O.; Schaefer, F.; Lochmüller, H.; et al. International Charter of principles for sharing bio-specimens and data. *Eur. J. Hum. Genet.* **2015**, *23*, 721–728. [CrossRef] [PubMed]
9. The World Medical Association-WMA. Declaration of Helsinki—Ethical Principles for Medical Research Involving Human Subjects. 2013. Available online: https://www.wma.net/policies-post/wma-declaration-of-helsinki-ethical-principles-for-medical-research-involving-human-subjects/ (accessed on 22 April 2024).
10. Council for International Organizations of Medical Sciences-CIOMS; World Health Organization-WHO. International Ethical Guidelines for Health-Related Research Involving Humans. 2016. Available online: https://cioms.ch/publications/product/international-ethical-guidelines-for-health-related-research-involving-humans/ (accessed on 22 April 2024).
11. Council of Europe. Additional Protocol to the Convention on Human Rights and Biomedicine, Concerning Biomedical Research. 2005. Available online: https://www.europeansources.info/record/additional-protocol-to-the-convention-on-human-rights-and-biomedicine-concerning-biomedical-research/ (accessed on 22 April 2024).

12. European Commission. Ethical Considerations for Clinical Trials on Medicinal Products Conducted with the Pediatric Population. 2017. Available online: https://health.ec.europa.eu/document/download/c1f2ff4c-63d0-4118-a6d6-a78197f04922_en (accessed on 22 April 2024).
13. Regulation (EU) No 536/2014 of the European Parliament and of the Council of 16 April 2014 on Clinical Trials on Medicinal Products for Human Use, and Repealing Directive 2001/20/EC. Available online: http://data.europa.eu/eli/reg/2014/536/oj/eng (accessed on 22 April 2024).
14. Magnin, A.; Iversen, V.C.; Calvo, G.; Čečetková, B.; Dale, O.; Demlová, R.; Blaskó, G.; Keane, F.; Kovacs, G.L.; Levy-Marchal, C.; et al. European survey on national harmonization in clinical research. *Learn Health Syst.* **2021**, *5*, e10220. [CrossRef] [PubMed]
15. Attar, S.; Price, A.; Hovinga, C.; Stewart, B.; Lacaze-Masmonteil, T.; Bonifazi, F.; Turner, M.A.; Fernandes, R.M. Harmonizing Quality Improvement Metrics Across Global Trial Networks to Advance Paediatric Clinical Trials Delivery. *Ther. Innov. Regul. Sci.* **2024**, *58*, 953–964. [CrossRef] [PubMed] [PubMed Central]

MDPI AG
Grosspeteranlage 5
4052 Basel
Switzerland
Tel.: +41 61 683 77 34

Healthcare Editorial Office
E-mail: healthcare@mdpi.com
www.mdpi.com/journal/healthcare

www.ingramcontent.com/pod-product-compliance
Lightning Source LLC
Chambersburg PA
CBHW041947260926
51850CB00018B/1803
* 9 7 8 3 7 2 5 8 5 8 4 1 5 *